Demographic Transformation and Socio-Economic Development

Volume 16

This dynamic series builds on the population and development paradigms of recent decades and provides an authoritative platform for the analysis of empirical results that map new territory in this highly active field. Its constituent volumes are set in the context of unprecedented demographic changes in both the developed—and developing—world, changes that include startling urbanization and rapidly aging populations. Offering unprecedented detail on leading-edge methodologies, as well as the theory underpinning them, the collection will benefit the wider scholarly community with a full reckoning of emerging topics and the creative interplay between them. The series focuses on key contemporary issues that evince a sea-change in the nexus of demographics and economics, eschewing standard 'populationist' theories centered on numerical growth in favor of more complex assessments that factor in additional data, for example on epidemiology or the shifting nature of the labor force. It aims to explore the obstacles to economic development that originate in high-growth populations and the disjunction of population change and food security. Where other studies have defined the 'economy' more narrowly, this series recognizes the potency of social and cultural influences in shaping development and acknowledges demographic change as a cause, as well as an effect, of broader shifts in society. It is also intended as a forum for methodological and conceptual innovation in analyzing the links between population and development, from finely tuned anthropological studies to global, systemic phenomena such as the 'demographic dividend'. Reflecting the boundary-blurring rapidity of developing nations' socio-economic rise, the editors are actively seeking studies relating to this sector, and also to Russia and the former Soviet states. At the same time as addressing their underrepresentation in the literature, the series also recognizes the critical significance of globalization, and will feature material on the developed world and on global migration. It provides everyone from geographers to economists and policy makers with a state-of-the-art appraisal of our understanding of demographics and development.

Christophe Z. Guilmoto
Editor

Atlas of Gender and Health Inequalities in India

Springer

Editor
Christophe Z. Guilmoto
Centre des Sciences Humaines/IRD
(CEPED)
New Delhi, India

ISSN 2543-0041 ISSN 2543-0068 (electronic)
Demographic Transformation and Socio-Economic Development
ISBN 978-3-031-47846-8 ISBN 978-3-031-47847-5 (eBook)
https://doi.org/10.1007/978-3-031-47847-5

This Springer imprint is published by the registered company Springer Nature Switzerland AG
The registered company address is: Gewerbestrasse 11, 6330 Cham, Switzerland

Paper in this product is recyclable.

"We actually made a map of the country, on the scale of a mile to the mile!
—Have you used it much? I enquired.
—It has never been spread out, yet, said Mein Herr, the farmers objected: they said it would cover the whole country, and shut out the sunlight! So we now use the country itself, as its own map, and I assure you it does nearly as well."

Lewis Carroll, *Sylvie and Bruno Concluded,* 1894

A map is not the territory, or is it?

Michael Batty, *Environment and Planning B,* 2019

Foreword

Intersections between geography and gender are well established in India. Indeed, a broad north-south distinction exists in kinship systems, with the northern region far more patriarchal, patrilineal, and patrilocal than the southern region. Wide differences have been identified in marriage practices (timing of marriage, spouse selection and the role of family elders, dowry practices, for example), inheritance norms, son preference, and unbalanced sex ratios and female seclusion norms, with women in the northern states far more disadvantaged than those in the southern region, although exceptions could exist. Deviation from established norms incurred heavy penalties not only on the individual but also on his or her family; hence, few dared to cross the line, resulting in the maintenance of the status quo over generations. In comparison to those from the north, women in the south of India have traditionally had a greater say in their own lives—they marry later, have decision-making authority in spouse selection, are less likely to espouse son preference, do not practice strict seclusion norms, and generally have closer spousal bonds with their husbands (Karve, 1965).

Over the years, evidence from censuses and surveys reiterated the persistence of this divide and its effects on both women's agency and demographic and reproductive behaviors. In an analysis of census data up to 1961 of factors underlying the unbalanced sex ratio of the population of India, for example, Visaria (1967; 1968) concluded that it was the female disadvantage in mortality that was largely responsible for the excess of males and that this disadvantage was most marked in the northern states and may be attributed to the "often overt but occasionally subtle discrimination against female children and the neglect of females even at adult ages." In their analysis, using indicators derived from censuses and surveys, of kinship structure, female autonomy, and demographic behavior, Dyson and Moore (1984) describe large differences in patterns of female agency, as measured by female seclusion (purdah), son preference, and educational attainment levels, as well as such demographic outcomes as sex ratios, infant and child mortality, fertility, child marriage, and contraceptive prevalence. A similar regional divide in female agency and reproductive behaviors was observed in a more micro-study using data from the

Status of Women and Fertility survey that sought to explain the association between female agency and reproductive behavior, comparing samples of women in two districts (one more and one less developed) in each of two states, namely Uttar Pradesh and Tamil Nadu (Jejeebhoy, 2001). Findings highlight a clear regional divide in both indicators of women's agency, as measured by women's reported decision-making authority, mobility, control over economic resources, and freedom from spousal violence, as well as in their reproductive behavior as measured by fertility and contraception. Jejeebhoy concludes that contextual factors, notably region as a proxy for gender systems and, less consistently, levels of development and religion, powerfully condition the impact of female agency on reproductive behavior. In short, the suggestion of all of these analyses is the centrality of gender systems and the culture of patriarchy, as defined by region in defining indicators of female agency and reproductive behaviors.

A serious limitation of using the state as the unit of analysis in discussions of the broad north-south divide is that the state is at too high a level of aggregation to enable a granular interpretation of sociocultural disparities within-state and within-region. Karve acknowledged, for example, that the broad north-south divide masked many exceptions at sub-regional levels: "[. . .] and yet no region has the same kind of kinship pattern [. . .] a description can give but a generalized picture, [. . .] and it is necessary to understand the variety and mode of the changes which are found in each linguistic region or in each case to understand well the implications of a social structure" (1965: 378).

This volume, *The Atlas of Gender and Health Inequalities in India*, takes off from and goes beyond previous work in multiple ways. For one, much has changed since earlier investigations were conducted, and this volume provides a view of the contemporary situation using data drawn from the NFHS and the wealth of demographic and female agency indicators that the NFHS incorporates. More importantly, it has overcome the limitation of the state as too high a level of aggregation by its use of the district as its unit of analysis, relying on data reflecting smaller units of analysis—India's 707 districts. Districts are likely more homogeneous than states, allowing researchers to better establish the extent to which a given indicator conforms to or deviates from the broad north-south divide pattern. The availability of the plethora of indicators reflecting the current scenario allows for investigation into intersections between geography, gender, and health across a range of outcomes.

Using factor analysis, this Atlas partitions India into four broad and seven specific clusters, refining but roughly retaining the familiar north-south divide observed earlier. A glance at the findings, moreover, confirms that geography continues to play a major role in the structure of gender and health outcomes in India. As others have suggested, this Atlas concurs that even today, geographic variation is more pronounced than other socio-demographic variations. While the north-south divide may be blurring in some indicators, the north-south gap persists in many indicators, especially those indicators reflecting the situation of women—underweight women, female under-five mortality, land ownership, anemia, land ownership, son preference, as well as such reproduction-related indicators as fertility and modern contraception, for example. In other indicators, such as cesarean section deliveries, diabetes/hypertension, and overweight, it is the southern districts that are disadvantaged compared to those in other parts of the country, the obvious result of lifestyle changes taking place among women in more gender egalitarian settings.

This Atlas has mapped the persistence of regional inequalities in gender and health and calls on further research to place geography at the core of the analysis of inequality in India. It opens a slew of questions for deeper analysis, for example: Why have regional patterns persisted in spite of the rapid demographic and development changes taking place in the country? What are the factors underlying deviations from the state- or region-level norm in some indicators in some districts? Which are the last mile districts, and what are the factors—programmatic and other—that account for their poor outcomes? In short, while this volume has showcased prevailing geographic inequalities, its findings invite further research to delve into explaining factors underlying these inconsistencies in various geographies.

Director, Aksha Centre for Equity and Wellbeing, Mumbai, India
Shireen J. Jejeebhoy

Distinguished Visiting Faculty, International Institute for Population Sciences, Mumbai, India

President, International Union for the Scientific Study of Population, Aubervilliers, France

References

Dyson, T., & Moore, M. (1984). On kinship structure, female autonomy, and demographic behavior in India. *Population and Development Review*, *9*, 1: 35–60.

Jejeebhoy, S. J. (2001). Women's autonomy and reproductive behaviour in India. In Sathar, Zeba A., & James F. Phillips (Eds.), *Fertility transition in South Asia*, Oxford University Press.

Karve, I. (1965). *Kinship organisation in India*. Asia Publishing House.

Visaria, P. (1968). *The sex ratio of the population of India*. Census of India 1961, v. 1, Monograph 10, Office of the Registrar General.

Visaria, P. (1967). The sex ratio of the population of India and Pakistan and regional variations during 1901–61. In Bose, A. (Ed.), *Patterns of population change in India, 1951–61*. Allied Publishers.

Preface

The connection between health, gender, and space may appear evident in India since the discussion of many distinctive features of India's modernity—from son preference to the overuse of C-sections or lack of health facilities—is inevitably cast in regional terms as if the location (Punjab, South India, the Northeast, etc.) by itself were the "explanation" for gender or health outcomes. However, the connection was impossible to establish without a solid empirical basis that only disaggregated statistics can provide. With the emergence of new data from the fourth National Family Health Survey (NFHS) conducted in 2015–16, it is now feasible to reconsider the existing evidence linking gender and health outcomes with India's intricate geography. As the microdata from the next NFHS wave were subsequently made available in 2022, we even have figures that may, to some extent, replace the delayed 2021 census to portray India's demographic and health situation at the beginning of the 2020s.

The ambition of this volume is to provide an empirical update on India's gender and health scenario with the help of India's most recent set of statistics and to walk the readers through India's intricate maps of inequalities across its 707 districts. Despite previous efforts to document gender and health inequalities in the recent past, no single volume has focused on the extent and regional contours of the considerable disparities in demographic and health outcomes, primarily for want of adequate statistical sources. For the first time, the last two rounds of the National Family Health Survey have offered statistical materials to investigate the socioeconomic and regional variations of a wide range of gender, health, and demographic indicators. By examining outcomes as varied as son preference, child morbidity, healthcare utilization, nutrition, menstrual hygiene, or women's health behavior, we show how the health status diverges across the country. The focus is here on women rather than men since gender and health dimensions are closely intertwined, as the analyses will demonstrate.

This Atlas represents the first initiative to investigate gender and health dimensions through multiple, locally estimated indicators while relying on a single nationally representative dataset, namely the fifth NFHS round conducted in 2019–21 over a population of 2.8 million people. Given the diversity of the dozens of dimensions reviewed, the volume has been divided into four parts, allowing for related chapters that refer to different gender, health mechanisms, and behavioral features to be read in succession. Each chapter can also be consulted independently of the rest of the Atlas, as they are centered on one or two dimensions of gender and health. The chapters' format and size are almost identical, and they all focus on one or two maps of the phenomenon under study plotted at the district level, along with the corresponding cluster maps highlighting regional concentrations of high and low values. Trend analysis and disaggregation by socioeconomic status have been added in some chapters. When included, statistical analyses—mostly logistic regressions of health and gender outcomes—have been simplified and summarized via a forest plot of odds-ratio coefficients. References to the existing literature and discussion of findings by other authors have also been kept to a minimum.

The topics covered in this Atlas may occasionally appear skewed toward specific questions (e.g., reproductive behavior) or, conversely, silent on others (e.g., gender violence). However, the selection of these themes was determined by a host of factors such as the perceived priority of some issues (e.g., son preference) and their novelty (e.g., hysterectomy), the availability of scholars working on them, and finally, the possibility to harness reliable and significant NFHS-5 data for a disaggregated analysis.

In addition, the book also includes two distinct chapters. The first chapter ("Sources, Maps, and Spatial Analysis") introduces the statistical sources and mapping methods used throughout the Atlas. It must be read as a methodological companion to all other chapters, as it provides necessary information about the origin of data (the fifth round of the NFHS), the methods used for mapping health and gender indicators, and the purpose and methods of the spatial analysis tools used in this volume. The last chapter ("The Geography of Gender and Health Inequalities in India") is an epilogue written once the Atlas was completed. It summarizes the findings by offering a unified perspective on India's current diversity of gender and health situations. This chapter encapsulates, in particular, the long-term persistence of these health and gender variations in India and their inherently spatial patterns. It should, however, remain clear to readers that the Atlas cannot do justice to all aspects of the heterogeneity of gender and health behavior. It does not pretend to be exhaustive but rather analytical, providing essential cues and clues for future research, especially when new, better data will be available.

The starting point for the volume was a series of two workshops held in Delhi in 2018 and 2019 and organized by the Centre des Sciences Humaines and Jawaharlal Nehru University. The first meeting in December 2018 was titled "Population, Health, and Society in India through the Lens of the Latest NFHS Round." It brought together 23 participants from all over India who had started working on the NFHS microdata immediately after its release. The intention for this initial workshop was to share the first results and critically discuss the quality and reliability of this unique dataset. A second two-day workshop ("Mapping Gender Discrimination in India") was convened in December 2019 and brought together an even more significant number of scholars—a combination of health, gender, and population specialists who had already explored the deep resources of the NFHS-4. This second meeting was organized thanks to funding from the Institut du Genre in Paris and the Ceped, a joint research center of the French Research Institute for Development and Université Paris Cité. I acknowledge the additional support from the Centre des Sciences Humaines and Jawaharlal Nehru University for organizing and hosting this second event. The 19 original papers presented in Delhi in 2019 ranged over a great diversity of topics; still, they all had in common the choice to follow a disaggregated regional with district-level statistical samples derived from NFHS-4. Since then, some papers could unfortunately not be turned into chapters, but several more authors joined us later and enriched the project with new studies on unexplored gender or health dimensions. The COVID-19 pandemic slowed down our work in 2020 and 2021, and the first manuscript draft was completed at the beginning of 2022—coinciding with the release of the NFHS-5 microdata by the International Institute of Population Sciences (IIPS). It was then decided to revise all chapters—analyses, maps, and tables—during the next 12 months to incorporate the 2019–21 figures. These episodes delayed the preparation of this Atlas but gave us the privilege of using the most recent data.

The book has been a long time in the making, and the contributors must be thanked for their patience. I am indebted to the 32 authors who contributed to this volume following the strict deadlines and waited patiently for publication. From the beginning, Nandita Saikia was part of the editorial team but had to withdraw because of other professional commitments. The thought and time she gave to the volume are greatly appreciated and have helped reshape many chapters. The initial workshops would not have taken place without substantial financial and logistical assistance from the Institut du Genre and the Centre des Sciences Humaines. Special thanks are also due to Nicolas Gravel and Amit Arora for their efficient support in Delhi during these events. At the time of the completion of this book, I was affiliated with the Centre des Sciences Humaines in Delhi and was also an invited professor at the Centre of Demography of Gender at the IIPS in Mumbai. I thank Profs Odile Henry, Abhishek Singh, and K.S. James for their hospitality and support. In addition, all authors benefited from the formidable efforts of the NFHS-5 team to complete the surveys in an epidemiologically and politically difficult period and to release the raw data within a year, without which this Atlas would not have been possible. A final word of thanks is due to Yoann Doignon, Sébastien Oliveau, and Eric Opigez for their initial advice on the volume's cartography, to Prof. Shireen Jejeebhoy for her foreword, and to Yves Charbit, Dharmalingam Arunachalam, and Evelien Bakker for their editorial enthusiasm and support.

New Delhi, India
August 2023

Christophe Z. Guilmoto

Contents

Contributors

Jayanta Kumar Bora VART Consulting, Mumbai, India

Bandita Boro Centre for the Study of Regional Development, Jawaharlal Nehru University, New Delhi, India

Aparajita Chattopadhyay International Institute for Population Sciences, Mumbai, India

Bhaswati Das Centre for the Study of Regional Development, Jawaharlal Nehru University, New Delhi, India

Moradhvaj Dhakad University of Vienna, Vienna, Austria
International Institute for Applied Systems Analysis, Laxenburg, Austria
Wittgenstein Centre for Demography and Global Human Capital (IIASA, VID/OAW, WU), Vienna, Austria

Mathieu Ferry Laboratoire Printemps, Université de Versailles Saint-Quentin-en-Yvelines, Versailles, France

Kirti Gaur Salaam Bombay Foundation, Mumbai, India

Dipti Govil International Institute for Population Sciences, Mumbai, India

Christophe Z. Guilmoto Centre des Sciences Humaines/IRD (CEPED), New Delhi, India

Ismail Haque Jamia Millia Islamia (A Central University), New Delhi, India

William Joe Institute of Economic Growth, Delhi, India

Mary E. John Formerly with the Centre for Women's Development Studies, New Delhi, India

Kunal Keshri International Institute for Population Sciences, Mumbai, India

Junaid Khan Vivekananda College, Kolkata, India

Ashish Kumar Upadhyay International Institute for Population Sciences, Mumbai, India

Abhishek Kumar Institute of Economic Growth, Delhi, India

Gulshan Kumar Kashi Sahu College, Seraikela, India

Rakesh Kumar Institute of Economic Growth, Delhi, India

Aditi Kundu Centre for the Study of Regional Development, Jawaharlal Nehru University, New Delhi, India

Bertrand Lefebvre French Institute of Pondicherry, Pondicherry, India

Thomas Licart Université de Strasbourg, Strasbourg, France

Raman Mishra College of Health Science, Korea University, Seoul, South Korea

Basant Kumar Panda Population Council Consulting, New Delhi, India

Sunil Rajpal FLAME University, Pune, India

Md Juel Rana G.B. Pant Social Sciences Institute, Prayagraj, India

Koyel Sarkar New York University, Abu Dhabi, United Arab Emirates

Abhishek Singh International Institute for Population Sciences, Mumbai, India

Akancha Singh International Institute for Population Sciences, Mumbai, India

Angad Singh Office of Registrar General of India, New Delhi, India

M. Sivakami Tata Institute of Social Sciences, Mumbai, India

Ankita Srivastava Centre for the Study of Regional Development, Jawaharlal Nehru University, New Delhi, India

About the Editor

Christophe Z. Guilmoto is a Senior Fellow in demography at the French *Institut de recherche pour le développement* (IRD) attached to the CEPED research unit in Paris. In France, he taught at Université Paris Descartes and EHESS. He joined in 2021 the *Centre de Sciences Humaines*, New Delhi, to work on the demography of inequalities.

He was trained initially in Mathematics and Sociology. After staying at the Madras institute of Development Studies in Chennai and the Institute of Economic Growth in Delhi, he received a Ph.D. in Demography in 1989 at Paris I University for a dissertation on India's historical demography. He then worked in Senegal in the early 1990s and published extensively on international migration. From 1997 to 2002, he was based at the French Institute of Pondicherry and worked primarily on fertility decline in India. Over the last decade, his research mainly focused on prenatal sex selection from Albania to China. He has since then organized several conferences, panels, and training sessions on sex imbalances at birth in Europe and Asia and wrote more than ten monographs on gender-biased sex selection in countries of Asia and Eastern Europe, including the global report on sex imbalances at birth published by the UNFPA in 2012.

His last book was *Demographic Transformation in China, India, and Indonesia* (coedited with Gavin Jones, Springer 2016). His recent work appeared notably in *Population Studies*, *Population and Development Review*, *Population, The Conversation, PLoS-One*, *JAMA*, *Lancet Global Health, The History of the Family,* and *BMJ Global Health*.

Abbreviations

ACMI	Aggregate Crude Migration Intensity
ANC	Antenatal Care
BMGF	Bill and Melinda Gates Foundation
BMI	Body-Mass Index
CAB	Clinical, Anthropometric, and Biochemical
CAPI	Computer-Assisted Personal Interviewing
CBR	Crude Birth Rate
CDC	Centre for Disease Control and Prevention
CI	Confidence Interval
CPR	Contraceptive Prevalence Rate
CRS	Civil Registration System
DBP	Diastolic Blood Pressure
DFID	The United Kingdom Department for International Development
DHS	Demographic and Health Survey
DLHS	District Level Health Survey
EAG	Empowered Action Group
EPI	Expanded Program on Immunization
FABM	Fertility Awareness-Based Method
GBD	Global Burden of Disease
HIV/AIDS	Human Immunodeficiency Virus/Acquired Immune Deficiency Syndrome
IFSS	Internet File Streaming System
IHDS	India Human Development Survey
IIPS	International Institute for Population Sciences
IUD	Intra-Uterine Devices
LAM	Lactational Amenorrhea Method
LISA	Local Indicator of Spatial Association
MCEB	Mean Children Ever Born
MCV	Measles-Containing Vaccines Coverage
MDG	Millennium Development Goals

MMR	Maternal Mortality Ratio
MOHFW	Ministry of Health and Family Welfare
MWCD	Ministry of Women and Child Development
NACO	National AIDS Control Organizations
NARI	National AIDS Research Institute
NCD	Non-Communicable Diseases
NFHS	National Family Health Survey
NNM	National Nutrition Mission
NPCDCS	National Program for Prevention and Control of Cancer, Diabetes, Cardiovascular Diseases, and Stroke.
NRHM	National Rural Health Mission
NSSO	National Sample Survey Office
OBC	Other Backward Classes
OLS	Ordinary Least Square
OR	Odds Ratio
ORGI	Office of Registrar General India
POSHAN	Prime Minister's Overarching Scheme for Holistic Nutrition
PPIUCD	Post-Partum Intrauterine Contraceptive Devise
PSUs	Primary Sampling Units
SBP	Systolic Blood Pressure
SCs	Scheduled Castes (Dalits)
SDG	Sustainable Development Goal
SR	Spatial Regression
SRS	Sample Registration System
STs	Scheduled Tribes (Adivasis)
TFR	Total Fertility Rate
U5MR	Under-Five Mortality Rate
UNFPA	United Nations Fund for Population Activities
UNICEF	United Nations Children's Fund
USAID	United States Agency for International Development
UT	Union Territory
WHO	World Health Organization

List of Figures

List of Tables

Chapter 1
Sources, Maps, and Spatial Analysis

Christophe Z. Guilmoto

The National Family Health Survey

Since the early 1990s, successive rounds of the National Family Health Survey have been conducted in India by the International Institute for Population Sciences (IIPS), Mumbai, under the Ministry of Health and Family Welfare (MOHFW) of the Government of India. The NFHS surveys replicate the framework of Demographic and Health Surveys conducted in 90 countries in Africa, Asia, Europe, Oceania, Latin America, and the Caribbean. DHS surveys aimed to generate high-quality data on population and health differentials and trends, addressing notably the lack of accurate demographic data from vital statistics or hospital records.

In India, the NFHS rounds provide national and state estimates for domains such as fertility, family planning, mortality, maternal and child health, nutrition, healthcare quality, and gender. They provide in particular information and microdata on demographic behavior and reproductive health that are not available from other sources existing in India, such as the civil registration system, the Sample Registration Scheme (SRS), the decennial censuses, or the national Sample Surveys (NSS).

In India, the NFHS surveys play a significant role in informing and monitoring population, health, and nutrition programs. They have modernized data availability on population and health, enabling interventions and improvements at the local level. The data collected through these surveys have been used to assess trends, evaluate programs, and guide policy-making in various health and family welfare areas. In the absence of data from the 2021 Census of India, which the government has postponed till 2024 or 2025, the latest NFHS round provides unique updated

C. Z. Guilmoto (✉)
Centre des Sciences Humaines/IRD (CEPED), New Delhi, India
e-mail: christophe.guilmoto@ird.fr

C. Z. Guilmoto (ed.), *Atlas of Gender and Health Inequalities in India*, Demographic Transformation and Socio-Economic Development 16,
https://doi.org/10.1007/978-3-031-47847-5_1

information on some basic sociodemographic such as age and sex distribution, age at marriage, and education attainment.

Below, I summarize the main features of the previous NFHS rounds:

- NFHS-1: Conducted in 1992–93, this first round included a nationally representative sample of 88,562 households and 89,777 ever-married women aged 13–49 years in 24 states and the National Capital Territory of Delhi. Similar to other DHS surveys conducted worldwide, it collected information on marriage, fertility, family planning, maternal and child health, and knowledge about HIV/AIDS.
- NFHS-2: Conducted in 1998–99, the second NFHS round was based on a sample of over 91,000 ever-married women aged 15–49 across all 26 states of India. It also collected data on population health components, health and family welfare services, reproductive health problems, women's status, and domestic violence.
- NFHS-3: Conducted in 2005–06, the third NFHS round included a sample of slightly bigger size, with 230,431 women aged 15–49 and 74,369 men aged 15–54. Besides the previous items, the NFHS-3 covered emerging issues such as perinatal mortality, male involvement in health and family welfare services, adolescent reproductive health, high-risk sexual behavior, family life education, safe injections, and knowledge about tuberculosis.
- NFHS-4: Conducted in 2015–16 after a gap of 10 years, this fourth round had a much larger sample size of 699,686 women aged 15–49 and 122,051 men aged 15–54 from all states and union territories. It aimed to provide indicators at the district level. It also expanded the scope of the NFHS by covering additional health issues through clinical, anthropometric, and biochemical (CAB) data collection.

The source of this Atlas is the fifth NFHS-5 round, conducted from 2019 to 2021, i.e., before and after the period affected by the COVID-19 outbreak in India that claimed millions of lives. Its primary aim was like that of the previous rounds of NFHS.[1] Its sample included 724,115 women aged 15–49 and 101,839 men aged 15–54 across India. NFHS-5 also provides district-level estimates for many essential indicators and covers new subject matters such as preschool education, disability, access to toilet facilities, death registration, bathing practices during menstruation, and safe abortion methods and reasons. Some data were, however, collected only at the state level (e.g., questions on gender violence) and cannot be estimated at the district level.[2]

The response rate in NFHS-5 was satisfactorily high at 98% among households, 97% among eligible women, and 92% among eligible men. Household response rates were over 94% in every state and union territory except Chandigarh (88%).

[1] More information on the surveys, the questionnaires, and the sampling design can be found in the report published by the IIPS (IIPS and ICF, 2022).

[2] See, however, the recent attempts at deriving district-level estimates of gender violence prevalence from state-level NFHS-4 figures (Srivastava et al., 2023).

Chandigarh's example illustrates the growing difficulty in surveying urban areas in India due to greater mobility, availability constraints, and privacy concerns. Computer-assisted personal interviewing (CAPI) significantly fastened data transmission, verification, and compilation. This new process explains why raw data were made available within a year in 2022. It should be added that some results derived from the NFHS-5 round (e.g., related to toilets or anemia) have proved politically unpalatable, and it remains to be seen whether raw data will remain entirely accessible in the next round.[3]

The most crucial dimension of the last two NFHS rounds relates to expanding the sample to provide district-level estimates, a historical breakthrough in data granularity. It should be noted that no other socioeconomic sample survey in India—such as the India Human Development Surveys or the National Sample Surveys—provides district-level estimates. The only comparable data source is the District-Level Household and Facility Survey (DLHS), the latest round of which was conducted in 2012–13. The DHLS was, however, much more limited in its scope than the NFHS surveys. Other sources of district-level statistics come from the Census of 2011 and the civil registration system for vital statistics (the latest report is available for 2020). A promising new source on reproductive health is the HMIS (Health Management Information System), which provides a yearly series of district-level estimates. However, the HMIS still needs a systematic quality assessment and regular statistical updates.[4]

The data used in this Atlas follow two distinct formats: on the one hand, district- or state-level weighted averages or, on the other hand, microdata at the individual or household level. The former is used for the spatial analysis, i.e., mapping and geostatistical analysis described in the next section. In contrast, the latter is used in the regression analysis found in several chapters.

As a summary of computations, I have added the table of variables used in this Atlas, with state-level averages (Table 1.1). These average values have also been computed and compared to the average for India's 707 districts for the 30 variables mapped in the different chapters of this Atlas. The complete definition of each variable will be found in individual chapters.

Microdata have also been used for the regression models. All these statistical models follow the same frame: multivariate logistic modeling of the outcome under study (occurrence of child anemia, female land ownership, etc.) against a set of demographic and socioeconomic variables (wealth, caste, marital status, etc.) and an additional set of control variables (region, age, etc.). The models have been tested on the entire weighted sample for India. Rather than providing the details of each statistical model in complex tables, I have opted for synthetic charts of odds ratios

[3] In July 2023, the director of IIPS was suspended reportedly due to the publication of unfavorable NFHS-5 results (see *Frontline* August 24, 2023).

[4] Since the Covid-19 epidemic and the controversy on its impact, disaggregated HMIS data are no longer available online.

Table 1.1 State-level average for the main variables used in the Atlas

	State	AND	AP	ARU	AS	BI	CD	CHH	DEL	DNH	GOA	GUJ	HAR	HP	J&K	JHA	KAR	KER	LAD	India
	Units																			
Underweight	%women	9.4	14.8	5.7	17.7	25.6	13.0	23.1	10.0	25.1	13.8	25.2	15.1	13.9	5.2	26.2	17.2	10.1	4.4	**18.7**
Overweight	%women	38.1	36.3	23.9	15.2	16.0	44.0	14.1	41.4	26.9	36.1	22.7	33.1	30.4	29.4	11.9	30.2	38.2	28.3	**24.0**
Vegetarianism	%women	0.7	3.2	0.4	0.6	12.8	40.8	15.4	28.1	20.0	3.0	58.4	70.1	41.2	12.0	6.0	16.5	1.1	2.4	**25.3**
Fish eaters	%women	93.5	56.5	62.9	81.0	36.8	6.3	31.0	21.2	36.6	92.4	13.8	3.4	3.5	16.2	40.8	35.5	88.4	10.5	**35.7**
Hypertension	%women	14.4	12.1	17.8	11.4	7.8	13.7	12.8	14.7	8.8	14.0	9.3	11.1	11.1	10.5	8.0	13.2	11.7	11.6	**10.8**
Hyperglycemia	%women	10.4	10.3	5.4	8.3	6.9	10.3	4.9	5.6	8.6	10.1	8.5	5.8	6.6	3.3	5.3	7.2	10.7	1.5	**7.2**
Anemia	%children	40.1	64.2	56.2	70.3	70.4	53.7	68.1	69.6	77.1	53.5	80.1	70.8	55.0	72.7	69.3	66.4	39.4	94.4	**68.0**
Anemia	%women	57.5	58.8	40.3	65.9	63.5	60.3	60.8	49.9	62.5	39.0	65.0	60.4	53.0	65.9	65.3	47.8	36.3	92.8	**57.0**
Under-5 mortality	p.1000 births	20.4	31.2	15.8	31.6	56.5	35.1	47.7	36.1	42.2	7.5	38.0	36.1	24.3	14.8	41.2	25.0	6.7	25.0	**42.0**
Landownership	%women	22.4	19.1	18.2	7.1	7.0	5.0	11.6	12.1	16.0	13.9	9.3	9.6	15.6	6.0	8.9	15.1	28.1	10.4	**10.8**
Patrilocality	%married children	83.2	91.7	90.8	96.8	95.5	97.5	96.9	97.0	92.6	95.4	97.5	99.3	98.0	97.3	95.6	91.4	87.9	93.9	**95.6**
Son preference	%women	35.6	39.8	44.4	44.2	64.7	52.8	55.6	53.5	64.3	44.6	58.1	65.8	54.5	45.2	59.1	47.1	31.5	35.6	**52.0**
Girl-only families	%women	22.1	17.3	9.0	14.7	4.3	9.6	10.1	10.5	7.8	18.1	8.4	5.3	9.0	8.2	7.0	14.6	22.6	10.7	**10.0**
Missing girl-only families	%women	13.0	19.4	48.1	28.5	65.2	53.1	41.7	46.9	56.9	28.7	57.6	72.7	59.7	55.1	55.1	31.4	1.4	45.3	**45.6**
Migrant husband	%women	2.6	3.0	4.2	3.4	25.4	2.1	1.7	1.4	3.4	6.7	3.5	3.4	12.7	0.6	14.9	3.3	17.6	0.8	**8.5**
Child marriage	%women	18.2	33.1	20.5	32.0	40.3	8.5	15.5	13.3	27.9	7.2	20.6	15.6	7.2	5.5	34.7	23.1	7.6	5.8	**24.7**
Menstrual hygiene	%women	98.9	85.2	92.0	67.0	59.2	94.5	69.0	97.1	94.3	96.8	66.9	93.5	92.0	74.5	75.1	84.6	93.3	79.1	**77.6**
Antenatal care	%births	83.6	67.5	36.6	50.7	25.2	79.4	60.4	77.8	86.2	93.0	77.2	60.9	70.6	81.1	38.7	70.9	81.4	78.9	**58.5**
Institutional deliveries	%births	98.9	96.5	79.2	84.1	76.2	96.9	85.7	91.8	96.5	99.7	94.3	94.9	88.2	92.4	75.8	97.0	99.8	95.1	**88.6**
Cesarean deliveries	%inst births	30.2	44.0	18.6	21.6	12.7	32.3	17.7	25.7	23.7	39.6	22.3	20.5	23.8	45.1	16.9	32.5	39.0	39.5	**24.3**
Hysterectomy	%women	2.0	8.7	1.9	1.1	6.0	0.9	1.7	1.7	1.9	1.9	3.9	2.4	2.0	2.7	2.6	3.4	2.0	3.6	**3.3**
Health insurance	%households	1.8	80.2	29.3	66.7	17.4	32.2	71.4	25.0	56.6	73.1	44.4	25.7	38.9	13.8	50.3	31.8	57.8	17.1	**41.0**
Mean number of children	children	1.3	1.7	1.7	1.7	2.3	1.6	1.7	1.6	1.7	1.1	1.7	1.7	1.6	1.3	2.0	1.6	1.5	1.2	**1.7**
Childlessness	%women	6.0	4.5	3.2	6.1	1.5	3.6	4.2	2.0	5.5	9.2	4.0	1.7	2.6	2.4	3.2	5.9	5.6	2.5	**3.8**
Only one child	%women	19.5	9.0	8.7	12.0	2.8	7.6	7.3	7.5	6.4	22.4	9.0	5.8	8.0	6.3	5.6	13.7	13.6	9.4	**9.7**
Full immunization	%children	78.5	72.2	63.8	65.9	70.8	80.2	79.6	75.5	94.9	81.1	76.0	77.2	88.9	86.8	73.4	84.1	77.6	86.8	**76.2**
Sterilization	%women	39.3	70.1	18.2	9.1	34.9	19.3	48.3	18.2	41.8	29.9	36.1	33.3	41.1	21.4	37.7	57.4	46.7	17.1	**38.2**
Modern contraception	%contraceptors	87.8	99.6	79.8	74.5	79.6	71.8	91.0	75.5	88.0	88.5	82.1	82.8	85.5	87.8	80.2	99.2	87.0	93.5	**84.6**

States: *AND* Andaman & Nicobar, *AP* Andhra Pradesh, *ARU* Arunachal Pradesh, *AS* Assam, *BI* Bihar, *CD* Chandigarh, *CHH* Chhattisgarh, *DEL* Delhi, *DNH* Dadra & Nagar Haveli & Diu, *GOA* Goa, *GUJ* Gujarat, *HAR* Haryana, *HP* Himachal Pradesh, *J&K* Jammu & Kashmir, *JHA* Jharkhand, *KAR* Karnataka, *KER* Kerala, *LAD* Ladakh

	State	LAK	MAH	MAN	MEG	MIZ	MP	NAG	ODI	PUD	PJB	RAJ	SIK	TN	TLG	TRI	UP	UK	WB	India
	Units																			
Underweight	%women	8.0	20.8	7.2	10.9	5.3	23.0	11.1	20.8	9.0	12.7	19.6	5.8	12.6	18.8	16.2	19.0	13.9	14.8	**18.7**
Overweight	%women	33.5	23.5	34.1	11.5	24.2	16.6	14.5	23.0	46.3	40.8	12.9	34.8	40.5	30.1	21.6	21.4	29.8	22.8	**24.0**
Vegetarianism	%women	0.0	24.3	0.2	0.5	0.1	50.5	0.1	5.2	2.3	59.7	67.1	8.1	3.0	3.9	0.6	38.9	24.0	0.9	**25.3**
Fish eaters	%women	97.1	30.7	67.3	57.4	26.2	11.5	30.7	66.3	82.2	3.6	4.5	56.8	61.3	18.6	87.5	15.3	13.7	87.8	**35.7**
Hypertension	%women	9.8	10.9	13.7	15.0	11.9	10.1	14.1	12.1	10.2	17.1	7.4	25.2	12.2	13.5	13.1	9.6	13.2	10.7	**10.8**
Hyperglycemia	%women	9.0	5.7	7.1	5.4	7.9	4.9	5.4	8.8	9.8	6.4	3.0	7.6	11.1	7.6	12.2	5.1	5.7	11.7	**7.2**
Anemia	%children	43.0	69.9	43.0	44.3	48.3	73.5	42.9	65.3	64.0	71.5	71.5	55.3	57.6	70.2	64.4	67.0	59.1	69.0	**68.0**
Anemia	%women	25.8	54.2	29.4	53.8	34.8	54.7	28.9	64.3	55.1	58.7	54.4	41.9	53.4	57.6	67.2	50.4	42.6	71.4	**57.0**
Under-5 mortality	p.1000 births	0.0	26.5	23.4	34.1	23.6	44.5	27.8	36.3	5.3	33.4	35.5	10.5	20.1	29.4	38.7	59.5	41.6	21.3	**42.0**
Landownership	%women	48.4	12.8	13.6	87.6	14.2	10.0	12.6	6.8	12.5	8.7	7.7	12.4	12.7	20.6	13.0	9.6	14.0	7.5	**10.8**
Patrilocality	%married children	21.0	97.3	94.8	19.7	92.8	97.7	91.6	94.9	83.8	98.5	99.0	92.5	89.5	92.3	92.7	98.2	98.6	94.9	**95.6**
Son preference	%women	31.8	51.4	44.8	22.4	27.1	64.2	49.3	47.9	31.7	60.6	68.2	32.1	41.0	43.0	30.3	60.7	58.7	40.2	**52.0**
Girl-only families	%women	19.3	11.4	11.3	12.8	13.2	6.4	9.7	13.9	22.7	8.0	4.9	23.2	17.8	15.1	22.1	6.3	7.6	17.5	**10.0**
Missing girl-only families	%women	4.0	46.5	37.3	16.5	20.6	62.4	37.2	35.1	6.9	63.4	70.6	14.8	21.4	25.8	16.3	55.7	57.2	27.2	**45.6**
Migrant husband	%women	29.4	1.9	5.8	2.4	1.9	3.5	3.6	9.1	4.6	5.7	8.1	6.6	8.5	3.6	4.2	13.2	11.0	6.0	**8.5**
Child marriage	%women	3.8	23.6	14.7	19.2	8.9	25.3	6.7	22.2	8.1	10.1	24.5	14.6	13.3	27.3	39.1	18.8	14.2	42.3	**24.7**
Menstrual hygiene	%women	98.3	85.3	83.4	65.3	91.0	60.9	80.6	81.7	99.1	93.3	84.3	86.3	98.4	93.4	69.1	72.9	91.5	83.4	**77.6**
Antenatal care	%births	92.1	71.4	79.4	52.2	58.1	57.5	20.7	78.1	87.4	59.8	55.4	58.4	90.6	70.5	55.2	42.5	61.8	76.7	**58.5**
Institutional deliveries	%births	99.6	94.7	79.9	58.1	85.8	90.7	45.7	92.2	99.6	94.3	94.9	94.7	99.6	97.0	89.2	83.4	83.2	91.7	**88.6**
Cesarean deliveries	%inst births	31.4	26.8	32.0	14.1	12.6	13.3	11.4	23.4	36.5	40.9	10.9	34.6	45.1	62.6	28.1	16.4	24.5	35.5	**24.3**
Hysterectomy	%women	1.2	3.0	1.8	0.7	1.5	2.8	1.8	1.9	1.6	3.2	2.1	0.8	2.5	8.2	1.7	2.6	2.1	2.7	**3.3**
Health insurance	%households	67.7	22.4	16.4	69.0	50.3	38.1	22.0	47.9	30.1	25.2	87.8	28.0	66.5	69.2	36.4	15.9	62.5	33.7	**41.0**
Mean number of children	children	1.3	1.6	1.6	2.0	1.5	1.9	1.6	1.6	1.4	1.5	1.8	1.1	1.5	1.7	1.5	1.9	1.8	1.6	**1.7**
Childlessness	%women	7.1	3.9	9.1	4.5	9.6	2.2	6.1	5.5	2.9	2.1	1.7	7.4	4.8	4.7	3.9	2.0	1.9	4.4	**3.8**
Only one child	%women	15.9	11.2	9.2	7.4	12.4	4.9	8.1	10.2	12.0	10.0	4.1	26.8	12.8	8.2	19.6	4.5	4.4	17.5	**9.7**
Full immunization	%children	85.2	73.6	69.9	63.2	72.6	77.0	56.6	90.6	82.3	75.5	80.2	79.6	88.6	79.3	68.4	69.2	82.0	88.1	**76.2**
Sterilization	%women	20.7	49.5	3.7	5.6	13.0	52.6	14.4	28.3	54.1	23.2	42.6	16.2	57.9	63.8	10.5	17.0	26.6	29.5	**38.2**
Modern contraception	%contraceptors	57.3	96.4	29.7	82.1	98.6	91.3	79.0	65.8	94.2	75.8	85.9	79.5	95.5	97.9	69.0	71.2	81.7	81.7	**84.6**

States: *MP* Madhya Pradesh, *MAH* Maharashtra, *MAN* Manipur, *MEG* Meghalaya, *MIZ* Mizoram, *NAG* Nagaland, *DEL* Delhi, *ODI* Odisha, *PUD* Puducherry, *PJB* Punjab, *RAJ* Rajasthan, *SIK* Sikkim *TN Tamil Nadu*, *TLG* Telangana, *TRI* Tripura, *UP* Uttar Pradesh, *UK* Uttarakhand, *WB* West Bengal

using "forest plots." Forest plots visually display the "odds ratios" of each explanatory variable: these ratios (centered on one and displayed with their confidence interval) sum up the strength of the association with the outcome variable. Odds ratios below (above) one are shown on the left (right) and correspond to a negative (positive) correlation. Odds ratios are displayed on a log scale for comparison since a negative odds ratio of 0.5 is the exact inverse of an odds ratio of two.

Mapping Districts

When NFHS-5 was conducted, India had 707 districts, i.e., 65 more than during the previous round following the 2011 census administrative division. The number has already jumped to over 780 by the beginning of 2024. Because of these continuous administrative changes, it is impossible to compare NFHS-5 figures with other district-level sources, including the 640 districts of the 2011 census. In the absence of an official vector file for these districts, I have generated a provisional map for the 707 districts using online cartographic information, including online maps of the new districts created since 2011.[5]

A critical administrative change occurred in 2019 when the government removed Jammu and Kashmir from its status as a state and converted it into two union territories (Jammu and Kashmir, and Ladakh). The two union territories of Daman and Diu and Dadra and Nagar Haveli were also merged a few months later into a single union territory (Dadra and Nagar Haveli and Daman and Diu). We follow this new regional administrative division for all maps and data. We endeavor to refer to places by their latest appellation, keeping in mind that many well-known localities, such as Gurgaon (now Gurugram) or Allahabad (now Prayagraj), have changed names recently.

The district-level maps were prepared based on the original NFHS-5 data by computing regional weighted averages. The classifications used for map data were systematically based on 6, 7, and 8 classes. The classification's first and last classes are often open-ended, allowing for outliers. Intervals are of the same range and are based on round numbers to allow easy comparison and ranking of districts. The classification may not be perfectly regular when the original data do not follow the expected Gaussian distribution. This is the case of the patrilocality variable—which hovers around 95% in most of North India but also records low values in matrilineal areas.

The color ramps follow suggestions from the www.colorbrewer2.org website developed by Cynthia A. Brewer. The saturation of the color used relates to the intensity of the variables used, with lighter shades for low-intensity areas. These

[5]There is today only one website providing some state- and district-level data from NFHS-5, but without the corresponding district base map (Riddhi Management Services, 2022). For an updated listing of existing districts, see: https://igod.gov.in

color schemes provide sequential chromatic patterns that are most efficient for communication (Harrower & Brewer, 2003). However, we sometimes wanted to highlight the lowest and the highest values. To do this, we resorted to diverging schemes based on two opposite colors: red for low intensity and blue for high intensity, with lighter shades for mid-range cases close to the national average. This method was used to map cesarean births (see Chap. 14). In this instance, we wanted to draw readers' attention to areas where women are deprived of access to surgical deliveries (e.g., Bihar) and to areas with a severe overuse of cesarean deliveries (e.g., Telangana). All final maps were prepared with QGIS 3.18 (Zürich version).

Spatial Autocorrelation and Clusters

Maps of health and gender features would be meaningless if the values were randomly distributed across Indian districts. With no spatial regularity, maps would turn into multicolored patchworks devoid of geographic interpretation. Nevertheless, socioeconomic features are never randomly distributed, and spatial patterns systematically emerge. This regularity is now the focus of demographic research (Matthews & Parker, 2013).

According to Tobler's first law of geography, "Everything is related to everything else, but near things are more related than distant things" (Miller, 2004). In other words, neighboring areas tend to share many social and economic features beyond common geography, and this homogeneity is evident in spatial patterns illustrated by maps. For instance, high values of a given variable often cluster in specific parts of India. Such a concentration is, for example, visible for the proportion of women married to a migrant, an indirect measure of male outmigration: their proportion is extremely low across India, except for a few (male) "migration pockets" visible, for instance, in Purvanchal and Bihar (see Chap. 10). For a less clustered phenomenon such as vegetarianism, the map displays a very regular gradient, with the proportion of vegetarian adult women regularly declining from 70% in Northwest India to close to zero along the eastern littoral (see Fig. 3.3). The first law of geography (NB: there is no second law) is so pervasive that the absence of notable spatial features points unquestionably to potential measurement issues.

What is "spatial dependency," and how do we know that geographic proximity affects the distribution of values of given characteristics? The primary indicator of spatial dependency is spatial autocorrelation, computed as the correlation between values in neighboring localities (see computational definition below). We are resorting here to Moran's *I*, the standard indicator of spatial autocorrelation implemented as the measure of the correlation between each observation and the averaged values of the "neighboring" observations. A zero value means that the estimates of adjacent districts are uncorrelated, while an *I* value of one corresponds to total spatial uniformity. An important issue relates to defining what makes up "neighbors." Given India's district distribution, the easiest method is to consider districts with common boundaries as neighbors, a technique referred to as "queen proximity of the first order."

I have compared the results with other definitions of the contiguity matrix, using notably second-order contiguity (counting adjacent districts of adjacent districts as neighbors). The resulting measures of spatial dependence are significantly weaker, and this is due to the wide variation in district size. "Neighbors of neighbors" (i.e., second-order contiguity) may lie at a considerable distance from the original district. For instance, district size in Western Rajasthan or Ladakh is immense and "neighbors of neighbors" of a given district may often be several hundred kilometers away. Inversely, in densely populated areas such as Delhi or West Bengal, where the surface area of districts tends to be comparatively minuscule, neighbors of neighbors are almost adjacent and may lie a few kilometers apart. For similar spatial reasons, a strictly geographical definition of distance in kilometers—in which districts would be considered neighbors if lying within a fixed distance of each other—is not applicable. The minimal distance between districts used in such calculations would indeed be huge as it would be based on the most isolated district (e.g., Lakshadweep, lying over 300 kilometers away from the closest district in Kerala) or on oversized and low-density districts such as Kutch, Jaisalmer, or Leh located along international borders.

Using first-order contiguity has, nonetheless, a few limitations. As explained earlier, the meaning of contiguity varies: a fringe district such as Kutch (Gujarat) is 500 kilometers away from the adjacent district of Jalor (Rajasthan). This "contiguity" corresponds to a 10-h drive between the two districts' headquarters. Sometimes, districts are not strictly contiguous (e.g., because of a waterway separating them), so I extended the tolerance in the definition of contiguity to one kilometer. With this revised definition of contiguity, districts have an average number of 5.5 neighbors, with a maximum of 11, as in Senapati in Manipur. However, there are still two insular units with no contiguous district (Lakshadweep and Nicobar) and eight more districts with only one neighbor, such as "edge districts" (e.g., Tawang in Arunachal Pradesh or Mumbai) or districts within a district (e.g., Hyderabad surrounded by Rangareddy). Spatial autocorrelation cannot be computed on isolated districts without neighbors, and its estimation is also less reliable for districts with one neighbor. The spatial autocorrelation can be calculated on 697 districts. They include 642 districts with four or more neighbors, accounting for 92% of the district sample.

Measuring Spatial Autocorrelation

The definition of spatial autocorrelation used here is Moran's I statistic. Moran's I is probably the most common measurement of overall spatial autocorrelation. To compute Moran's I, we start with a variable v and compute its deviation from the mean, i.e., v_i in locality i. Moran's I is then calculated as the cross-product of this variable v_i and its spatial lag (the average value of its neighbors v_j). The spatial autocorrelation of variable v over n districts is finally computed as:

$$I = \frac{\sum_{i,j} w_{ij}.v_i.v_j / S_0}{\sum_i v_i^2 / n}$$

In this equation, w_{ij} are the weights of the contiguity matrix, and S_O is the sum of all w_{ij}. Individual weights w_{ij} are equal to one only when districts i and j are neighbors (and zero otherwise). After row standardization of the weights ($S_O = n$), the formula simplifies to:

$$I = \frac{\sum_{i,j} w_{ij}.v_i.v_j}{\sum_i v_i^2}$$

The computation can also be illustrated by Moran's scatterplot (Fig. 1.1), in which district values of a given variable are shown against the spatial lag. Moran's I is indeed almost identical to the definition of standard linear regression, and its value is equal to the correlation coefficient of the regression of spatial lagged district values ($w_{ij}.v_j$) to original values (v_i) of district i. Moran's I vary from 0 (no autocorrelation) to 1 (perfect autocorrelation). With 707 districts in NFHS-5, the indicator significantly differs from zero when greater than 0.1. Nevertheless, 0.1 corresponds to an exceptionally low spatial autocorrelation level; Moran's I above 0.5 values are far more common and frequently exceed 0.7.

I use here as an illustration the proportion of women using hygienic methods during menstruation (see Chap. 12). The corresponding scatterplot with normalized values is shown in Fig. 1.1. The chart contrasts the original measurements of this variable in each district ("HYGIENIC," shown on the X-axis) with its spatial lag measured as the average value of adjacent districts ("lagged HYGIENIC," shown on the Y-axis). It demonstrates the strong correlation between measurements in districts and their neighbors, with Moran's I attaining 0.721. This value is one of the top spatial autocorrelation levels of this Atlas, and it means that the average values of neighboring districts account for over 70% of the variance of menstrual hygiene in a district.

The scatterplot is centered on zero as the original variables are standardized. It determines four quadrants with values below or above the mean for districts and their spatial lag. These four quadrants are further used to identify some critical characteristics of spatial distributions. For instance, the top-right quadrant includes districts with values above the mean and whose neighbors also record values above the mean. Conversely, the bottom-left quadrant points to districts with lower-than-average values surrounded by districts that also show lower-than-average values. After statistical testing (see below), these districts, when significant, will be identified as "hotspots" (or "high-high districts") and "cold spots" ("low-low districts"), respectively. Finally, in the remaining two quadrants, we have a smaller number of districts

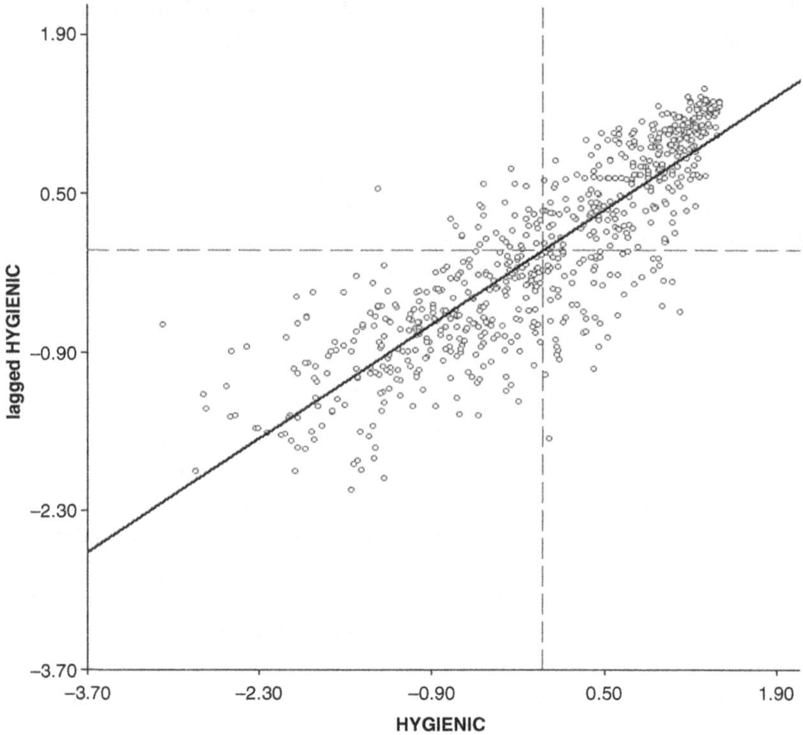

Fig. 1.1 Moran scatterplot for menstrual hygiene
Note: normalized district values on the X-axis and average values of neighboring districts on the Y-axis

whose individual values differ from those of their spatial lags. These are spatial outliers ("low-high districts" and "high-low districts").

The next step is to confirm the significance of these spatial patterns by randomized permutations. In this analysis, we have set the significance level at 5% after 999 permutations. Several hundred districts shown in the scatterplot are not significantly different from the mean distribution. As a result, they will appear on the cluster map neither as "hotspots" (in red) nor as "cold spots" (in blue).

This analysis leads to maps of clusters for all variables under study. For instance, the map (Fig. 1.2) shows India's spatial clustering of menstrual hygiene based on the same district-level variable. This map is drawn directly from the GeoDa 1.18 software (Anselin et al., 2010) used to compute spatial autocorrelation and identify Moran clusters. Lakshadweep and Nicobar are not included in the analysis for lack of immediate neighbors. In South and Northwest India, red districts exhibit a high frequency of menstrual hygiene, with similar values observed in surrounding districts. Conversely, blue districts are characterized by poor hygiene practices. Districts with less frequent antenatal care cluster around a large chunk of Central India,

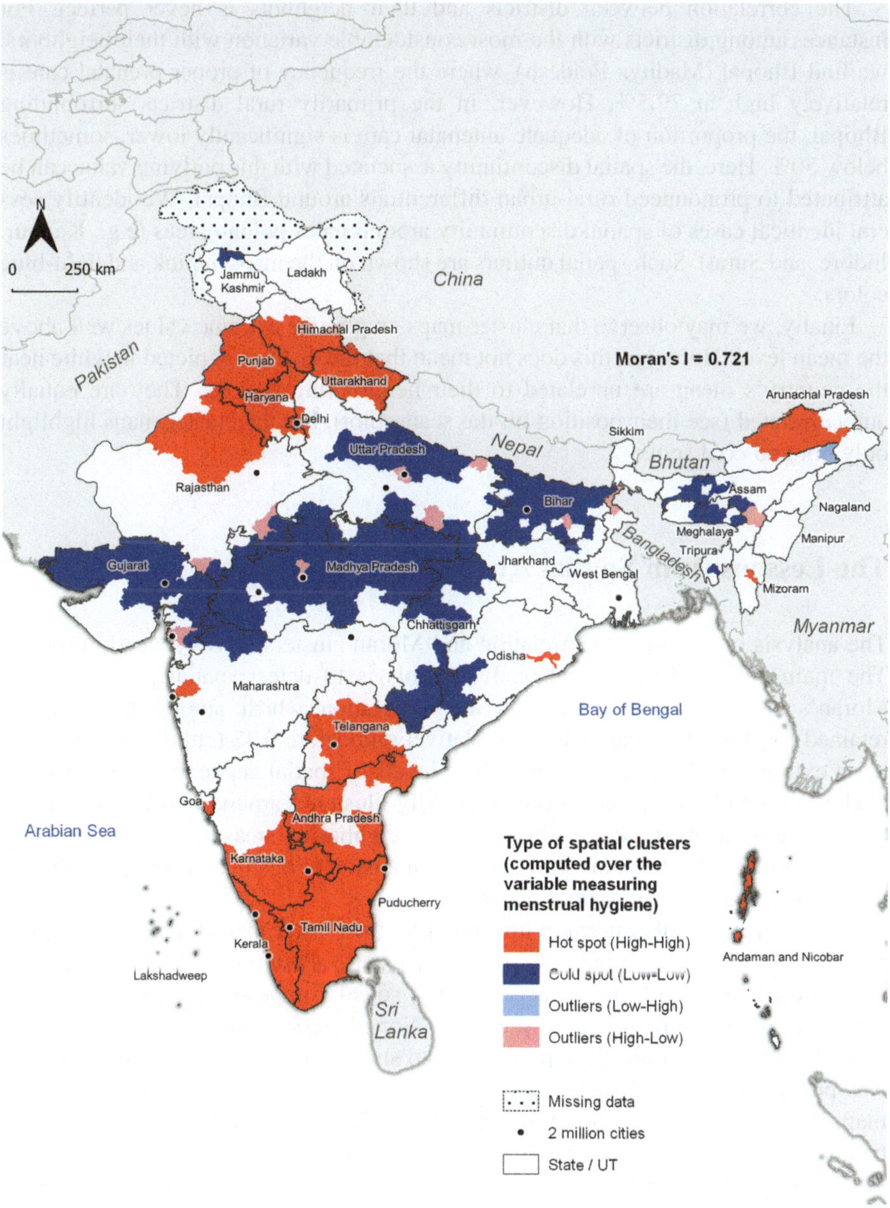

Fig. 1.2 Moran clusters for menstrual hygiene
See text for definition
Source: NFHS-5, 2019–21
The map is for illustrative purposes and may not represent official boundaries

extending from Gujarat to Bihar. In addition, we can detect smaller isolated territories characterized by poor menstrual hygiene on the map.

The correlation between districts and their neighbors is never perfect. For instance, among districts with the most considerable variation with their neighbors, we find Bhopal (Madhya Pradesh), where the frequency of proper prenatal care is relatively high at 79.5%. However, in the primarily rural districts surrounding Bhopal, the proportion of adequate antenatal care is significantly lower, sometimes below 50%. Here, the spatial discontinuity associated with this outlying value can be attributed to pronounced rural-urban differentials around Bhopal. We identify several identical cases of spatial discontinuity around metropolitan areas (e.g., Kanpur, Indore, and Surat). Such spatial outliers are shown on the maps in pink and light-blue colors.

Finally, we may observe that cluster maps emphasize extreme values well above the mean level. However, this does not mean that the districts depicted in white near the country's mean are unrelated to their neighboring regions. They are equally autocorrelated (see their position on the scatterplot), but the cluster maps highlight only hot and cold spots.

The Lessons from Spatial Analysis

The analysis of spatial autocorrelation and Moran clusters serves several purposes. The main aim of these spatial analysis tools is to detect spatial patterns. First, Moran's *I* tells us the strength of the autocorrelation, which, among the indicators retained for this Atlas, varies from a relatively moderate 0.42 (child immunization) to an extreme 0.92 (vegetarianism). Such levels of spatial dependency suggest that health and gender outcomes are substantially clustered around specific regions of high and low intensity, and the influence of neighboring areas on each district may be considerable. As the Atlas shows, each dimension of health and gender studied in this Atlas reveals unique spatial patterns.

Second, the spatial patterning illustrated by the cluster maps forces the reader to envisage factors accounting for specific clusters. Common explanatory frames (standard of living, education, accessibility, social composition, exposure to risk, etc.) are often used for that purpose. Nonetheless, local patterns often go unexplained. For example, the previous map showed that better menstrual hygiene was prevalent in central Arunachal Pradesh, emerging as a separate cluster on the map. However, there is no obvious explanation for this clustering. It is also important to stress that geographic patterns highlighted by the maps only partly align with state boundaries. Moreover, they often do not precisely coincide with India's conventional geography of development or urbanization.

A third lesson from the spatial analysis is entirely different. As we expect reasonably high spatial autocorrelation, we have become wary of cases of weak spatial autocorrelation. A low Moran's *I* could very well mean that this feature described by the indicator under study is poorly spatially autocorrelated, but, as I said earlier, this is relatively uncommon among social phenomena. A more plausible explanation relates to the poor quality of the measurement used. Such measurement deficiency may stem from two factors. One factor is the sampling itself and the resulting district-level sample size. While each district of the NFHS-5 survey includes about 1000 households, measurements sometimes apply to a much smaller subsample. For instance, some fertility measurements are based on women in their forties. Sampling issues may be another cause for measurement bias. The second factor relates directly to the quality of the measure itself. Such limitations may be due to a poorly worded or translated item in the NFHS-5 questionnaire, the lack of familiarity of interviewers or interviewees about specific items, or imperfect measurement by field workers. The volatility of imperfect measurement increases when two weak indicators are combined when based, for instance, on the ratio of two indirect indicators.[6]

A rule of thumb used here is to handle with care variables that demonstrate a Moran's *I* lower than 0.5. With low levels of spatial autocorrelation, the resulting map of the variable is inevitably complex to interpret, and the corresponding cluster map is limited to smaller and more scattered clusters. As a result, several maps were ultimately rejected from the Atlas, as we had serious doubts about the robustness of the indicator used. Beyond its use to measure spatial dependency, Moran's *I* provides a reliable indicator of inaccurate measurement, even if this is not the primary goal of spatial autocorrelation estimation.

References

Anselin, L., Syabri, I., & Kho, Y. (2010). GeoDa: An introduction to spatial data analysis. In *Handbook of Applied Spatial Analysis* (pp. 2115–2123). Springer.

Harrower, M., & Brewer, C. A. (2003). ColorBrewer.org: An online tool for selecting colour schemes for maps. *The Cartographic Journal, 40*(1), 27–37.

International Institute for Population Sciences (IIPS) and ICF. (2022). *National Family Health Survey (NFHS-5), 2019–21: India.* IIPS.

Matthews, S. A., & Parker, D. M. (2013). Progress in spatial demography. *Demographic Research, 28*, 271.

Miller, H. J. (2004). Tobler's first law and spatial analysis. *Annals of the Association of American Geographers, 94*(2), 284–289.

Riddhi Management Services. (2022). *User's Guide, NFHS-5 GIS India.* Riddhi Management Services. http://nfhs5.indiagis.org/nfhs5

Srivastava, S., Kumar, K., McDougal, L., Kannaujiya, A. K., Sikarwar, A., Raj, A., & Singh, A. (2023). Spatial heterogeneity in intimate partner violence across the 640 districts of India: A secondary analysis of a cross-sectional, population-based survey by use of model-based small-area estimation. *The Lancet Global Health, 11*(10), e1587–e1597.

[6] The sex ratios of several health and mortality indicators were found to be statistically unstable and, therefore, were not retained in the final version of the Atlas.

Part I
Nutrition and Morbidity

Chapter 2
Underweight and Overweight Prevalence Among Indian Women

Rakesh Kumar, Abhishek Kumar, Sunil Rajpal, and William Joe

Nutrition has highly instrumental and intrinsic relevance for individuals as well as population health and well-being. It has emerged as a fundamental global health concern in recent years, with ever-increasing policy attention in various national and international forums, including the Sustainable Development Goals (SDGs). The global burden of undernutrition is disproportionately borne by women and children in the low-and middle-income countries, further reinforcing the intergenerational undernourishment cycle. Worldwide, 9.4% of women (240 million) are estimated to be underweight (Global Nutrition Report, 2020). Targeted policy efforts are therefore necessary to accelerate progress in reducing nutritional deprivation.

While undernutrition continues to be a prominent contributor to disease burden, developing countries are also increasingly concerned about rising trends in the prevalence of overweight and obesity among adults (McDonald et al., 2010; Swaminathan et al., 2019). These trends are driven by developmental processes and are associated with rapid changes in diets and activity patterns (Popkin, 2001). The global burden of overweight (including obesity) is much more pronounced than the underweight problem and is also concentrated among women (Global Nutrition Report, 2020). Estimates suggest that 39.2% (1.02 billion) of women globally are overweight or obese, a proportion almost four times higher than among men (284.1 million or 11.1%). A simultaneous manifestation of both underweight and overweight among communities and populations is an emerging concern referred to as the double burden of malnutrition (Popkin, 2001).

R. Kumar · A. Kumar · W. Joe (✉)
Institute of Economic Growth, Delhi, India
e-mail: william@iegindia.org

S. Rajpal
FLAME University, Pune, India

C. Z. Guilmoto (ed.), *Atlas of Gender and Health Inequalities in India*, Demographic Transformation and Socio-Economic Development 16,
https://doi.org/10.1007/978-3-031-47847-5_2

Low- and middle-income countries such as India are grappling with the dual problems of underweight and rising overweight prevalence, particularly among women in the reproductive age groups (Kulkarni et al., 2017; Subramanian et al., 2009). In 2005–06, 35.6% and 12.6% of these women were underweight and overweight (including obese), respectively. In 10 years, the prevalence of underweight has declined to 22.9%, whereas overweight prevalence has increased to 20.7% (IIPS and ICF, 2021). Keeping in mind these contrasting trends, we present in this chapter an analysis of district-level estimates of underweight and overweight among women (aged 15–49 years) in India, and we identify the main geographical clusters of high and low prevalence for policy targeting and prioritization.

Data and Methods

The analysis is based on India's data from the National Family Health Survey (2019–21). Anthropometric information on heights (in meters) and weights (in kilograms) of women aged 15–49 years is used to estimate the body mass index (BMI). Following the WHO reference standards, individuals are categorized as underweight (BMI <18.5 kg/m^2), normal, or overweight (BMI >25.0 kg/m^2) for analytical purposes (IIPS and ICF, 2021).[1]

NFHS-5 is the sole and most recent data source yielding estimates of the prevalence of female underweight and overweight in India at the district level. Other surveys, such as the India Human Development Survey (IHDS), capture this information, but the survey is not designed to provide district-level estimates. Similarly, government databases such as the ICDS-CAS (Integrated Child Development Services—Common Application Software) provide information limited to pregnant and lactating women, and their data are not in the public domain for analysis. The NFHS-5 sample comprises 636,699 households and 724,115 women, with BMI estimates available for 658,896 women aged 15–49.[2]

We apply various inequality indicators such as the variance, the coefficient of variation, and the Gini coefficient to describe inter-district inequality in prevalence levels. We also use the generalized entropy class of indicators to decompose the disparity in prevalence level into the within-state and between-state components. Finally, we also utilize the hierarchical nature of data to present a variance partitioning analysis whereby the surveyed individuals in a primary sampling unit (village/wards) were nested within a district and further nested within a state. The analysis is based on a multilevel logistic regression (null model) with four levels, depicting individual women, PSU, district, and state. The variance estimates of the random part of the model provide insights into between-group differences in

[1] The original NFHS dataset and the spatial analysis methodology are described in detail in Chap. 1.

[2] Women who were pregnant at the time of the survey or had given birth in the preceding 2 months are excluded from the sample.

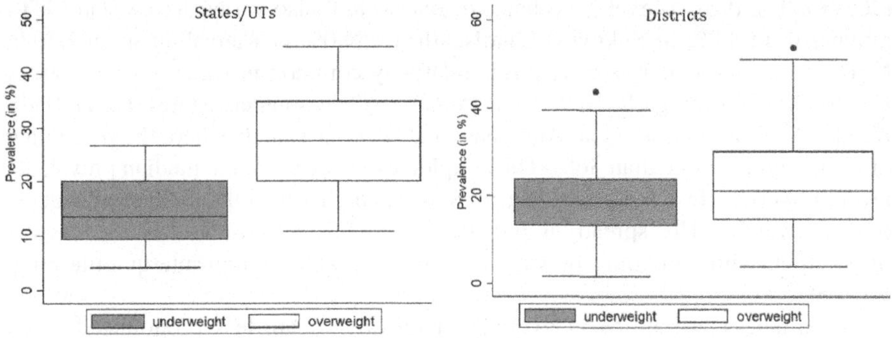

Fig. 2.1 Boxplot of underweight and overweight prevalence among women aged 15–49 years spread across states/UTs and districts
Source: computed from NFHS-5, 2019–21

underweight and overweight outcomes attributable to each level. The statistical analysis is performed through the *runmlwin* routine using MLwiN 2.28 and Stata SE 15.1 software.[3]

Results

In India, 18.7% of women aged 15–49 have a BMI lower than 18.5 kg/m^2 and are categorized as underweight (thin). Underweight prevalence is higher in rural India (21.3%) than in urban India (13.3%). The underweight prevalence differs across states and Union Territories (UTs). Jharkhand has the highest underweight prevalence, at 26.2%, whereas Ladakh has the lowest prevalence, at 4.4%.

Figure 2.1 boxplots display the spread of underweight outcomes across states and UTs. The median underweight prevalence across states/UTs is 13.9%, with an overall prevalence range of 21.9% and an interquartile range of 9.3%. The prevalence spread of underweight outcomes widens as we shift focus from the state/UTs level to the districts. The median underweight prevalence across districts is 18.0%, but the prevalence level ranges from a low 1.2% in Tawang (Arunachal Pradesh) to a record 43.6% in Bijapur (Chhattisgarh), a district in which more than two third of the women is underweight. The district-level prevalence range is 42.5%, whereas the district-level interquartile range is 10.4%. In no less than 130 districts in India, the proportion of underweight women exceeds 25%. This figure reflects both the intensity and the regional spread of the country's malnourishment issue in 2019–21.

At the same time, 24.0% of Indian women aged 15–49 years have a BMI above 25.0 kg/m^2 and are therefore categorized as overweight or obese. The prevalence of overweight and obesity is notably higher in urban areas (33.0%) than in rural areas

[3]For details on the methods and the routine used, see Leckie and Charlton (2012).

(20.0%). The district-level prevalence of overweight also varies across states/UTs, ranging from 3.8% in Sukma (Chhattisgarh) to 53.0% in Kanyakumari in Kerala. NFHS-5 data show that overweight is relatively common in some northern states/ UTs such as Chandigarh, Delhi, and Punjab, and in southern states Tamil Nadu, Kerala, Andhra Pradesh, Goa, Andaman, and Nicobar Islands where the percentage of overweight is more than 36%. The boxplot also shows that the median prevalence level of overweight across states/UTs (28.8%) is higher than the median prevalence of underweight. The spread in prevalence level is also higher in the case of overweight, with an overall prevalence range of 34.8% and an interquartile range of 13.6%.

Nevertheless, variations in overweight prevalence are less pronounced at the district level than with underweight outcomes (Fig. 2.1). The median overweight prevalence across districts is 21.3%, ranging from a low 3.8% in Sukma (Chhattisgarh) to the highest level of 53.0% in Kanyakumari in Kerala, where more than women are classified as overweight or obese. The district-level range in overweight prevalence is 24.0%, whereas the interquartile range is 15.3%. Overall, 65 districts in India have an overweight prevalence of below 10%, whereas 178 districts have a prevalence rate above 30%.

Figure 2.2 displays district-level variations in the prevalence of underweight. Underweight is widespread across Indian districts, and few districts report low prevalence. Low underweight prevalence tends to cluster in a few pockets in South India (Kerala and parts of Tamil Nadu), in the northern tip of India (Himachal Pradesh, Jammu and Kashmir, Ladakh, and parts of Punjab), as well in several states in the Northeast (Arunachal Pradesh, Manipur, Mizoram, Sikkim). Apart from northeastern districts, the lowest underweight rates are found in some of the most prosperous districts of India. In contrast, underweight prevalence is common in a much larger part of the country. However, its peak levels are concentrated in Central and East India. Specific clusters can be identified, such as the borders between Rajasthan, Madhya Pradesh, Gujarat, and Maharashtra, as well as in a region extending from Madhya Pradesh to Bihar to the north and Chhattisgarh, Vidarbha, and Odisha to the south. These areas broadly correspond to the Adivasi-inhabited parts of Central India.[4]

Moran's I statistic of 0.73 suggests high district-level spatial clustering of underweight prevalence in India, as reflected on the map. The hotspots of underweight in India described above correspond to about 150 districts, where both local and adjacent district-level prevalence is distinctly higher than the Indian average. This spatial concentration indicates that malnutrition is not an isolated phenomenon and affects a handful of adjoining districts.

Figure 2.3 replicates the same analysis for overweight estimates. The corresponding map reveals that overweight and obesity are primarily concentrated in South India, particularly South Karnataka, Kerala, Tamil Nadu, Puducherry, and

[4]For a spatial analysis of nutrition following a slightly different procedure, see Striessnig and Bora (2020).

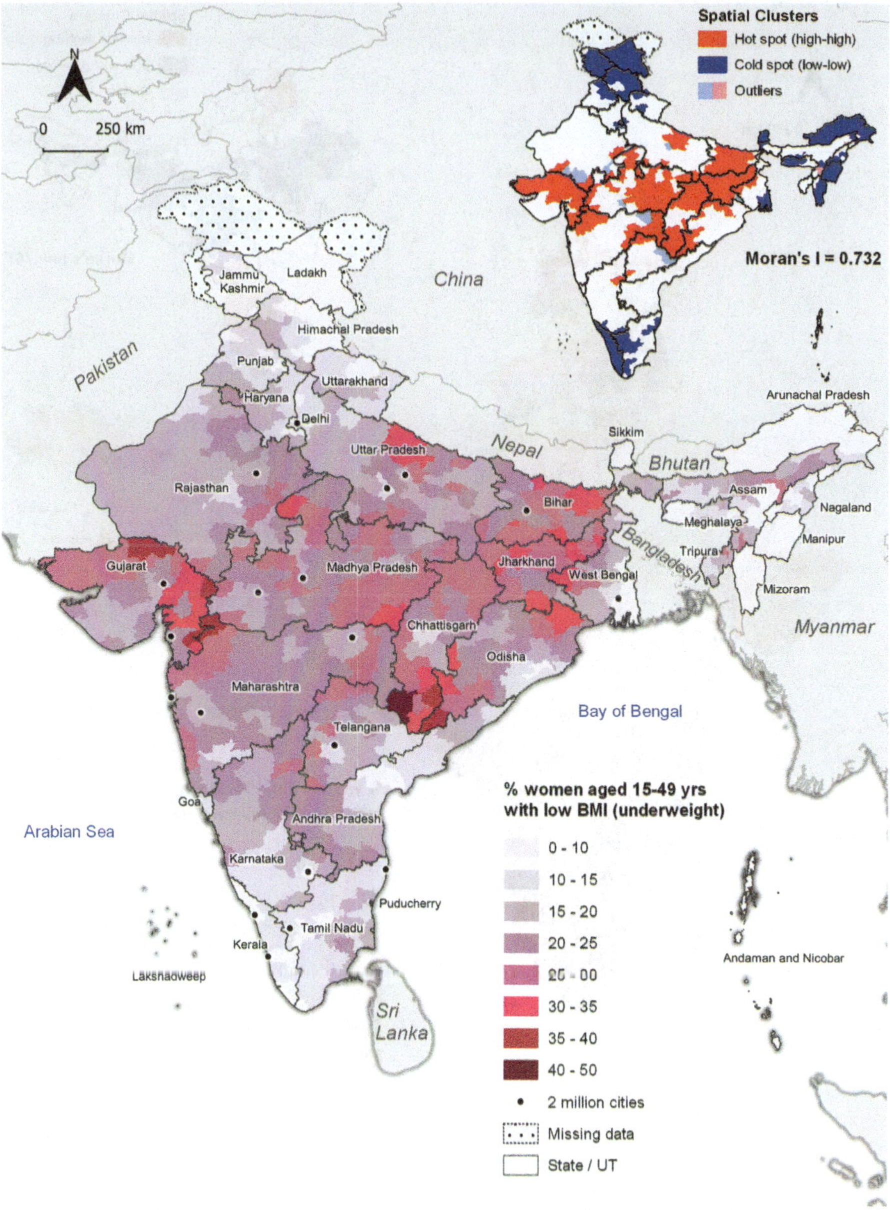

Fig. 2.2 Percentage of underweight women aged 15–49 years
Source: NFHS-5, 2019–21
The map is for illustrative purposes and may not represent official boundaries

Andhra Pradesh, where districts record prevalence levels greeter than 35%. In the rest of India, overweight and obesity prevalence is clustered in a region centered on Punjab and Haryana, as well as in smaller pockets in coastal Odisha, Sikkim, or around metropolitan areas such as Mumbai, Hyderabad, Pune, Delhi, or Kolkata.

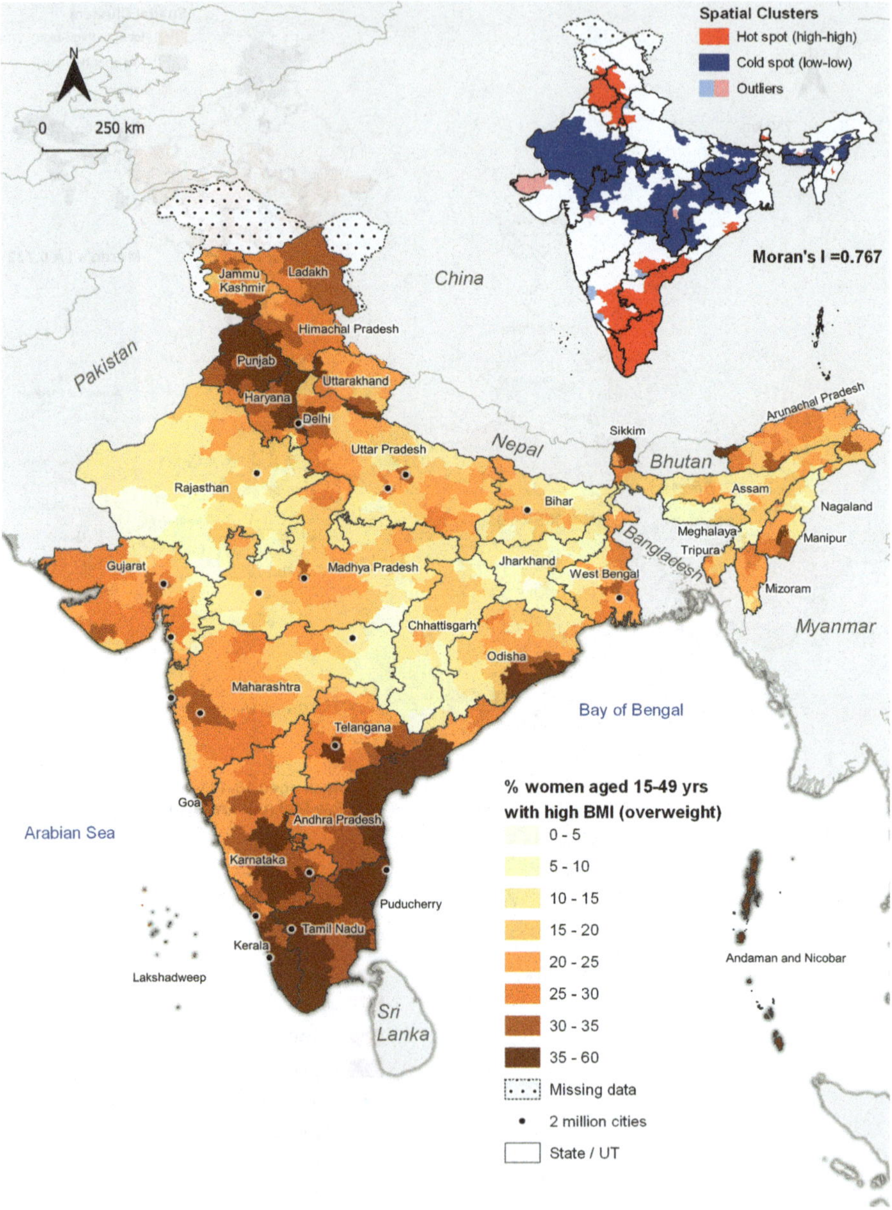

Fig. 2.3 Percentage of overweight women aged 15–49 years
Source: NFHS-5, 2019–21
The map is for illustrative purposes and may not represent official boundaries

To a large extent, this map reflects socioeconomic inequalities, with wealthier districts reporting almost inevitably higher prevalence levels of female overweight and obesity. We may relate the prevalence of overweight to other types of health behavior reviewed in this volume. This is notably the case of C-sections (see

Chap. 14 in this Atlas), as overweight and the apparent overuse of cesarean deliveries appear to peak in Telangana. The degree of spatial autocorrelation of overweight prevalence is extremely high (Moran's $I = 0.77$), confirming the strong spatial patterning of BMI indicators.

Comparing underweight and overweight indicators, we may notice a strong convergence between the low prevalence of underweight and the high prevalence of overweight. This similarity reflects the current nutrition transition that takes the population from relatively high levels of malnutrition in Central India to emerging overnutrition and unbalanced diets in more prosperous areas. These maps, however, are not simply inverted pictures of each other. In several mountainous regions of North and Northeast India, low levels of underweight have not given way to high levels of overweight.

Following a more statistical approach,[5] the inter-district variations in underweight prevalence are also high, as measured by indicators such as coefficient of variation (0.415) and Gini coefficient (0.230). An inequality-decomposition exercise based on the generalized entropy (GE) class of indices suggests that 76% of these variations are attributable to states, whereas 24% are within states. We get higher estimates related to variations in overweight prevalence, with the coefficient of variation and Gini coefficient for inter-district disparities in overweight prevalence estimated at 48% and 27%, respectively. Overweight appears more concentrated across some districts, whereas underweight tends to be more widespread in comparison.

The GE decomposition reveals that 38% of the variability in overweight prevalence is within states/UTs (between districts), whereas 62% is between states/UTs. Compared to underweight levels, a higher degree of within-state variability is noted in overweight, thus indicating more significant intrastate imbalances in diets and development patterns.

Finally, we utilize the unit-level hierarchical nature of NFHS data and apply multilevel logistic regression analysis to decompose the variance in underweight outcomes attributable to individuals, village/ward, district, and state levels (see Table 2.1). This analysis reveals that the bulk of variations in underweight are noted at the individual level (81.8%), whereas 9.2%, 2.5%, and 6.5% of the variation is because of between-villages, between-districts, and between-states variations. The variance partition coefficients (VPC) are also computed, excluding the individual-level variation. The analysis based on overweight prevalence provides similar inferences but suggests more significant individual-level variability in the prevalence of high BMI.

The final analysis highlights the close relationship between nutritional status (underweight and overweight) and household socioeconomic status (NFHS-5 wealth index).

Figure 2.4 shows that the concentration of underweight prevalence is higher among women from the poorest households (28.0% underweight), with a distinct negative gradient. In contrast, there appears to be a strong positive association

[5] Results in the following two paragraphs are based on the NFHS-4 district-level estimates.

Table 2.1 Multilevel logistic regression-based variance partition coefficients (VPC) for underweight and overweight women (15–49 years) across states/UTs and districts

Levels	Underweight (BMI < 18.5)		
	Var (95% CI)	VPC	% contribution
State	0.26	6.5%	35.5%
95% CI	[0.13–0.39]		
District	0.101	2.5%	13.8%
95% CI	[0.09–0.11]		
Village/Ward	0.371	9.2%	50.7%
95% CI	[0.36–0.38]		
Individual (level 1)	3.29	81.8%	
	Overweight (BMI > 25.0)		
	Var (95% CI)	VPC	% contribution
State	0.245	6.5%	49.1%
95% CI	[0.13–0.36]		
District	0.086	2.3%	17.2%
95% CI	[0.08–0.1]		
Village/Ward	0.168	4.4%	33.7%
95% CI	[0.16–0.17]		
Individual (level 1)	3.29	86.8%	

Source: computed from NFHS-5, 2019–21
Note: The 95% confidence interval is reported in [ ]; *See Leckie and Charlton (2012)

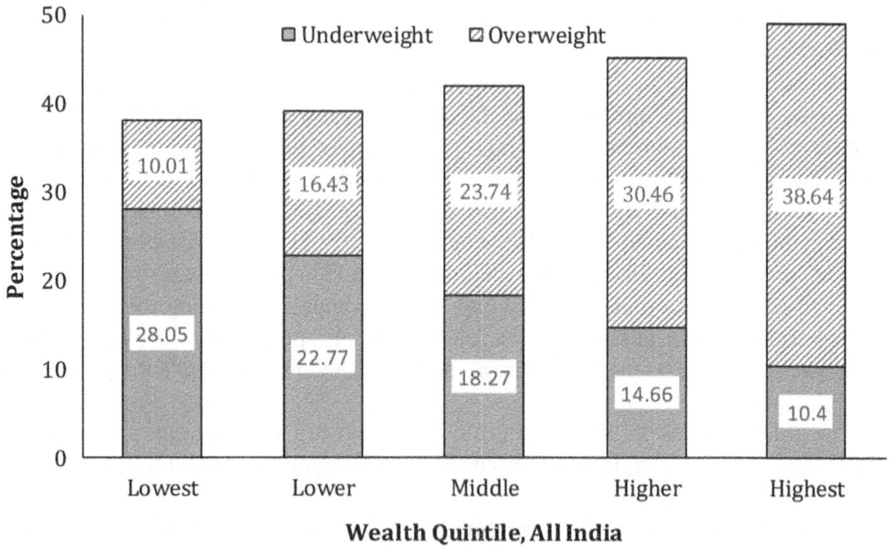

Fig. 2.4 Prevalence of underweight and overweight women aged 15–49 years by wealth quintile
Source: computed from NFHS-5, 2019–21

between household wealth and overweight and obesity, with average prevalence levels rising from 10.0% among the poorest quintile to 38.6% among the richest. This rise in overweight among wealthier groups contradicts the more encouraging results about the progress of dietary diversity linked to household wealth and maternal education measured from the NFHS-4 survey (Agrawal et al., 2019). Furthermore, this chart exemplifies the shift from being underweight to being overweight as the socioeconomic status of women improves. Worryingly, it also demonstrates that the rise in the proportion of overweight women is much faster than the decline in the proportion of underweight as we move up the income ladder.

The range of variations in nutrition levels observed across wealth quintiles appears quite pronounced. It does not precisely overlap regional variations since we find poor and rich households in each district—however, wealthy district households may be on average. Nutrition is, therefore, a health issue in which both spatial and socioeconomic differentials determine large variations across households.

Discussion and Conclusion

Underweight among women has declined worldwide since the 2000s, but its prevalence has not vanished: it affects 9.7% of women aged 20–49 and 5.7% of adolescent girls aged 15–19 (Global Nutrition Report, 2020). At the same time, overweight and obesity have increased globally over the same period. As for India, it is still facing the problem of undernutrition, which is inextricably linked to mass poverty. Nevertheless, a new trend has emerged in the country, with increased obesity in urban areas among people of better socioeconomic status.

The present study focuses on the district-level underweight and overweight prevalence patterns among women aged 15–49 in India. Several research studies establish the association of underweight and overweight with socioeconomic and other demographic indicators (Kulkarni et al., 2017; Subramanian et al., 2009). This chapter represents the first study identifying the district-wise prevalence of underweight and overweight through both statistical and spatial analysis. The geographical distribution patterns of health indicators can help us understand the dynamics of spatial determinants of the outcome variable. We observe that most of Jharkhand, Bihar, Rajasthan, Maharashtra, Odisha, and Uttar Pradesh display the highest prevalence of underweight in India.

In contrast, more than half of the districts in South India, notably in Andhra Pradesh, Tamil Nadu, and Kerala, display high proportions of overweight women. Districts with a high prevalence of undernutrition or overweight among women warrant urgent attention. Further, there is a need to study block- or village-level intervention programs, especially for Chhattisgarh (predominantly tribal belts) and Bihar (mainly in the northern district), to understand why some districts face a dual burden of health outcomes with a significant proportion of overweight and underweight.

There are a few caveats to this study. First, results of the multilevel model show that variation at the sub-district level is higher than at other geographic levels. Future endeavors must examine the difference in prevalence and inequalities below the district level. Second, the estimates provided in this study are crude and are not corrected by socioeconomic status. Local cultural features and socioeconomic status appear to be strong predictors of dietary habits and account for a large share of the variations in the prevalence of undernutrition and overweight. Third, NFHS does not hold much information on risk factors—such as physical activity level, sleeping patterns, or stress levels—which could account for these differentials in nutrition outcomes.

The findings of this study indicate that the dual burden of malnutrition is now considerable in India, affecting both the underprivileged and the most affluent sections of the population. This analysis confirms that pockets of nutritional deprivation within districts must be identified and prioritized for policy action. There is a further need to sensitize women about risk factors to reduce the prevalence of undernutrition and overweight. Furthermore, lifestyle changes can reduce a large part of the dual burden. Identifying the regions based on prevalence is only the first step. Focusing on villages and wards within districts and specific social groups is a natural progression required to target vulnerable populations better and improve the design of interventions.

References

Agrawal, S., Kim, R., Gausman, J., Sharma, S., Sankar, R., Joe, W., & Subramanian, S. V. (2019). Socio-economic patterning of food consumption and dietary diversity among Indian children: Evidence from NFHS-4. *European Journal of Clinical Nutrition, 73*(10), 1361–1372.

Global Nutrition Report. (2020). *Global nutrition report: Action on equity to end malnutrition*. Development Initiatives.

IIPS and ICF. (2021). *National Family Health Survey (NFHS-5), 2019–21, India*. International Institute for Population Sciences (IIPS).

Kulkarni, V. S., Kulkarni, V. S., & Gaiha, R. (2017). "Double burden of malnutrition": Re-examining the coexistence of undernutrition and overweight among women in India. *International Journal of Health Services: Planning, Administration, Evaluation, 47*(1), 108–133. https://doi.org/10.1177/0020731416664666

Leckie, G., & Charlton, C. (2012). Runmlwin: A program to run the MLwiN multilevel modeling software from within Stata. *Journal of Statistical Software, 52*(11), Article 11. https://doi.org/10.18637/jss.v052.i11

McDonald, S. D., Han, Z., Mulla, S., & Beyene, J. (2010). Overweight and obesity in mothers and risk of preterm birth and low birth weight infants: Systematic review and meta-analyses. *BMJ, 341*, c3428. https://doi.org/10.1136/bmj.c3428

Popkin, B. M. (2001). The nutrition transition and obesity in the developing world. *The Journal of Nutrition, 131*(3), 871S–873S. https://doi.org/10.1093/jn/131.3.871S

Striessnig, E., & Bora, J. K. (2020). Under-five child growth and nutrition status: Spatial clustering of Indian districts. *Spatial Demography, 8*(1), 63–84.

Subramanian, S., Perkins, J. M., & Khan, K. T. (2009). Do burdens of underweight and overweight coexist among lower socioeconomic groups in India? *The American journal of clinical nutrition, 90*(2), 369–376. https://doi.org/10.3945/ajcn.2009.27487

Swaminathan, S., et al. (2019). The burden of child and maternal malnutrition and trends in its indicators in the states of India: The global burden of disease study 1990–2017. *The Lancet Child and Adolescent Health, 3*(12), 855–870. https://doi.org/10.1016/S2352-4642(19)30273-1

Chapter 3
Vegetarianism and Non-Vegetarian Consumption in India

Mathieu Ferry

Compared to food diets globally, non-vegetarian consumption appears to be much lower in India than elsewhere. For example, take the case of meat: on average, a person worldwide consumed 43 kg of meat in 2020 when it was barely 4.6 kg in India.[1] This variation is striking since the global consensus is that meat consumption increases with the standard of living, but this is scarcely the case in India. Indeed, the food transition model assumes a positive correlation between meat consumption levels and GDP per capita (Popkin, 1993). Confronted with the "exception" of more than one billion Indian inhabitants in this theoretical model, social scientists have called for including sociocultural factors in the analysis of non-vegetarian consumption (Landy, 2009). The health implications are notable since stunting appears less common among children from vegetarian households (Headey & Palloni, 2020), while anemia proves higher in Indian states which have banned beef consumption (Dasgupta et al., 2023).

Overall, the trends of India's nutritional per capita levels, which reduced in the 1980s and 1990s (Deaton & Drèze, 2009), are puzzling and have led geographers to highlight the possible cultural and spatial factors behind this phenomenon. Beyond socioeconomic status, the social composition of local populations and the place of residence are critical dimensions for understanding the diversity in food diet—particularly the prevalence of vegetarianism on the Indian subcontinent, as illustrated by a recent study (Natrajan & Jacob, 2018).

[1] These annual estimates are computed from the Food Balance Sheet, 2020, provided by the Food and Agriculture Organization.

M. Ferry (✉)
Laboratoire Printemps, Université de Versailles Saint-Quentin-en-Yvelines, Versailles, France
e-mail: mathieu.ferry@uvsq.fr

C. Z. Guilmoto (ed.), *Atlas of Gender and Health Inequalities in India*, Demographic Transformation and Socio-Economic Development 16,
https://doi.org/10.1007/978-3-031-47847-5_3

This chapter completes and engages with these previous analyses by documenting geographic patterns of vegetarianism at the district level and by analyzing the consumption frequency of non-vegetarian items, namely meat, egg, and fish.

Data and Measurement

Data on food consumption from the NFHS may appear limited compared to the information collected in other surveys (India Human Development Survey, NSSO Consumer Expenditure Survey). NFHS-5 data were also collected differently.[2] Standard household-level units are generally used in large-scale surveys to inquire about the quantity and cost of a wide range of food items consumed during the past month (or the past week). The objective is to reconstruct a somewhat exhaustive food basket. The NFHS collects data on the consumption frequency (daily, weekly, occasionally, never) of selected food items (in the NFHS-5, nine items are surveyed). This strategy was introduced in the NFHS-2 and continued in the following rounds, in which both women (aged 15–49 years) and men (aged 15–54 years) were surveyed. NFHS is the only large-scale survey that can capture individual food diversity among households since several individuals are surveyed in each household—allowing for the analysis of individual factors of food consumption, particularly those related to gender differences.

Two critical limits of these data should be kept in mind. First, meat is not a simple food item: the consumption of chicken, mutton, goat, pork, beef, or buffalo varies over time and even more across social groups, depending on the economic cost and the social acceptability of these different types of meat. These variations are better captured with the data from the NSSO Consumer Expenditure Survey (Ferry, 2020). Second, besides socioeconomic differentials, caste is often an essential determinant of foodways, but it is never identified correctly in large-scale surveys or by the census. Whereas the previous round of the NFHS made it possible to quantify caste based on self-identification (Ferry, 2019), the corresponding data have not yet been released for NFHS-5 and could not be used for this study.

This chapter examines vegetarianism's frequency and spatial spread across India. The data on vegetarianism will be further disaggregated by states, districts, and social groups. Meat, fish, and egg consumption frequency is also analyzed separately. We focus on the female population, for which data on meat consumption is available at the district level, but data on male consumption are also used for comparative purposes.

[2] The original NFHS dataset and the spatial analysis methodology are described in detail in Chap. 1.

Findings and Discussion

The data on vegetarianism in India derived from the NFHS rounds point to a prolonged decline. 28% of women aged 15–49 were vegetarian in 1998, as against 27% in 2015 and 25.3% in 2021. Male vegetarianism declined slowly between 2005 and 2015, decreasing from 20% to 18%, but dropped to 13.4% in 2021. The first question relates to the higher prevalence of vegetarianism among women in India. This significant variation may be due to two different factors. First, one argument that could be put forward is that consuming non-vegetarian products provides nutritional resources appropriated by men at the expense of women within households. This explanation resonates with the general idea of "son preference" (Purewal, 2010) prevailing in India's patriarchal context. Several maps in this Atlas document the intensity of son preference and its regional variations across the country (see notably Chaps. 8 and 9). Women are more marked by malnutrition and underweight, and their lower consumption of non-vegetarian products could partly result from discrimination and lead to their vulnerable nutritional status. Nevertheless, as the analysis will show, vegetarianism also reflects compliance with social norms in specific religious and caste groups and may affect women in specific ways.

The second explanation emphasizes that the higher level of vegetarianism among women reflects gendered social roles (Natrajan & Jacob, 2018), where non-vegetarianism is more associated with masculinity, a social norm not specific to India (Fournier et al., 2015). Women act as "gatekeepers" of the adherence to vegetarianism in the household, a social role favored by their lower labor force participation. They are relegated to the management of the domestic economy. In contrast, men enjoy greater freedom from the social norm of vegetarianism. Male non-vegetarianism also partly results from their food consumption outside of the household. They enjoy outdoor paid meals about four times more often than women do.[3]

We find marked regional disparities in vegetarianism and the vegetarian gender gap. The highest levels of vegetarianism are observed in the northwestern states, where more than half of the female population reports the avoidance of meat-eating. This geographical concentration primarily concerns Rajasthan (67.1%), Haryana (70.1%), Gujarat (58.4%), and Punjab (59.7%). Still, vegetarianism sharply drops as we move from rural to metropolitan areas—down to 40.8% in Chandigarh and 28.1% in Delhi. Conversely, vegetarianism is least common in the Northeast, where less than 1% of women are vegetarian, and in states along the southern and eastern coasts, where vegetarianism ranges from 0% to 5%. Moreover, in three regions (Lakshadweep, Nagaland, and Mizoram), only one out of a thousand women reports

[3]Overall, the proportion of men and women aged 18–60 years enjoying food outdoors is 6.7 and 1.8% respectively. These figures are computed from the "Consumer Expenditure Survey" 2011–2012 in the National Sample Survey Office. Surveys, however, fail to document the extent of indoor versus outdoor non-vegetarian consumption.

being vegetarian. These gaps illustrate how deceptive the national average of 25.3% of vegetarian women can be and how it conceals huge variations across regions.

Interestingly, the gender gap in vegetarianism is also clustered in the northwestern states, i.e., in regions of entrenched vegetarianism. The most striking of these variations in meat avoidance can be seen in Punjab (59.7% among females against 35.4% among males) and Haryana (70.1% against 42.8%). The aforementioned metropolitan areas also stand out regarding gender gaps in vegetarianism in Delhi (28.1% for females against 14.8% for males) and in Chandigarh (40.8% versus 16.8%). Elsewhere in India, this gender gap is significantly smaller. For example, the difference between female and male rates is negligible in Kerala or Telangana.

Figure 3.1 displays the proportion of vegetarian women against that of men at the state level. The fitted regression line (with a slope of 0.64) reveals that male vegetarianism increases slower than female vegetarianism and that the gap between

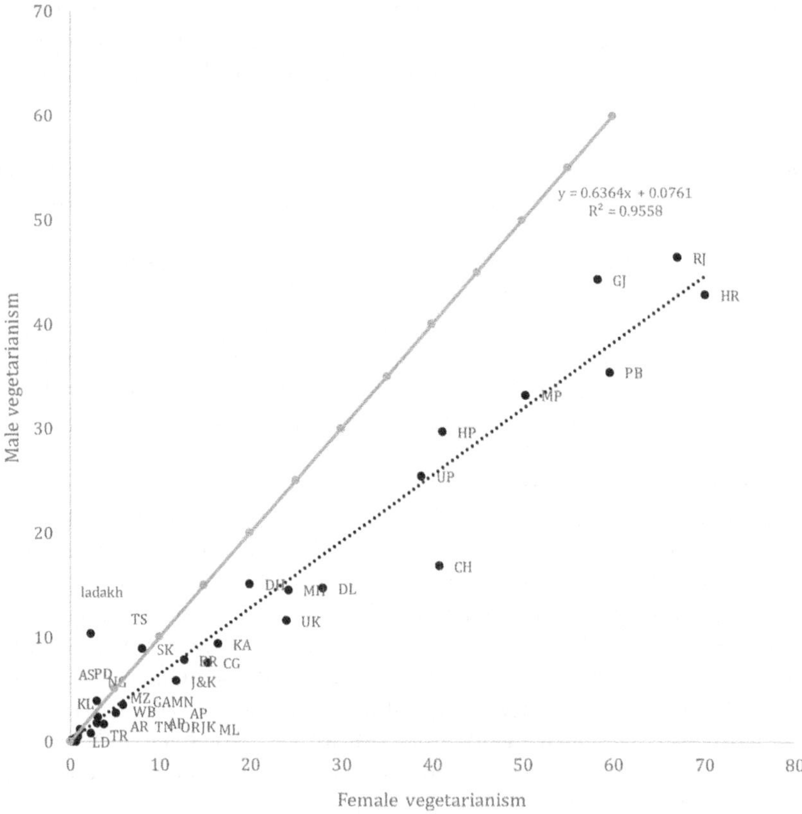

Fig. 3.1 Vegetarianism among women aged 15–49 years and men aged 15–54 years
Note: The solid line is the equality line (with equal female and male vegetarianism levels), and the dotted line is the linear regression line fitted to the data

female and male vegetarianism tends to increase proportionally in areas where female vegetarianism is more frequent.[4]

The same spatial analysis is replicated at the district level for women (data on men are unavailable at this scale). The resulting map (Fig. 3.2) plots female vegetarianism locally for India's 707 districts. This map confirms the apparent spatial patterning of vegetarianism across the country. We distinguish, in particular, a broad triangular cluster of highly vegetarian districts that extends from Punjab to Gujarat to the south and from Western Madhya Pradesh to the east. Twenty-five districts report a maximal prevalence of female vegetarianism above 75%: they are located in Rajasthan, Gujarat (including Botad in Saurashtra, where no less than 87% of women are vegetarian), Haryana, and Madhya Pradesh. If we examine this cluster of vegetarianism in the northwest, we may discern a sharp gradient in the north. Female vegetarianism brutally drops from above 50% to less than 20% as we move about 100 km north of Punjab towards the semi-mountainous areas of Jammu and Kashmir, Himachal Pradesh, and Uttarakhand.

The spatial distribution remains highly regular, as the gradual decline in female vegetarianism as we move from northwest to east attests. This explains why Moran's I is close to one ($I = 0.92$), the highest spatial autocorrelation level recorded for any indicator examined in this Atlas.[5] The high degree of spatial dependence highlighted by Moran's index confirms India's substantial regional homogeneity of foodways. If we search for spatial outliers (i.e., individual districts significantly different from their neighbors), the only example may be found in the Mewat region of Haryana, where vegetarianism drops to 22%. Noticeably, Mewat (now Nuh District) stands out from the adjacent districts by its social composition since Muslims account for almost 80% of Mewat's population, and literacy rates are significantly lower than neighboring districts such as Gurugram or Alwar.

Karnataka and Maharashtra display contrasting figures for the coastal and inland districts, with a proportion of vegetarian women significantly lower along the littoral than inland. We can recognize the influence of the Konkan culture extending from North Maharashtra to Kerala. It may also be noted that state administrative boundaries are recognizable on the map despite vegetarianism being the product of century-old social practices. The most salient illustration of such discontinuity relates to Telangana, a distinctly non-vegetarian zone surrounded in the north and the west by districts of Karnataka and Maharashtra, where rates are often higher by 20 percentage points. However, as the cluster analysis shows (Fig. 3.2), the core of non-vegetarianism in India (with fewer than 10% of vegetarian women) corresponds to a coastal strip running from Kerala to West Bengal and extending to the entire Northeast. This region covers Kerala, Tamil Nadu, Andhra Pradesh, Odisha, West Bengal, and all northeastern states, as well as the insular UTs.

[4]The former Union Territory of Daman and Diu represents the only case of higher vegetarianism among men.

[5]As a matter of fact, we do not know of other measures of spatial autocorrelation for Indian districts above 0.9.

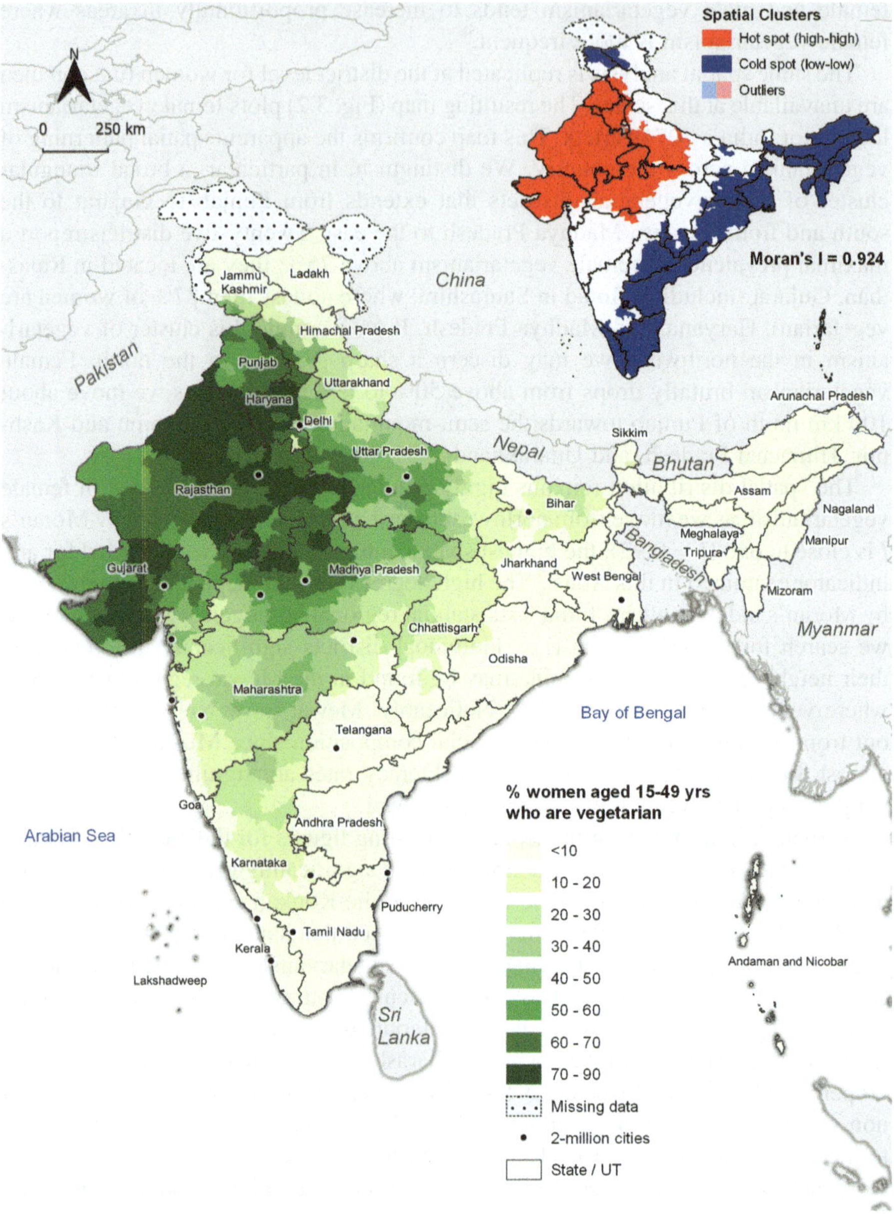

Fig. 3.2 Percentage of vegetarian women aged 15–49 years
Source: NFHS-5, 2019–21
The map is for illustrative purposes and may not represent official boundaries

Mewat and northeastern states illustrate that districts with a sizable non-Hindu population (notably Muslims or Christians) invariably record lower proportions of vegetarians among women. The same can be said of tribal (Adivasi) populations: the

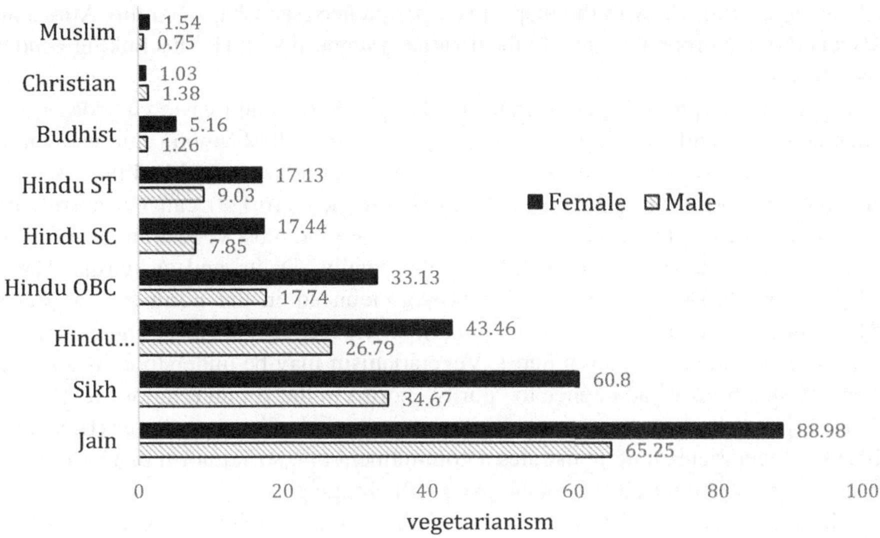

Fig. 3.3 Percentage of vegetarian women aged 15–49 years and men aged 15–54 years by religion, caste, and sex

border between Gujarat and Madhya Pradesh provides an example of areas where Adivasi populations (mostly Bhils) suddenly shrink the proportion of vegetarian women. This feature is confirmed by data discussed further in Fig. 3.3.

However, the local social composition is not the primary explanation for the regional variations depicted on the map since the share of vegetarianism can be extremely low in the districts of Tamil Nadu, Andhra Pradesh, or Odisha, populated mainly by Hindu non-tribal populations. Furthermore, the prevalence of vegetarianism also declines among Hindu women as we move away from the northwestern states.

Vegetarianism makes up a geographically coherent food lifestyle, and its unique spatial patterning can be only indirectly related to other variables such as wheat cultivation. The geographical distribution of vegetarianism is uncorrelated with wealth or urbanization—contrary to what the food transition hypothesis would have us assume. Vegetarianism and wealth are positively associated at the individual level: vegetarianism is much higher among the wealthiest individuals (36% of women and 21% of men) than among the poorest (17.3% of women and 7.9% of men), and rural-urban variations are almost negligible. Still, higher socioeconomic status conceals a crucial sociodemographic dimension in vegetarianism: caste and religion. Indeed, the wealthiest religious and caste groups are most prone to vegetarianism, and the association between vegetarianism and wealth is somewhat spurious. When we compare this unique map with other health and demographic features examined in this volume, the most surprising is the relative coincidence of female vegetarianism with the map of son preference (see Chap. 8 in this Atlas), an association that probably refers to local value systems among Hindus linking gender and food norms.

Figure 3.3 displays vegetarianism levels by religious and caste categories and illustrates the significant variations across groups (from 89% among Jain women to 17% among Dalits, and even lower values among Christians and Muslims). A third of Hindu women (29%) and a sixth of Hindu men (16.1%) can be considered vegetarian. Among them, Hindu forward castes are the most vegetarian group, and the proportion declines among OBCs, and finally, Dalits and Adivasis. These religious and caste differences are more pronounced in the northwestern states (Haryana, Rajasthan, Gujarat, and Punjab), where vegetarianism is higher than in other regions (data not shown here). Vegetarianism may be understood as a social marker that expresses adherence to "purity" norms in the Hindu religious realm and reflects specific culinary practices attached to caste and religious cultures (Baviskar, 2018).[6] Vegetarianism demonstrates a commitment to a social norm that is more or less salient depending on the social group of belonging.

Meanwhile, it should also be acknowledged that no religious or caste group, except perhaps for the Jains, totally adheres to vegetarianism. Religion, caste, gender, and socioeconomic status provide essential clues for deciphering Indian foodways but are insufficient when explaining their unique geography.

Going further with the information on food practices collected by the NFHS-5, *I* will now focus on individuals who declare consuming meat, fish, or eggs, for which we identify frequent consumers as those who report consuming specific items "daily" or "weekly" (and not simply "occasionally"). The mapping of each of these three items (not shown here) again highlights a potent form of spatial patterning. Moran's I is relatively high at 0.66 for frequent meat consumption, 0.71 for eggs, and 0.77 for fish (values computed over NFHS-4 district data). Meat consumption is most frequent in the southern states except Kerala, Sikkim, and the plains of the Northeast. Regular egg consumption is clustered in the same regions, with the addition of West Bengal.

With fish, high consumption frequency is restricted to the coastal districts in the south, West Bengal, Odisha, and the plains of the Northeast (Fig. 3.4). The corresponding map displays a pretty high level of spatial autocorrelation (Moran's $I = 0.88$). The supply factor predominates, as frequent fish consumption follows the littoral and the Brahmaputra Valley. Fish consumption remains, nevertheless, marginal in Gujarat, one of the leading fish producers in India.

Contrary to our expectations, a low frequency of non-vegetarian consumption is not associated with the northwestern vegetarian region. Occasional meat consumption (among meat eaters) is observed in parts of Rajasthan, Punjab, and Western Uttar Pradesh, but also in the Gangetic plains, Southeastern Uttar Pradesh,

[6] The tabulation of disaggregated caste data from the NFHS-4 would allow a more detailed analysis since specific caste groups such as Brahmins or Vaishyas (among forward castes) are more vegetarian, whereas Kshatriyas (also forward castes) tend to be non-vegetarian (Staples, 2014).

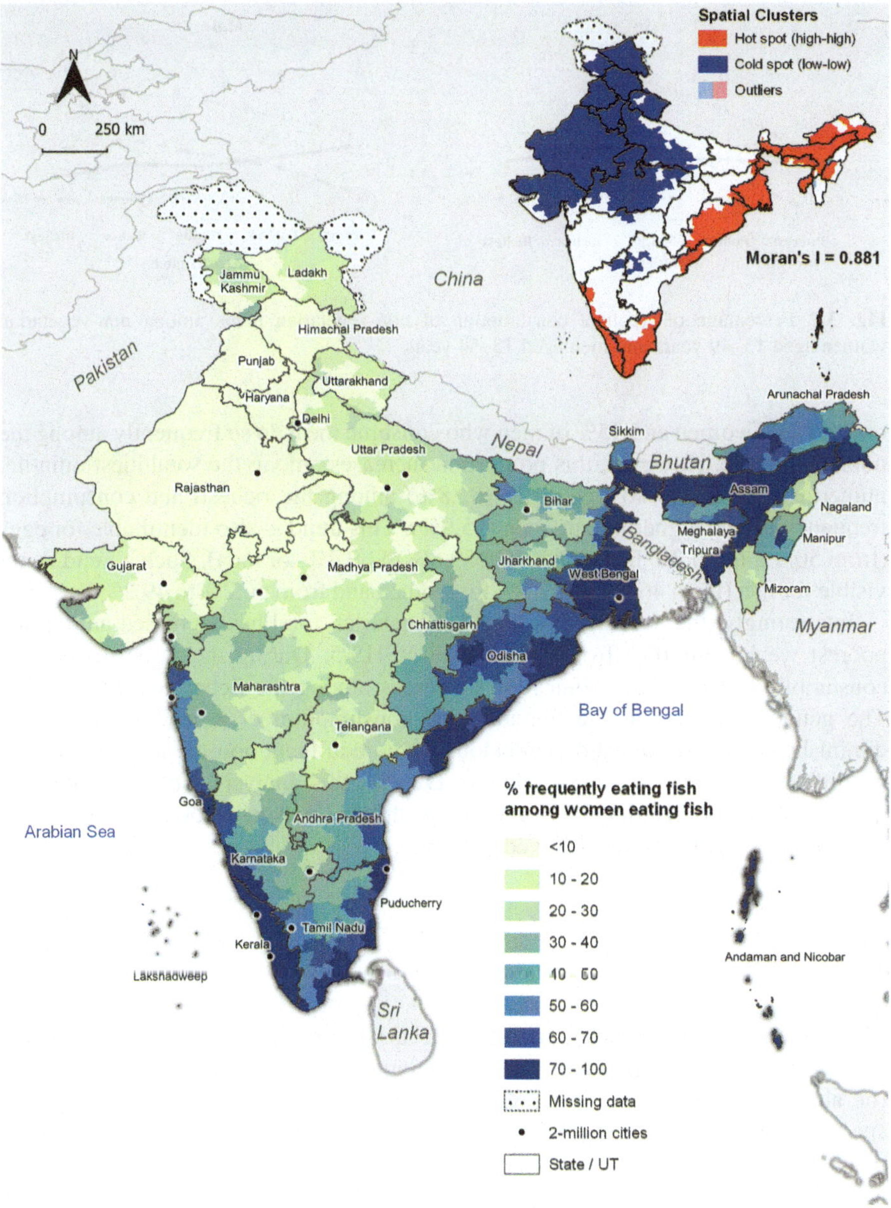

Fig. 3.4 Percentage of frequent fish eaters among women aged 15–49 years consuming fish
Source: NFHS-5, 2019–21
The map is for illustrative purposes and may not represent official boundaries

Northwestern Madhya Pradesh, Bihar, and North Jharkhand. Since these regions also present poorer populations, examining whether socioeconomic status affects non-vegetarian consumption is worthwhile. Data plotted in Fig. 3.5 indicate that

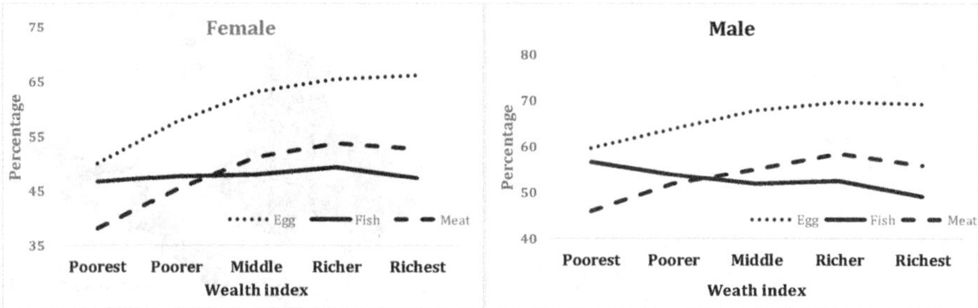

Fig. 3.5 Percentage of frequent consumption of non-vegetarian items among non-vegetarian women aged 15–49 years and men aged 15–54 years

only 38% of women and 45% of men who consume meat do so frequently among the poorest quintile. However, this proportion increases among the wealthiest quintile: numerous women do so frequently (52.8%) among the richest, and consumption frequency is also higher among men (55.9%). This trend is also identifiable for eggs (from 50.1% to 66.2% for women and 59.8% to 69.4% for men). Such a trend is not visible for fish (from 46.6% to 47.3% for women and from 56.7% to 49.2% for men).

Interestingly, the consumption of non-vegetarian food has increased among the poorest wealth quintiles from NFHS-4 to NFHS-5. During the same period, the consumption of non-vegetarian food decreases among the richest wealth quintile. The gender disparity in the frequency of consumption of non-vegetarian items diminishes when women and men belong to more affluent households, with almost no difference in the wealthiest quintile. Overall, this analysis shows that the frequency of non-vegetarian consumption is driven by socioeconomic status and geographic availability, as observed with fish.

Conclusion

The resilience of vegetarianism in India reflects the substantial impact of geographic, gender, and social disparities. This food regime is associated with the strength (or absence) of religious tenets and rules regarding meat consumption among specific groups, as illustrated, for example, by the differences between Jains, Christians, and Hindus. In a context where meat consumption is highly politicized, and abstinence from beef is mobilized as a vector of national belonging (Ferry, 2021), the analysis of the geography of food consumption shows the diversity of vegetarian food practices on the subcontinent. Still, the spatial heterogeneity of vegetarianism does not simply proceed from the social composition of Indian regions. The map indicates that vegetarianism should be understood as a food diet driven by local social norms, with gender, socioeconomic status, and caste superimposed on regional determinants. That said, the northwestern gradient of vegetarianism remains puzzling, and it should certainly be added to the numerous enigmas about trends and patterns of food consumption on the subcontinent (Deaton & Drèze, 2009).

Frequent consumption of non-vegetarian items, albeit partly reflecting this vegetarian geographic cluster, more evidently reflects spatial hotspots corresponding to more affluent regions. This feature is confirmed when examining individual socio-economic status, which increases the frequency of non-vegetarian consumption for those engaged in it and reduces the gender gap in food consumption. Far from turning everyone into non-vegetarians, food transition may emphasize more frequent non-vegetarian consumption for some while keeping vegetarian food diets for others, particularly for women.

References

Baviskar, A. (2018). New cultures of food studies. In S. Srivastava, Y. Arif, & J. Abraham (Eds.), *Critical themes in Indian sociology*. SAGE.

Dasgupta, A., Majid, F., & Orman, W. H. (2023). The nutritional cost of beef bans in India. *Journal of Development Economics, 163*, 103104.

Deaton, A., & Drèze, J. (2009). Food and nutrition in India: Facts and interpretations. *Economic and Political Weekly, 44*(7), 42–65.

Ferry, M. (2019). *Caste links: Quantifying social identities using open-ended questions* (OSC papers no. 2019–1). Observatoire Sociologique du Changement.

Ferry, M. (2020). What's India's beef with meat? Hindu orthopraxis and food transition in India since the 1980s. *Sociological Forum, 35*(2), 511–534. https://doi.org/10.1111/socf.12592

Ferry, M. (2021). *What goes around meat eating, comes around: Vegetarianism as a status marker in contemporary India.*, Ph.D. Dissertation, (p. 412). Sciences Po.

Fournier, T., Jarty, J., Lapeyre, N., & Touraille, P. (2015). L'alimentation, arme du genre. *Journal des Anthropologues, 140–141*(1), 19–49.

Headey, D. D., & Palloni, G. (2020). Stunting and wasting among Indian preschoolers have moderate but significant associations with the vegetarian status of their mothers. *The Journal of Nutrition, 150*(6), 1579–1589.

Landy, F. (2009). India, "cultural density" and the model of food transition. *Economic and Political Weekly, 44*(20), 59–61.

Natrajan, B., & Jacob, S. (2018). "Provincialising" vegetarianism: Putting Indian food habits in their place. *Economic and Political Weekly, LIII*(9), 54–64.

Popkin, B. M. (1993). Nutritional patterns and transitions. *Population and Development Review, 19*(1), 138–157. https://doi.org/10.2307/2938388

Purewal, N. K. (2010). *Son preference: Sex selection, gender and culture in South Asia*. Routledge.

Staples, J. (2014). Civilizing tastes: From caste to class in south Indian Foodways. In J. A. Klein & A. Murcott (Eds.), *Food consumption in global perspective: Essays in the anthropology of food in honour of Jack goody* (pp. 65–86). Palgrave Macmillan.

Chapter 4
Diabetes and Hypertension Among Indian Women

Moradhvaj Dhakad

India has been undergoing a rapid epidemiological transition in recent decades. A trend analysis of the causes of death shows that the country has transitioned from infectious, nutrition-related, and maternal and childhood diseases to noncommunicable diseases (NCDs), according to the national report on causes of death statistics, NCDs, like cardiovascular diseases, neoplasms, diabetes, and respiratory diseases, contributed in 2007–2013 to nearly half of the total deaths in India. Rapid urbanization and behavioral and biological risk factors such as tobacco and alcohol use, physical inactivity, overweight and obesity, increased fat and sodium intake, and low fruit and vegetable intake raised the prevalence of NCDs in India. The burden of NCDs is disproportionately high among adults aged 15–69 years and is continuously rising. Also, the NCD burden varies widely by geographical and administrative regions throughout the country.

Among all NCDs, there is an alarming growth in diabetes and hypertension among adults in India. With 69.2 million people (8.7% of the population) living with diabetes in 2015, India is often seen as a "diabetes capital" (WHO, 2016). Hypertension, a critical risk factor for cardiovascular diseases and other NCD-related deaths, is another serious public health concern in India (Reddy et al., 2005). About 207 million persons in the country live with hypertension, which was the cause of 1.63 million deaths in India in 2016 compared to 0.78 million in 1990, an increase of 108% (Gupta et al., 2019). Hypertension is responsible for 57% of deaths due to stroke and 24% of all coronary heart disease deaths in

M. Dhakad (✉)
University of Vienna, Vienna, Austria

International Institute for Applied Systems Analysis, Laxenburg, Austria

Wittgenstein Centre for Demography and Global Human Capital (IIASA, VID/OAW, WU), Vienna, Austria
e-mail: Moradhvaj@iiasa.ac.at

C. Z. Guilmoto (ed.), *Atlas of Gender and Health Inequalities in India*, Demographic Transformation and Socio-Economic Development 16,
https://doi.org/10.1007/978-3-031-47847-5_4

Table 4.1 Prevalence of diabetes and hypertension in various surveys, 2011–21

Period	Sex	2011–12	2015–16	2017–18	2019–21	2019–21
Diabetes	Male	0.9	1.9	0.4	2.7	9.0
Diabetes	Female	0.9	1.8	0.4	1.9	7.2
Hypertension	Male	1.1	Not available	0.3	3.3	16.1
Hypertension	Female	2.6	Not available	0.5	4.7	11.7
Method					Self-reported	Tested
Survey		*IHDS-1*	*NFHS-4*	*NSSO*	*NFHS-5*	*NFHS-5*

Note: figures in %

India (Gupta, 2004). The burden of diabetes and hypertension will likely increase further in the country because of the growing population, aging, urbanization, sedentary lifestyle, and lack of awareness.

Table 4.1 presents a comparative picture of diabetes and hypertension prevalence from three nationally representative Indian surveys: the National Family Health Surveys (NFHS-4 and NFHS-5), the India Human Development Survey (IHDS-I), and the seventy-fifth round of the National Sample Survey Office (NSSO), 2017–18. Data are classified by sex in view of the significant gender variations. The NFHS-4 did not collect the reported prevalence of hypertension, whereas NFHS-5 collected reported hypertension data. NFHS-5 also collected hypertension data based on anthropometric measurements (used for the primary analysis in the present chapter).

The self-reported diabetes prevalence rate is higher according to the most recent NFHS-5 figures (men: 2.7% and women: 1.9%) compared to those reported in IHDS (men: 0.9% and women: 0.9%) and NSSO (Men: 0.4% and women: 0.5%). Diabetes measured by a glucometer test is 9.0% among males as against 7.2% for women, according to NFHS-5 data. This result demonstrates a worrying level of under-reported and under-diagnosed diabetes in India (Claypool et al., 2020).

According to IHDS, the national level figures of hypertension were 1.1% and 2.6% among men and women, respectively, while NSSO reported about 0.3% and 0.5% for men and women, respectively. The difference between self-reported and measured hypertension in NFHS-5 for both genders is huge. The measured hypertension for males is 16.1% against the self-reported hypertension of 3.3%. For females, the measured hypertension is 10.7% against self-reported hypertension of 4.7%. As for diabetes, we recognize a high level of under-awareness around hypertension conditions in India again.

Diabetes and hypertension prevalence rates are higher among men than women nationally. Prevalence rates of the two diseases also vary according to data sources. Differences in survey estimates stem from their dates and reference periods and the way they collected information on diabetes and hypertension (e.g., based on medical or self-reported diagnosis). The NFHS-5 estimates may be more reliable as they derive from biomarker tests, whereas the other surveys' estimates are based on self-reported assessments. In addition, the recent NFHS figures rest on considerably larger samples, as detailed below.

Because of critical regional disparities in demographic, socioeconomic, dietary, and lifestyle factors, we should expect significant variations in diabetes and hypertension prevalence in India, as documented in NFHS-4 data (Ghosh et al., 2020). Therefore, identifying the regional patterns of diabetes and hypertension provides essential information for trend monitoring and interventions. This chapter investigates the regional patterns of hypertension and diabetes prevalence among men and women.

Data and Methods

The National Family Health Survey-5 conducted in 2019–21 provides samples of 101,839 eligible men aged 15–54 and 724,115 women aged 15–49.[1] The biomarker test is done among men and women above 15 in the selected households. Out of 1,410,154 males aged 15 and above, 694,996 males consented to a blood pressure test (for hypertension). Similarly, out of 1,433,580 females, 674,723 agreed to blood pressure tests. For the glucometer (diabetes) test, 677,582 males and 659,408 females gave consent to conduct the test.

In this chapter, we restrict the analysis to the population aged 15–49.[2] Our sample comprises 486,438 males and 539,737 females for hypertension, and 516,741 males and 567,323 females for diabetes. An *Omron Blood Pressure Monitor* was used to diagnose hypertension among eligible women and men. Blood pressure measurements for each respondent were taken three times with an interval of 5 min between readings. An individual is classified as suffering from hypertension if they have a systolic blood pressure (SBP) level of greater than 140 mm Hg or diastolic blood pressure (DBP) level of greater than or equal to 90 mm Hg or if they are currently taking antihypertensive medication to lower their blood pressure. For diabetes, random blood glucose was measured with a finger-stick blood specimen for eligible women and men using the *Accu-Check Performa* glucometer (an instrument for testing blood sugar levels) with glucose test strips.[3] An individual is classified as having high blood glucose (hyperglycemia) or diabetes if the respondent has a random blood glucose level of higher than 140 mg/dl.

We also performed two logistic regression analyses to investigate the association between the occurrence of hypertension/diabetes and selected socioeconomic characteristics at the individual level. The dependent variables are categorized as having hypertension/diabetes (yes = 1, no = 0).

[1] The original NFHS dataset and the spatial analysis methodology are described in detail in Chap. 1.

[2] Hypertension and diabetes prevalence rises fast with age, with rates that are several times greater than the adult average among the population above 70 years.

[3] Data for men are available only at the state level.

Results

At the national level, 16.2% of males aged 15–49 suffer from hypertension, against 10.7% of females of the same age. Over 20% of males suffer from hypertension in 13 states and UTs such as Chhattisgarh, Andhra Pradesh, Andaman and Nicobar, Tamil Nadu, Puducherry, Chandigarh, Telangana, Uttarakhand, Delhi, Manipur Punjab, Arunachal, and Sikkim. Around one-third of Sikkim's males suffer from hypertension (32.9%). Bihar, Rajasthan, Jammu and Kashmir, Lakshadweep, and West Bengal males have the lowest prevalence of hypertension, ranging between 11.2% and 12.0%. For females, we observe a higher level of hypertension prevalence in the same states and UTs, with a slight change in the state-level rank. Female hypertension rates range from 8.0% in Jharkhand to 25.2% in Sikkim.

Diabetes tends, on average, to be less common than hypertension. At the national level, diabetes affects 9.0% of men aged 15–49 years and 7.2% of women. More than 10% of women have diabetes in Andhra Pradesh, Kerala, and Tamil Nadu, in West Bengal and Tripura, as well as in Andaman and Nicobar Islands and Chandigarh. For males, diabetes prevalence follows a similar geography, with higher prevalence rates found in West Bengal and Tripura, Andhra Pradesh, Tamil Nadu, Goa, and Dadra and Nagar Haveli. Adults from the southern states are experiencing relatively higher diabetes rates than the northern states, with some exceptions like Chandigarh and West Bengal. These regional findings align with the estimates drawn from the Global Burden of Disease (GBD) study, which shows a similar regional pattern of diabetes (Tandon et al., 2018).

District-level patterns of female hypertension are mapped in Fig. 4.1. Prevalence levels are far from homogenous across the country, varying from levels below 5% to 30%. In 12 districts, more than a fifth of women suffer from hypertension. Inversely, 130 districts record a prevalence level below 8%. Moran's *I* value shows that hypertension prevalence across districts is characterized by a moderate level of spatial autocorrelation (Moran's $I = 0.54$). This value is one of the lowest levels of spatial autocorrelation measured in this Atlas, which seems to be due to the number of adjacent districts with high and low values. For example, sizable local variations can be identified in Punjab or Arunachal Pradesh. However, it is difficult to determine how far this apparent local heterogeneity between districts is real or whether it may be attributable to measurement issues such as small samples.

The cluster map for hypertension identifies several hotspots. The first is in Arunachal Pradesh but does not extend to adjacent states, barring Nagaland. Another hotspot is in Punjab, while the last covers South Karnataka (excluding Bengaluru). Sikkim constitutes a less visible pocket of acute female hypertension prevalence. All its four districts record levels above 20%; the North District (now renamed as Mangan) tops the list at 30.1%, the highest female hypertension prevalence recorded in 2020–21. High levels in the mountainous northeast corroborate the well-known link between hypertension and elevation (Narvaez-Guerra et al., 2018).

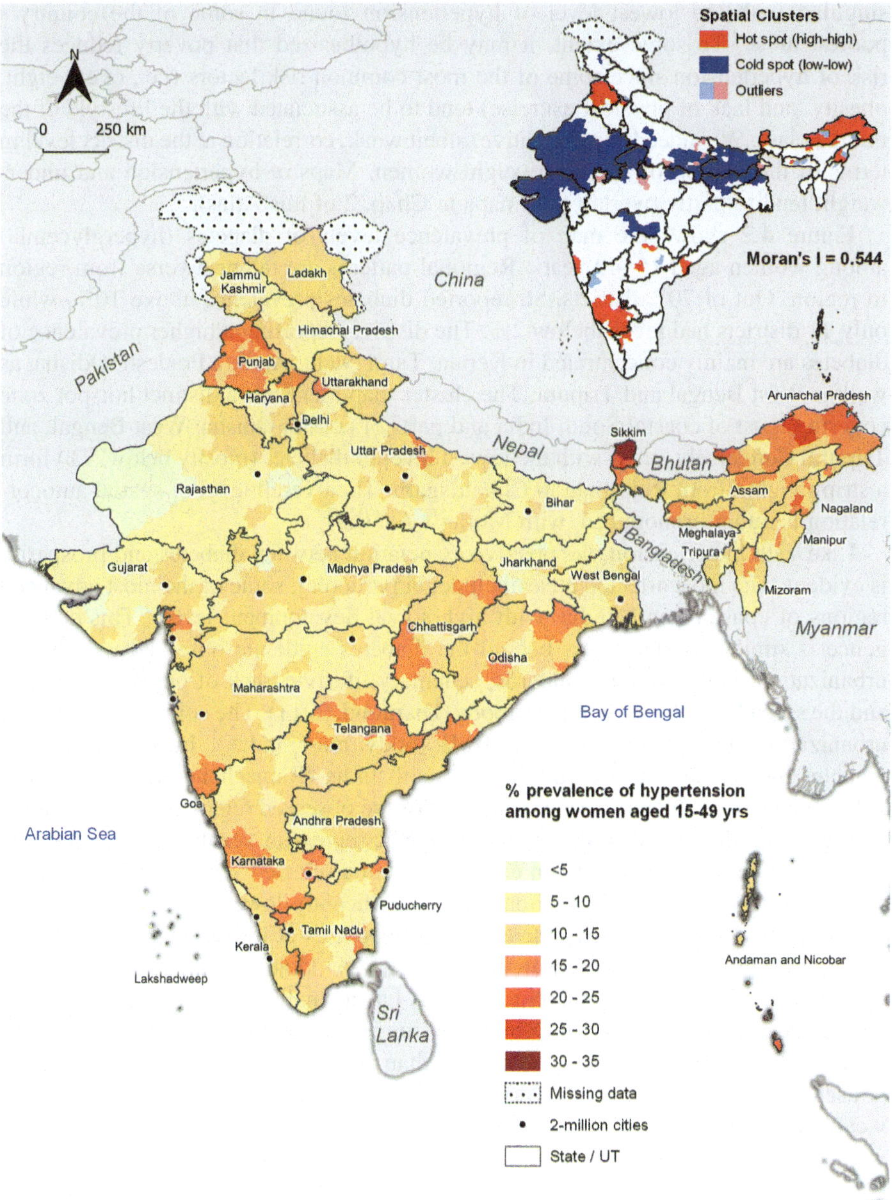

Fig. 4.1 Percentage of women aged 15–49 years with hypertension
Source: NFHS-5, 2019–21
The map is for illustrative purposes and may not represent official boundaries

On the contrary, low-prevalence districts are more clustered. We can notably identify the large low-hypertension region stretching over North India from Gujarat and Rajasthan to Uttar Pradesh, Bihar, and Jharkhand. In this region, the prevalence of hypertension is below 10%. The geography of hypertension appears somewhat singular, with the lowest level of hypertension found in some of the country's poorest areas. To some extent, it may be hypothesized that poverty reduces the risk of hypertension since some of the most common risk factors (i.e., overweight, obesity, and lack of physical exercise) tend to be associated with the lifestyle of the middle class. We indeed see a negative, albeit weak, correlation at the district level in terms of the proportion of underweight women. Maps of hypertension and underweight tend to partly overlap (see maps in Chap. 2 of this Atlas).

Figure 4.2 shows the map of prevalence levels of diabetes (hyperglycemia) among women aged 15–49 years. Regional patterns are rather diverse from region to region. Out of 707 districts, 86 reported diabetes prevalence above 10%, while only 11 districts had levels below 2%. The districts reporting a higher prevalence of diabetes are mainly concentrated in Kerala, Tami Nadu, Andhra Pradesh, Odisha, as well as West Bengal and Tripura. The cluster map identifies a distinct hotspot zone covering most of coastal South India and parts of coastal Odisha, West Bengal, and Tripura. Conversely, areas with the lowest level of diabetes (mostly below 5%) form a strip ranging from Rajasthan to Chhattisgarh. The overall level of spatial autocorrelation is rather pronounced, with Moran's I at 0.61.

Like with hypertension, the positive association between diabetes and prosperity is evident. The most affected areas include, in particular, some of the most advanced regions of coastal South India, with high social development levels. This convergence is similar to the factors behind the diabetes epidemic observed worldwide: urbanization, higher living standards, sedentary lifestyle, lack of physical exercise, and the spread of calorie-rich, fatty foods (Diamond, 2011). The connection between urbanization, higher income, high BMI (body mass index), hypertension, and diabetes has already been evidenced in South India (Ramachandran et al., 2008). Additional genetic factors may explain part of the observed regional concentrations.

Figure 4.3 displays the odds ratios of logistic regression results investigating the association between hypertension experience and a selected socioeconomic characteristic.[4] The likelihood of hypertension is significantly lower among females than among males. The risk of hypertension also increases at higher ages. The odds of hypertension increase 2.35 times in the age group 25–34 and 5.66 among adults aged 35–49. The educational attainment of adults has a smaller but positive association with hypertension: Adults who completed upper secondary schooling have 10% lower odds of suffering from hypertension than adults with no education. Inversely, household economic status has a positive effect since the adults from the wealthiest wealth quintile group have a higher risk of hypertension than adults from the poorest wealth quintile. Intriguingly, education and wealth appear to have inverse effects on the risk of hypertension. The social affiliation of the individual has an additional role in reporting hypertension. OBC adults have a lower risk of hypertension than other caste groups, while other religions (mostly Sikhs and Christians) are associated with higher risks.

[4]Odds ratios measure the strength of the correlation with the outcome variable. Values above (below) one correspond to a positive (negative) association.

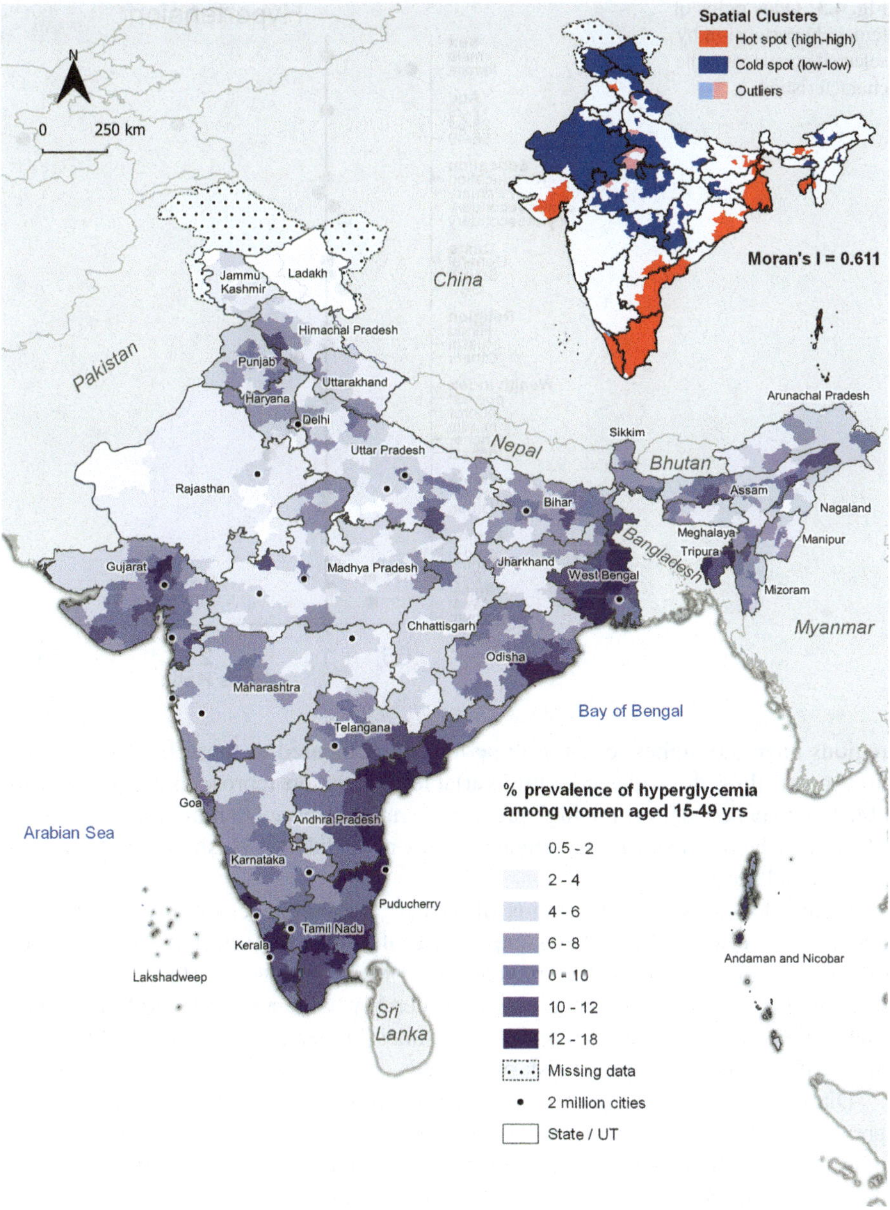

Fig. 4.2 Percentage of women aged 15–49 years with diabetes (hyperglycemia)
Source: NFHS-5, 2019–21
The map is for illustrative purposes and may not represent official boundaries

As expected, the regional factor is also significantly associated with hypertension suffering. Compared to adults living in the southern part of India, adults living in the Central and North-East have a lower risk of hypertension. The adults in western

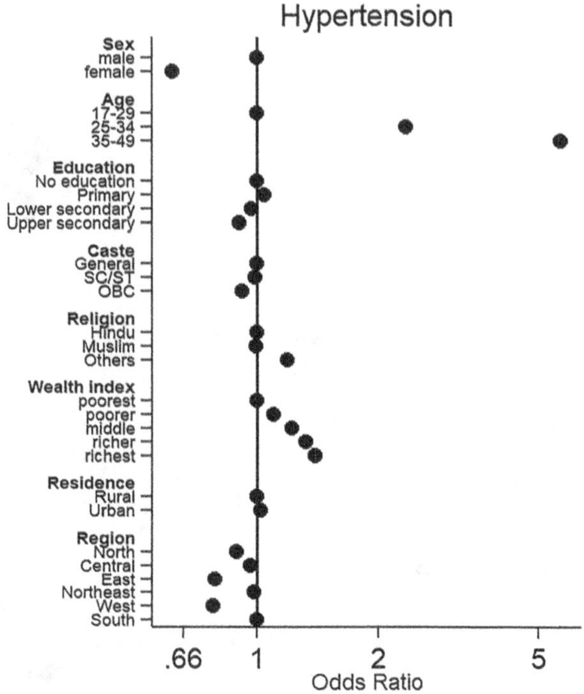

Fig. 4.3 Odds ratios of female hypertension by selected socioeconomic characteristics

regions have the highest odds of hypertension compared to those from other areas after controlling the socioeconomic variables. Elevation represents a missing variable that may account for the high prevalence rates observed in mountainous districts of the Northeast—even if hypertension rates in Ladakh or Kashmir do not appear exceptionally high.

Figure 4.4 plots the odds ratios of logistic regression results investigating the association between the diabetes experience of adults and selected socioeconomic characteristics. The risk of having diabetes is lower among females. As for hypertension, the risk of diabetes grows considerably with age. The odds of having diabetes in the age group 35–49 are five times higher than that of 15–24. SC/ST and OBC adults have a lower risk of diabetes.

Diabetes is more frequent among adults from the richest wealth quintile, as previously observed with hypertension rates. Each wealth quintile is more affected than the preceding one. Educational attainment has a limited positive impact on diabetes, with the highest rates estimated among adults with lower-secondary education. As illustrated by the previous map, the region patterning is most pronounced. Compared to the adults of North India, adults living in other regions have significantly higher odds of suffering from diabetes. The South, Northeast, and East regions record the highest prevalence of diabetes in the country, with odds ratios above two.

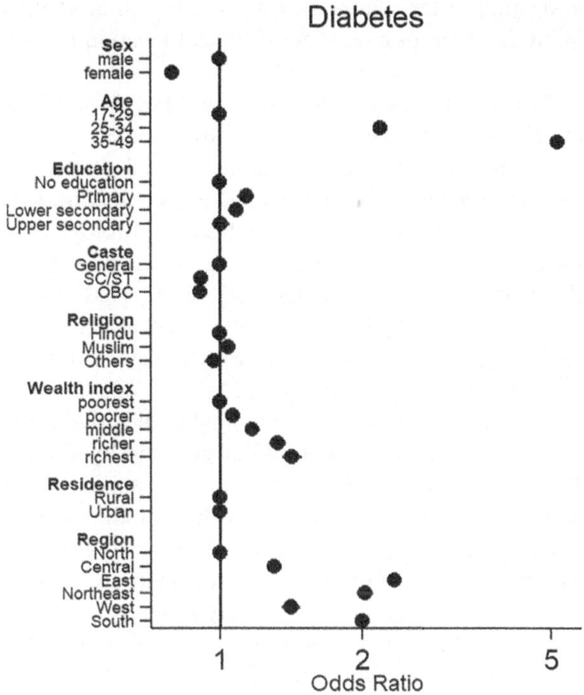

Fig. 4.4 Odds ratios of female diabetes by selected socioeconomic characteristics

Conclusion

Goal 3 of the UN's Sustainable Development Goals emphasizes the reduction of premature mortality from noncommunicable diseases by one-third by 2030. The level of premature mortality in India is high compared to that of some of its neighboring countries with similar levels of economic status.

The higher burden of NCD and consequent premature death also has numerous implications on household impoverishment, educational status of household members, disability, overall well-being, and quality of life (Jaspers et al., 2015). To prevent premature mortality, it is imperative to identify administrative and geographical areas reporting a high burden of non-communicable diseases, the leading causes of death. Such identification can help frame local-level policy and its implementation to reduce the burden of NCDs in India. Understanding NCDs is also crucial to evaluate the ongoing programs by the Government. In recent years, the Government of India launched in 2010 the National Program for Prevention and Control of Cancer, Diabetes, Cardiovascular Diseases, and Stroke (NPCDCS) in 100 districts across 21 states. In terms of program management, state NCD cells have been established in all 36 states/UTs, and district NCD cells have been set up in 390 (55%) of 719 district headquarters by March 2017, which means that nearly half of the country remains uncovered. Since disease prevalence and healthcare service utilization differ significantly by gender, an in-depth analysis of gender differences in NCDs regarding their geographical location is essential for policy and academic purposes.

Previous research across the world has documented the male-female differences in NCDs. Studies also report sex differences in hypertension and diabetes (Cutler et al., 2008). This study's findings reveal that hypertension prevalence is higher among men than women. Rich and higher caste adults and those from southern India have a higher risk of these two diseases. Biological and behavioral factors account for differences in hypertension and diabetes disease by sex (Sandberg & Ji, 2012). Behavioral risk factors include high body mass index (Brown et al., 2000; Hu et al., 2004) and lack of physical activity (Hu et al., 2004). Men and women differ in these critical behavioral risk factors, which leads to a disproportionate prevalence of the disease among men and women.

Our findings provide crucial input to the government program. The present study shows a substantial burden of diabetes and hypertension among Indian adults aged 15–49 years. The prevalence of diabetes and hypertension displays a unique geography, in which South India, Northwest India, and the Northeast appear especially vulnerable. Several affected states are in the advanced demographic and health transition stage. More research based on known risk factors (urbanization, smoking, sedentary lifestyle, obesity, hypertension, and hypercholesterolemia) is needed to understand better the socioeconomic, environmental, and genetic factors at the core of the growing burden of hypertension and diabetes in India.

References

Brown, C. D., et al. (2000). Body mass index and the prevalence of hypertension and dyslipidemia. *Obesity Research, 8*(9), 605–619.

Claypool, K. T., Chung, M. K., Deonarine, A., Gregg, E. W., & Patel, C. J. (2020). Characteristics of undiagnosed diabetes in men and women under 50 years in the Indian subcontinent: The National Family Health Survey (NFHS-4)/demographic health survey 2015–2016. *BMJ Open Diabetes Research and Care, 8*(1), e000965.

Cutler, J. A., Sorlie, P. D., Wolz, M., Thom, T., Fields, L. E., & Roccella, E. J. (2008). Trends in hypertension prevalence, awareness, treatment, and control rates in United States adults between 1988–1994 and 1999–2004. *Hypertension, 52*(5), 818–827.

Diamond, J. (2011). Diabetes in India. *Nature, 469*(7331), 478–479.

Ghosh, K., Dhillon, P., & Agrawal, G. (2020). Prevalence and detecting spatial clustering of diabetes at the district level in India. *Journal of Public Health, 28*, 535–545.

Gupta, R. (2004). Trends in hypertension epidemiology in India. *Journal of Human Hypertension, 18*(2), 73–78.

Gupta, R., Gaur, K., & Ram, C. (2019). Emerging trends in hypertension epidemiology in India. *Journal of Human Hypertension, 33*(8), 575–587.

Hu, G., Barengo, N. C., Tuomilehto, J., Lakka, T. A., Nissinen, A., & Jousilahti, P. (2004). Relationship of physical activity and body mass index to the risk of hypertension: A prospective study in Finland. *Hypertension, 43*(1), 25–30.

Jaspers, L., et al. (2015). The global impact of non-communicable diseases on households and impoverishment: A systematic review. *European Journal of Epidemiology, 30*(3), 163–188.

Narvaez-Guerra, O., Herrera-Enriquez, K., Medina-Lezama, J., & Chirinos, J. A. (2018). Systemic hypertension at high altitude. *Hypertension, 72*(3), 567–578.

Ramachandran, A., Mary, S., Yamuna, A., Murugesan, N., & Snehalatha, C. (2008). High prevalence of diabetes and cardiovascular risk factors associated with urbanization in India. *Diabetes Care, 31*(5), 893–898.

Reddy, K. S., Shah, B., Varghese, C., & Ramadoss, A. (2005). Responding to the threat of chronic diseases in India. *The Lancet, 366*(9498), 1744–1749.

Sandberg, K., & Ji, H. (2012). Sex differences in primary hypertension. *Biology of Sex Differences, 3*(1), 7.

Tandon, N., et al. (2018). The increasing burden of diabetes and variations among the states of India: The global burden of disease study 1990–2016. *The Lancet Global Health, 6*(12), e1352–e1362.

WHO. (2016). *Global report on diabetes* (p. 978). WHO Press.

Chapter 5
Anemia Among Children and Women in India

Ankita Srivastava and Bandita Boro

Anemia is a condition in which a person has insufficient red blood cells or hemoglobin. Hemoglobin is needed to carry oxygen. Hence, low or abnormal hemoglobin levels lead to a decreased capacity of the blood to carry oxygen to the body's tissues. The result is anemia, with symptoms such as fatigue, weakness, dizziness, and shortness of breath. The optimal hemoglobin concentration needed to meet physiologic needs varies by age, sex, residence elevation, smoking habits, and pregnancy status. The most common cause of anemia relates to nutritional deficiencies, particularly in iron, vitamins B12 and A, and folate.

Anemia represents a severe global public health problem concerning all ages, affecting an estimated 2.36 billion individuals worldwide (Stevens et al., 2013). In general, the prevalence rate is the highest among women and children. According to the WHO Global Database on Anemia, the estimated prevalence of anemia is about 25% of the general population globally, with higher percentages among children under 5 (42%) and pregnant women (40%). In low-income countries, the prevalence of anemia among pregnant women climbs to 51%.

Existing literature suggests that iron deficiency is the most critical cause of anemia among children in India, a deficiency attributable to inadequate nutritional iron intake and low iron bioavailability (WHO, 2011). Several adverse health outcomes have been associated with anemia, including maternal morbidity and mortality, perinatal and neonatal mortality, low birth weight, and poor cognitive development (Kozuki et al., 2012; Suryanarayana et al., 2017). Anemia affects human health, labor productivity, and earning capacity (Horton & Levin, 2001). Anemia in children affects cognitive and psychomotor development (Onyeneho et al., 2019). India carries a high disease burden despite having an anemia control

---

A. Srivastava (✉) · B. Boro
Centre for the Study of Regional Development, Jawaharlal Nehru University, New Delhi, India

C. Z. Guilmoto (ed.), *Atlas of Gender and Health Inequalities in India*, Demographic Transformation and Socio-Economic Development 16,
https://doi.org/10.1007/978-3-031-47847-5_5

program for the last 50 years. The fifth National Family Health Survey revealed that 57.0% of women aged 15–49 years and 68.0% of children aged 6–59 months in India were anemic.[1] Furthermore, previous research has already stressed the marked spatial patterning of anemia at the district level (Sharma et al., 2020).

Understanding the trends and patterns of anemia within the most vulnerable groups (i.e., women and children) is necessary for planning and policy interventions. This chapter aims to estimate trends in the complete distributions of hemoglobin concentration and anemia prevalence by severity for children aged 6–59 months and non-pregnant and non-lactating women by region. The objectives of the present chapter are twofold: (1) to examine changes in hemoglobin and anemia among non-pregnant women and children in India from 2006 to 2021 at national and district levels, and (2) to identify drivers of anemia and their respective contribution to observed variations in prevalence levels.

Data and Method

Normal hemoglobin for women is 12 grams per deciliter (g/dL); for children, 11 g/dL; and for men, 13 g/dL (WHO, 2011).[2] We examined changes in hemoglobin levels and anemia prevalence among non-pregnant and non-lactating women (15–49 age group) and children (6–59 months) in India from NFHS-2 to NFHS-5. We also identified some determinants of the anemic condition among women and children.

The three rounds of NFHS used the *HemoCue HB 201* method to estimate hemoglobin. The levels of severity of anemia were defined according to the World Health Organization hemoglobin (HB) cut-off (WHO, 2011). Severe anemia was defined as hemoglobin level < 8.0 g/dl for non-pregnant and non-lactating women; moderate anemia was defined as 8.0–10.9 g/dl; and mild anemia was defined as 11.0–11.9 g/dl. Any anemia was defined as a hemoglobin level below <12.0 g/dL in NP-NL women. Anemia for children was defined as mild (hemoglobin level 10.0–10.9 g/dl), moderate (hemoglobin level 7.0–9.9 g/dl), and severe (hemoglobin level < 7.0 g/dl). Any anemia level for children is <11.0 g/dl.

We computed the district-level prevalence of anemia for 707 Indian districts using the NFHS-5, based on a sample of 682,033 non-pregnant and non-lactating women aged 15–49 years, and 179,262 children aged 6–59 months ($n = 220{,}487$).

[1] Our computations slightly differ from the average levels (53.1% for women and 67.1% for children) reported in the NFHS-5 report due to the weighting method used.

[2] The original NFHS dataset and the spatial analysis methodology are described in detail in Chap. 1.

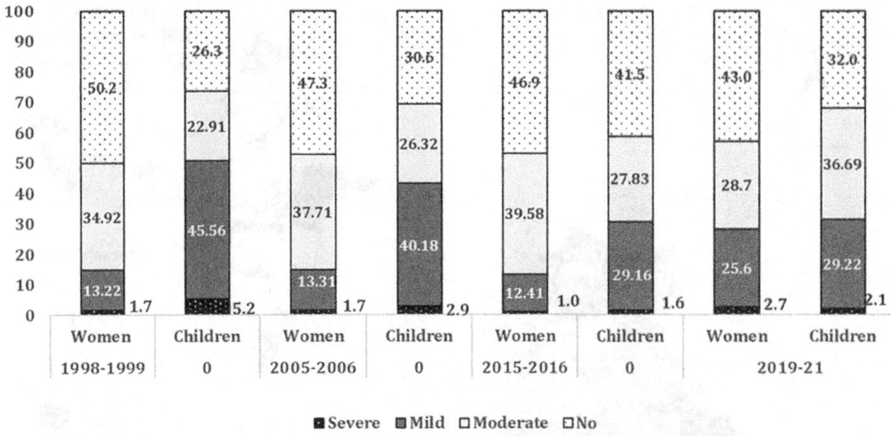

Fig. 5.1 Trends in anemia prevalence for women and children in 1998–21
Note: Computed for women aged 15–49 years and for children aged 6–59 months (6–35 months for NFHS-2)

Results

Figure 5.1 shows the trends in the percentage of anemia from 1998–99 to 2019–21 for women aged 15–49 years and children aged 6–59 months. It reveals that the percentage of children with severe anemia has reduced from 5.2% (NFHS-2) to 2.1% (NFHS-5). Moreover, the percentage of mild anemia decreased sharply, from 45.6% (NFHS-2) to 29.2% (NFHS-5), whereas moderate anemia increased from 22.9% (NFHS-2) to 36.7% (NFHS-5). The percentage of children without anemia has grown over the period (26.3%, NFHS-2 to 32.0% NFHS-5).

Available figures point, however, to a sharp increase in mild anemia among children between the last two NFHS rounds. As a result, children's anemia rate (in its moderate, mild, and severe forms) has unexpectedly escalated from 59.5 to 68.0% in less than 5 years.

Severe anemia has slightly increased from 1.7% (NFHS-2) to 2.7% (NFHS-5) for women. Mild anemia has also increased substantially from 13.2% (NFHS-2) to 25.6% (NFHS-5). The percentage of women without anemia has regularly decreased from 50.2% (NFHS-2) to 43.0% (NFHS-5). This result is partly due to the recent increase in the prevalence of mild anemia recorded by the NFHS-5 survey (25.6% in 2019–21 as against 12.4% 4 years earlier).

Figure 5.2 represents the prevalence of any type of anemia among children aged 6–59 months at the district level. The national average of any anemia (Hb < 11.0 g/dL) for children aged 6–59 months stands at 58%. In over six hundred districts, anemia rates exceed 50%. In 65 districts, more than 80% of children suffer from anemia. Affected areas cover a large part of the central India belt, starting from Gujarat, the southern portion of Rajasthan, north Madhya Pradesh, and parts of

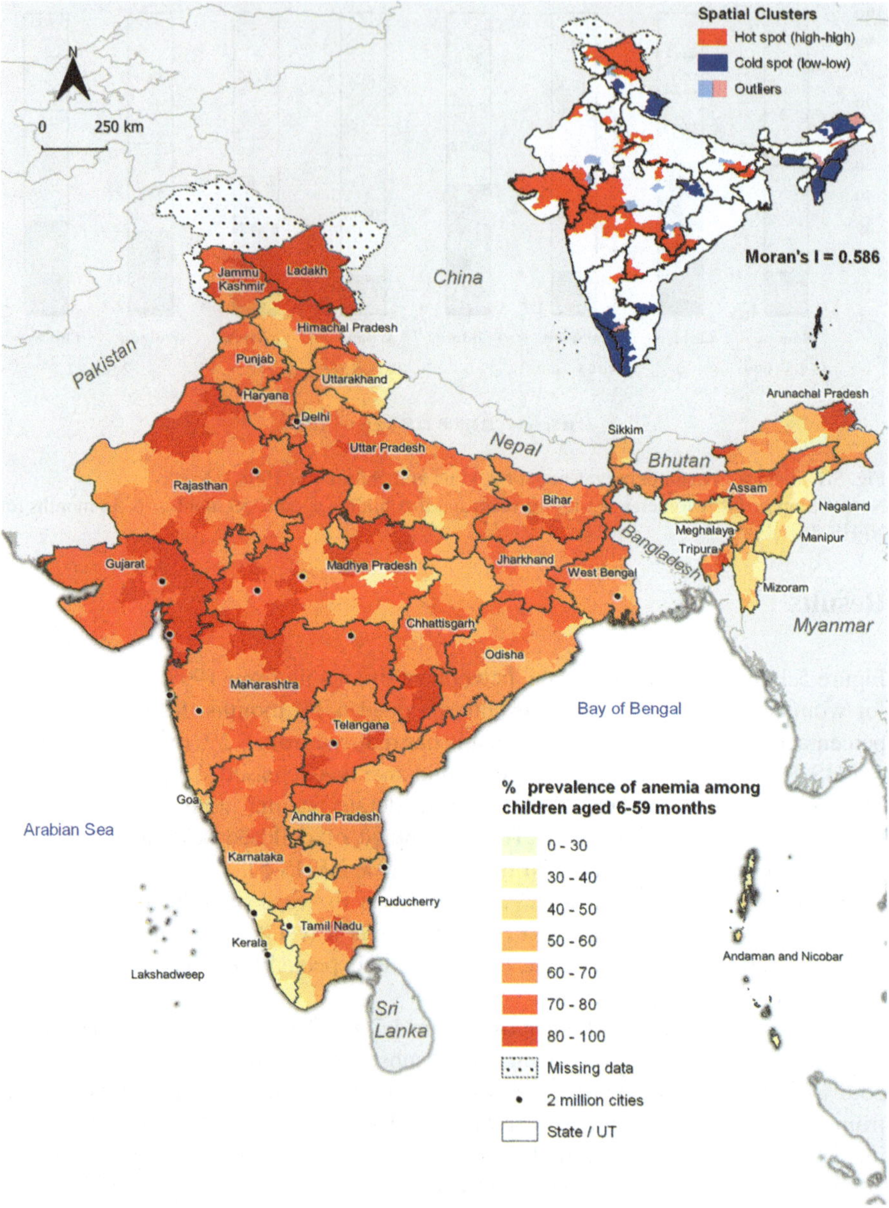

Fig. 5.2 Percentage of children aged 6–59 months with anemia
Source: NFHS-5, 2019–21
The map is for illustrative purposes and may not represent official boundaries

Telangana. Nevertheless, other areas register record levels of child anemia found almost anywhere in India, from Himachal Pradesh to Bihar, Assam, or even Tamil Nadu. The highest rates of child anemia in India are observed in Gujarat and Ladakh.

The Moran's I statistic is found to be 0.59 for child anemia, corresponding to a pronounced level of spatial autocorrelation. Even if the overall map is uneven, it confirms the main traits of spatial patterning of child anemia in India, with hotspots in a broad region running from Gujarat to South Odisha. In addition, several other sizable clusters emerge, one in Ladakh and North Himachal Pradesh, and smaller pockets of high anemia prevalence are visible in Bihar, Uttar Pradesh, and the Deccan. The second is along the Haryana-Uttar Pradesh border north of Delhi. Finally, smaller pockets of high child anemia are visible in Karnataka, Andhra Pradesh, and Jharkhand.

The map of the main concentrations of lowest child anemia prevalence is equally interesting to understand the progress accomplished. Two salient clusters are found in Kerala and bordering Tamil Nadu districts, as well as in the Northeast (except for Assam and Tripura). It may be observed that this regional distribution of child anemia does not coincide with local prosperity. Advanced regions registering high anemia, such as Gujarat, illustrate this discrepancy.

Figure 5.3 represents the prevalence of any anemia among non-pregnant and non-lactating women aged 15–49. The national average for anemia among women is 53%, but over a tenth of the districts record a high prevalence rate above 70%. They are notably located in Gujarat, Bihar, and West Bengal. The highest prevalence of female anemia at the district level is again found in Ladakh at a shocking level of 93.6%, followed by neighboring Kargil and individual districts of WB and Himachal Pradesh.

Our computations point to a solid spatial autocorrelation level (Moran $I = 0.68$). Hot and cold spots (areas of homogenous high and low anemia prevalence) are relatively dispersed across the country. Four major hotspots can be identified: (1) adjacent areas of West Bengal, Odisha, Jharkhand, and Bihar; (2) Ladakh and north Himachal Pradesh; (3) Gujarat-Maharashtra border; and (4) districts around Bastar in south Chhattisgarh. Once again, Kerala (along with coastal Karnataka) and several northeastern states emerge with the lowest prevalence of anemia. Another narrower cold-spot area in Kumaon along the Nepalese border in Uttarakhand can be identified

The overall geography of female anemia partly corresponds to that of child anemia. However, some regions exhibit low rates of anemia for both children and women, such as Kerala, south Karnataka, Kumaon, Manipur, Mizoram, and Nagaland, as well as parts of Arunachal Pradesh. In contrast, anemia prevalence is high for both children and women along the Gujarat-Maharashtra and Bihar-Jharkhand borders, around Bastar and Ladakh.

Figures 5.4 and 5.5 display the logistic regression results in which anemia among women and children was tested against selected background variables.[3] The female population is restricted to non-pregnant and non-lactating women aged 15–49. Our models estimate the odds ratio and 95% confidence intervals. The first model

[3]Odds ratios measure the strength of the correlation with the outcome variable. Values above (below) one correspond to a positive (negative) association.

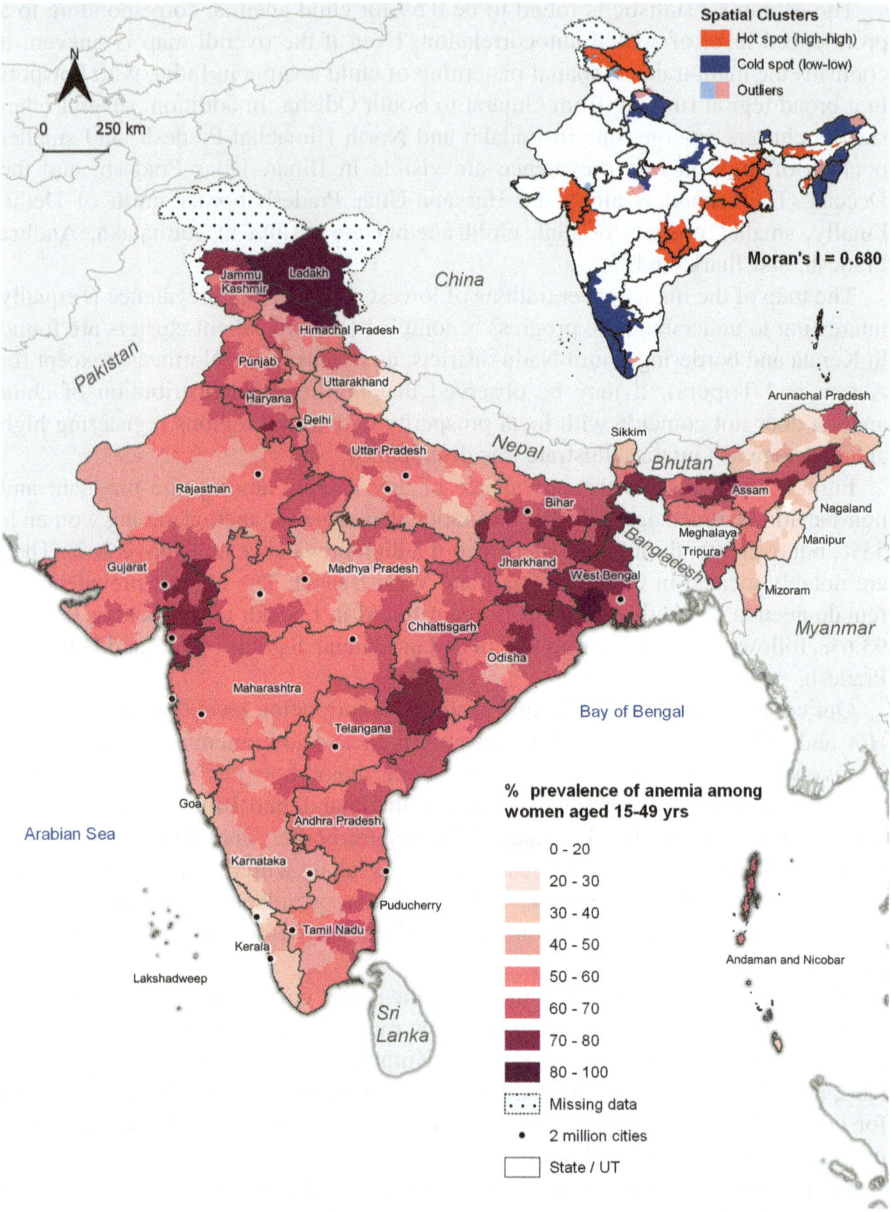

Fig. 5.3 Percentage of women aged 15–49 years with anemia
Source: NFHS-5, 2019–21
The map is for illustrative purposes and may not represent official boundaries

(Fig. 5.4) controls for demographic and socioeconomic characteristics such as residence, educational level, caste, religion, and wealth quintile. No significant difference in anemia status emerges between rural and urban women in this model. Still, compared to the general-category women, Dalit (SC) and Adivasi (ST) women

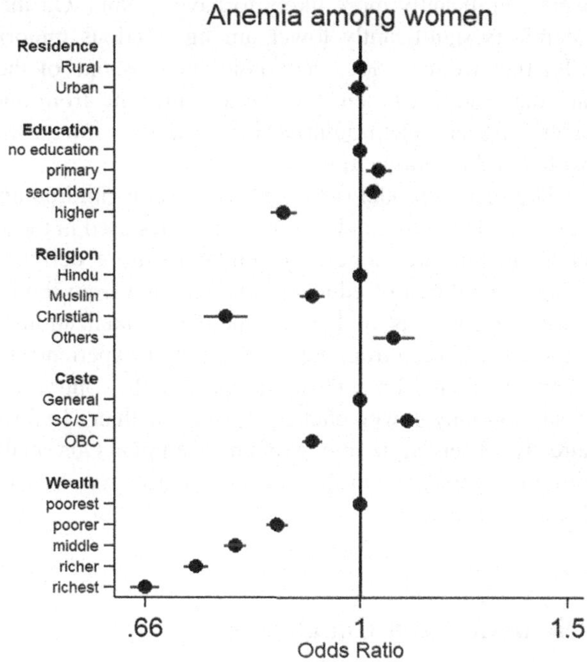

Fig. 5.4 Odds ratio of anemia among women of age 15–49 by selected background characteristics

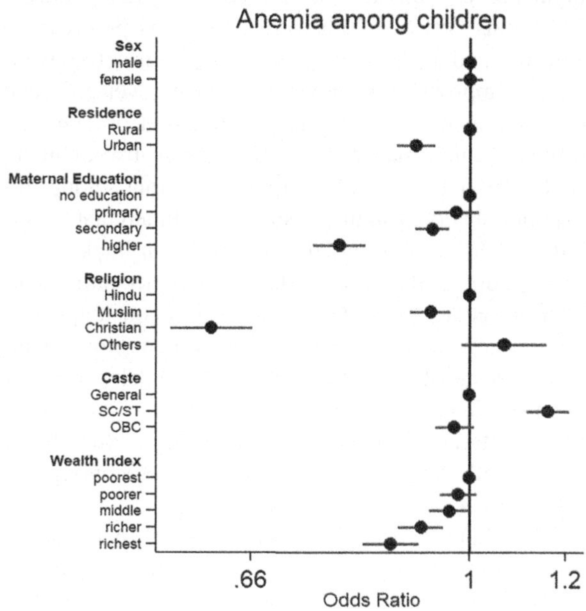

Fig. 5.5 Odds ratio of anemia among children aged 6–59 months by selected background characteristics

were significantly more likely to have anemia. On the contrary, the prevalence of anemia is significantly lower among religious minorities, surprisingly so among Christian women. Socioeconomic status is one of the most distinct correlates of anemia among women: the risk of suffering from anemia significantly decreases with a higher wealth quintile. It is also at its lowest for the most educated women, with an odds ratio below 0.7.

The second model (Fig. 5.5) focuses on children aged 6–59 months. It includes sex and all the other independent variables used in the previous model. Correlates of child anemia are somewhat similar to those derived from the analysis of adult women. Children of educated mothers and from the higher wealth quintile experienced lower odds of having anemia. Urbanization also reduces anemia among children. Children from the ST/SC groups experienced a distinctly higher likelihood of anemia than the rest of the sample. On the contrary, Christian children experience a substantially lower chance of anemia than Hindu children—a striking feature already observed in the women's sample. Our analysis cannot tell us if these religious variations in anemia prevalence may be linked to food habits or other behavioral factors.

Discussion and Conclusion

India has considerably improved in reducing anemia among children aged 6–59 months between 2006 and 2016. This progress can be attributed to improving nutrition and health interventions in children (Nguyen et al., 2018). However, most of this improvement appears to have reversed, according to the latest NFHS-5 figures. Anemia has gradually increased among non-pregnant and non-lactating women, which may be more likely because of inadequate policy focus (Nguyen et al., 2018). Reported high rates of anemia among Indian women are primarily due to poor nutritional status. A study concluded that the decrease in coarse cereals in the Indian diet has substantially reduced iron intake without compensation from other food groups, particularly in states where rice rather than wheat replaced coarse grains (DeFries et al., 2018). Hence, increased consumption of coarse cereals could reduce anemia prevalence among Indian women, along with other interventions. Overall, women's nutritional status is determined by access to healthcare, resources, and income (Bentley & Griffiths, 2003). A study also showed that compared to non-vegetarians (38%), more vegetarians (65.9%) were anemic (Verma et al., 1998). Still, the maps of anemia prevalence only partly match those of a vegetarian diet (see Chap. 3 in this Atlas).

This chapter also brings a district-level spatial analysis and regression analysis of anemia indicators. It showed stark spatial variations in the prevalence of anemia across districts. Overall, poorer communities record a higher prevalence of anemia. In addition, childhood anemia is highly prevalent among the poorest households of Ladakh, Rajasthan, Gujarat, Madhya Pradesh, and Telangana (Liou et al., 2020).

According to the National Rural Health Mission, India, poor environmental sanitation, unsafe drinking water, and inadequate personal hygiene contribute to anemia prevalence. Another study also demonstrated that child health outcomes are the worst in Central, Eastern, Northern, and Northeastern India because of the poor quality of healthcare infrastructure (Puri et al., 2020). The highest predicted frequencies of anemia were found in Central India (Hockham et al., 2018). The robust clustering of high anemia rates for children or women points to several regions on which to focus attention in the future. As depicted by the maps, the rise of anemia rates observed in some relatively prosperous areas, such as West Bengal or Gujarat, requires more investigations to understand the underlying reasons for this unexpected finding.

Our findings have several important policy implications. We have highlighted the unique geographies of anemia prevalence among children and women, which should target resources and relevant programs for populations in greatest need. The study's findings suggest that more attention is required to improve the conditions of women in the areas where anemia among women is high. Strategies to minimize childhood anemia should target nutritional intake and address maternal anemia, poverty, and food insecurity.

India has made several large-scale efforts to prevent and treat anemia. Most notably, the National Nutritional Anemia Prevention Programme has provided free iron and folic acid supplements for children, expectant and nursing mothers, and women who attend family planning services through primary healthcare facilities since they were launched in 1970 (Anand et al., 2014). In 2013, the National Iron Plus Initiative extended the provision of free iron and folic acid supplements to boys aged 10–19 years. However, the few existing evaluations of the National Nutritional Anemia Prevention Programme suggest it has not successfully reduced anemia prevalence in any age group (Kapil & Singh, 2014). In 2018, POSHAN Abhiyaan (National Nutrition Mission, NNM) was launched. The Ministry of Women and Child Development's flagship program aimed to make India malnutrition-free by 2022 by ensuring holistic development and adequate nutrition for pregnant women, mothers, and children. More than 100 million people are expected to benefit from this program.

The Anemia Mukt Bharat (Anemia Free India) has also strengthened the earlier Iron Plus Initiative by fostering new strategies for tackling anemia. It focuses on six target beneficiary groups through six interventions and six institutional mechanisms to achieve the envisaged target under the POSHAN Abhiyaan. It combines several strategies to prevent and treat anemia, including iron and folic acid supplementation, deworming, food fortification in schools, and malaria screening. Anemia Mukti Bharat was projected to reach 450 million beneficiaries by 2022 (GOI, 2018). While these programs may have favorable impacts on the further reduction of anemia among children and women, it is necessary to monitor and evaluate the success of such programs in India, given the recent deterioration of the situation reflected by the NFHS-5 estimates.

References

Anand, T., Rahi, M., Sharma, P., & Ingle, G. K. (2014). Issues in the prevention of iron deficiency anemia in India. *Nutrition, 30*(7), 764–770. https://doi.org/10.1016/j.nut.2013.11.022

Bentley, M. E., & Griffiths, P. L. (2003). The burden of anemia among women in India. *European Journal of Clinical Nutrition, 57*(1), 52–60. https://doi.org/10.1038/sj.ejcn.1601504

DeFries, R., Chhatre, A., Davis, K. F., Dutta, A., Fanzo, J., Ghosh-Jerath, S., Myers, S., Rao, N. D., & Smith, M. R. (2018). Impact of historical changes in coarse cereals consumption in India on micronutrient intake and anemia prevalence. *Food and Nutrition Bulletin, 39*(3), 377–392. https://doi.org/10.1177/0379572118783492

GOI. (2018). Ministry of Health and Family Welfare Intensified National Iron Plus Initiative (I-NIPI): Operational guidelines for program managers.

Horton, S., & Levin, C. (2001). Commentary on "Evidence That Iron Deficiency Anemia Causes Reduced Work Capacity.". *The Journal of Nutrition, 131*(2), 691S–696S. https://doi.org/10.1093/jn/131.2.691S

Hockham, C., Bhatt, S., Colah, R., Mukherjee, M. B., Penman, B. S., Gupta, S., & Piel, F. B. (2018). The spatial epidemiology of sickle-cell anemia in India. *Scientific Reports, 8*(1), 17,685. https://doi.org/10.1038/s41598-018-36077-w

Kapil, U., & Singh, A. B. (2014). National Iron-plus Initiative guidelines for control of iron deficiency anemia in India, 2013. *The National Medical Journal of India, 27*(1), 27–29.

Kozuki, N., Lee, A. C., & Katz, J. (2012). Moderate to severe, but not mild, maternal anemia is associated with an increased risk of small-for-gestational-age outcomes. *The Journal of Nutrition, 142*(2), 358–362. https://doi.org/10.3945/jn.111.149237

Liou, L., Kim, R., & Subramanian, S. V. (2020). Identifying geospatial patterns in wealth disparity in child malnutrition across 640 districts in India. *SSM—Population. Health, 10*, 100,524. https://doi.org/10.1016/j.ssmph.2019.100524

Nguyen, P. H., Scott, S., Avula, R., Tran, L. M., & Menon, P. (2018). Trends and drivers of change in the prevalence of anemia among 1 million women and children in India, 2006 to 2016. *BMJ Globalization and Health, 3*(5), e001010. https://doi.org/10.1136/bmjgh-2018-001010

Onyeneho, N. G., Ozumba, B. C., & Subramanian, S. V. (2019). Determinants of childhood anemia in India. *Scientific Reports, 9*(1), 16,540. https://doi.org/10.1038/s41598-019-52793-3

Puri, P., Khan, J., Shil, A., & Ali, M. (2020). A cross-sectional study on selected child health outcomes in India: Quantifying the spatial variations and identifying parental risk factors. *Scientific Reports, 10*(1), 6645. https://doi.org/10.1038/s41598-020-63210-5

Sharma, H., Singh, S. K., & Srivastava, S. (2020). Socio-economic inequality and spatial heterogeneity in anaemia among children in India: Evidence from NFHS-4 (2015–16). *Clinical Epidemiology and Global Health, 8*(4), 1158–1171.

Stevens, G. A., Finucane, M. M., De-Regil, L. M., Paciorek, C. J., Flaxman, S. R., Branca, F., Pena-Rosas, J. P., Bhutta, Z. A., & Ezzati, M. (2013). Global, regional, and national trends in hemoglobin concentration and prevalence of total and severe anemia in children and pregnant and non-pregnant women for 1995–2011: A systematic analysis of population-representative data. *The lancet Globalization and Health, 1*(1), e16–e25. https://doi.org/10.1016/S2214-109X(13)70001-9

Suryanarayana, R., Chandrappa, M., Santhuram, A. N., Prathima, S., & Sheela, S. R. (2017). Prospective study on prevalence of anemia of pregnant women and its outcome: A community-based study. *Journal of Family Medicine and Primary Care, 6*(4), 739–743. https://doi.org/10.4103/jfmpc.jfmpc_33_17

Verma, M., Chhatwal, J., & Kaur, G. (1998). Prevalence of anemia among urban school children of Punjab. *Indian Pediatrics, 35*(12), 1181–1186.

WHO. (2011). *Hemoglobin concentrations for the diagnosis of anemia and assessment of severity. Vitamin and mineral nutrition information System.* World Health Organization.

Chapter 6
Female Under-Five Mortality in India

Jayanta Kumar Bora

Until recently, in all South Asian countries,[1] females have had a survival disadvantage compared to males, particularly young females. Gender disparity in mortality indicators results from the complex interplay of biological differences between males and females and discrimination in healthcare and nutrition linked to gender inequality. Earlier studies conducted in different South Asian countries have documented excess female mortality in childhood as a reflection of bias towards female children (Bhattacharya, 2006; D'Souza & Chen, 1980; Guilmoto et al., 2018; Gupta, 1987). Other studies found that girls are treated less favorably than boys in nutrition, breastfeeding, and healthcare treatment (Borooah, 2004; Chen et al., 1981; Fledderjohann et al., 2014; Raman, 1998).

Gender disparities in health and mortality have been the subject of intensive research in India, focusing on prenatal sex selection, excess female mortality at a young age, gender disparity in immunization, breastfeeding, nutrition, healthcare access, and health finance in India. Researchers showed, in particular, a keen interest in examining the dynamics of sex differentials in under-five mortality in the past decades. It has been documented that, until recently, despite an advantage in life expectancy at birth by females in India, female children bear an extra burden of death than their male counterparts in all states of India (Canudas-Romo et al., 2015). Guilmoto et al. (2018) estimated about 0.24 million excess deaths of girls annually around 2003 due to gender discrimination. Nevertheless, recent Million Deaths Study findings revealed that India had significantly reduced child mortality and excess mortality among girl children (Collaborators, 2010).

[1]With the exception of Sri Lanka which has never experienced excess female mortality among children.

J. K. Bora (✉)
VART Consulting, Mumbai, India
e-mail: jayanta.bora@vartindia.com

C. Z. Guilmoto (ed.), *Atlas of Gender and Health Inequalities in India*, Demographic Transformation and Socio-Economic Development 16,
https://doi.org/10.1007/978-3-031-47847-5_6

The present study re-examines gender disparity in India's under-five mortality rates, employing more recent nationally representative data. It attempts to answer the following research questions: (1) What is the level of gender and regional disparity in under-five mortality in India? (2) What are the factors affecting under-five mortality in India by gender?

Data and Measurement

This study is based on the National Family Health Survey (NFHS) data. To see the trend of child mortality, we used NFHS-2 (1998–1999), NFHS-3 (2005–2006), NFHS-4 (2015–16), and NFHS-5 (2019–21).[2] To examine the level of gender inequality in child mortality at the district level and their associated factors, we used NFHS-5 data. Our computations are based on estimates of the U5MR (under-five mortality rate), which is the probability of dying between birth and the fifth birthday expressed per 1000 live births. We extended the reference period to 10 years before the survey to maximize the sample size needed to estimate the district mortality rate.

We applied direct methods of mortality-rate calculation using data on children's date of birth, their survival status, and the date and age at death of deceased children on women's complete birth history data. Rustein and Rojas described the synthetic cohort probability approach using complete birth history data of women aged 15–49 to estimate U5MR rates (Rutstein & Rojas, 2003). We used the Stata package "syncmrates" to allow full use of the most recent data. This method produces the U5MR for total, female, and male populations, as well as the corresponding 95% confidence interval and significance level.

Our estimates are restricted to districts for which (1) estimated mortality rates are statistically significant at a 10% significance level and (2) estimated mortality rates are greater than zero. The details of this method can be found in previous studies (Bora & Saikia, 2018; Rutstein & Rojas, 2003).

Our dependent variable for regression analysis is the mortality risk (coded as one for children who died before reaching their fifth birthday). In addition, upon reviewing the previous research, we have considered the following independent variables: sex, region (South, North, Central, East, West, Northeast), socio-religious groups (high caste Hindu, OBC Hindu, scheduled tribes, scheduled castes, Muslims, rest); mother's education (no education, primary education, secondary education, higher education); wealth index (poorest, poorer, middle, richer, richest); mother's age at birth (less than 20 years, 20–24 years, and 25 and above); type of fuel used for cooking (safe and unsafe); type of toilet (improved and not improved toilet); source of drinking water (improved and not improved), place of birth (home delivery and

[2]The original NFHS dataset and the spatial analysis methodology are described in detail in Chap. 1.

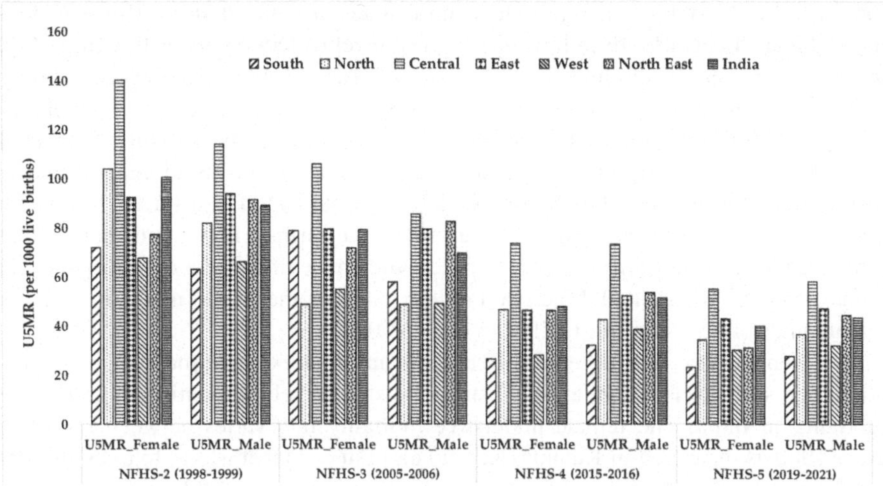

Fig. 6.1 Trends in under-five mortality rate in 1998–2021

institutional delivery); and the number of prenatal visits during the pregnancy of last birth (0, 1, 2–3, and 4 visits).

We also used community-level contextual characteristics such as maternal education, electric connection, poverty, institutional delivery, and distance to health facilities. These community-level variables are calculated as the average of each cluster's corresponding individual or household variables.

Findings and Discussion

Figure 6.1 presents the trends in under-five mortality rate (per 1000 live births) by region and gender from 1998 to 2021 for six major regions in India. These estimates highlight the speed of mortality reduction and direction of change in the child mortality scenario; under-five mortality rates have been reduced consistently from NFHS-2 to NFHS-5, with a noticeably sharper decline among girls.

Nevertheless, regional variations in under-five mortality remain wide in NFHS-5, with a similar rank maintained by the regions in all periods. For example, the southern region experienced the lowest under-five mortality from NFHS-2 to NFHS-5, while the central region experienced the highest mortality level in all rounds of NFHS. Interestingly, female U5MR was previously higher in central, northern, and southern regions during 1998–2006. Still, in 2020–21, female U5MR is now lower than male U5MR everywhere in India, a feature more in line with the excess male mortality in childhood observed worldwide.

At the state level, the highest female under-five mortality was observed among girls in Uttar Pradesh (59.5 per 1000 live births), followed by the state of Bihar

(56.5 per 1000 live births). While the central states of Uttar Pradesh, Bihar, Chhattisgarh, and Madhya Pradesh have the highest level of female under-five mortality, the southern states, including Kerala, Goa, and Tamil Nadu, experienced a pretty low level of under-five mortality rate. The lowest estimate pertains to Puducherry (5.3 per 1000 live births). Furthermore, northeastern states Sikkim, Arunachal Pradesh, Manipur, and Mizoram also experienced lower levels of female under-five mortality during the study period. Of 37 states and Union Territories, 14 met the under-five mortality SDG target (25 per 1000 live births). It is worth noting that female under-five mortality is equal to or less than male under-five mortality rates in Uttar Pradesh, Bihar, and Madhya Pradesh, states otherwise known for excess female under-five mortality (Guilmoto et al., 2018).

We then explore district-level differentials and first examine the statistical variations across districts. There exist substantial district-level differentials in under-five mortality in India. The female under-five mortality rate varies between less than 2 per 1000 as measured in Kannur (Kerala) and Pune (Maharashtra) to over 100 per 1000 estimated for Hardoi and Kanshiram Nagar (now Kasganj) districts that are in Uttar Pradesh. This range of U5MR estimates represents a variation by a factor of 50. When using international estimates of U5MR, these levels correspond to those of Japan and Nigeria, respectively. The coefficient of variation of U5MR is considerable at 56%.

Figure 6.2 plots the district-level under-five mortality rate for females on the map of India.[3] The highest mortality levels are observed in north-central India, forming a belt running from east Rajasthan to Uttar Pradesh, Madhya Pradesh, Bihar, and north Jharkhand. Inversely, the lowest U5MR values are primarily found in South India, with a regional extension towards coastal Maharashtra and pockets of low under-five mortality in northwest India and parts of the Northeast and West Bengal.

The district-level analysis brings to the fore significant mortality variations within states. For instance, we can identify important disparities in mortality estimates inside Punjab, Maharashtra, or Odisha. State borders often remain detectable on the map, as illustrated between Maharashtra and Karnataka or between Tamil Nadu and Andhra Pradesh. This relative discontinuity points to the distinctness of regional demographics, be it the heritage of local social and gender structures or the impact of regional population policies and development dynamics. This heterogeneity explains why Moran's I is only 0.54 despite the clear spatial patterns, a low value that points to potential measurement issues of female under-five mortality on district samples.

Large areas of homogenous mortality levels emerge when we conduct a spatial cluster analysis based on spatial autocorrelation. Higher mortality is notably concentrated around Uttar Pradesh, the northern districts of Madhya Pradesh, and adjacent districts in Bihar and Chhattisgarh. In addition, a smaller hotspot of high mortality can be identified in South Odisha. As for low mortality areas, they mostly form one large region extending from southwest Maharashtra to Kerala and south

[3]The map of male U5MR is not distinguishable from that of female rates and, therefore, not shown here.

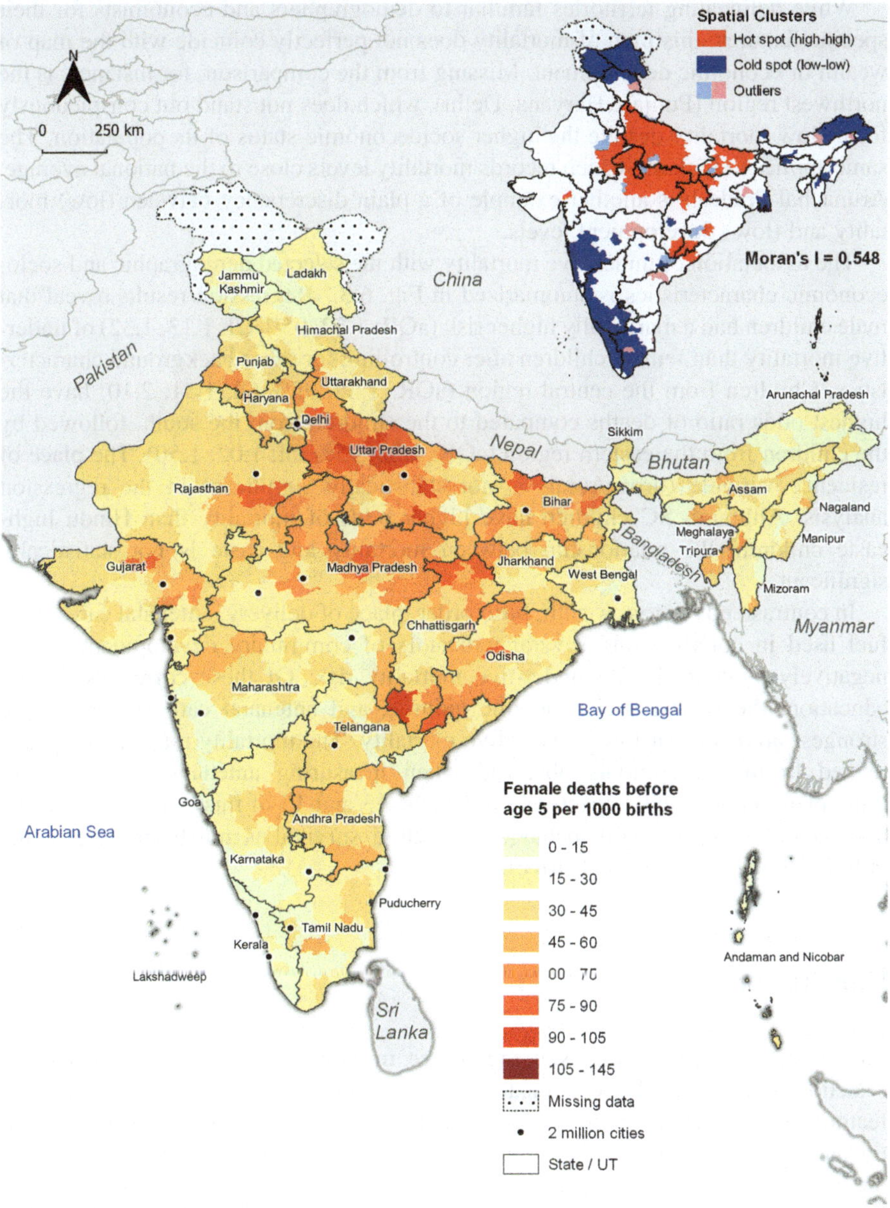

Fig. 6.2 Female under-five mortality rate
Source: NFHS-5, 2019–21
The map is for illustrative purposes and may not represent official boundaries

Tamil Nadu. Surprisingly, given their spatial isolation, two mountainous regions—in Arunachal Pradesh and around Jammu and Kashmir—emerge as a smaller cluster of low under-five mortality.

While delineating territories familiar to demographers and economists for their specific features, this map of mortality does not perfectly coincide with the map of wealth or economic development. Missing from the comparison, for instance, is the northwest region (Punjab, Haryana, Delhi), which does not stand out conspicuously for its low mortality despite the higher socioeconomic status of its population. The same applies to Gujarat, which records mortality levels close to the national average. Arunachal Pradesh is another example of a plain discrepancy between (low) mortality and (low) development levels.

The association of under-five mortality with the selected demographic and socioeconomic characteristics is summarized in Fig. 6.3.[4] Regression results reveal that male children had a marginally higher risk (aOR: 1.22, 95% CI: 1.13, 1.32) of under-five mortality than female children after controlling for other background characteristics. Children from the central region (aOR: 1.68, 95% CI: 1.41, 2.10) have the highest odds ratio of deaths compared to the children from the south, followed by the children from the eastern region (aOR: 1.23, 95% CI: 1.02, 1.50). The place of residence variable (urban/rural) is not statistically significant in the regression analysis. Although SC children have higher odds of mortality than Hindu high-caste children, the relationship between mortality and caste is not statistically significant.

In contrast, education, wealth, birth order, place of delivery, antenatal care, clean fuel used in cooking, and several indicators of community development are all negatively associated with under-five mortality risk. Of these correlates, higher education, the richest socioeconomic quintile, and antenatal care emerge as the strongest predictors of lower under-five mortality. The mortality map can be partly related to the differentials observed when measuring antenatal care and full immunization depicted respectively in Chaps. 13 and 15 of this Atlas—even if the association between health behavior and child survival is much stronger at the individual level than at the district level.

Conclusion

Earlier studies showed that son preference in India leads to both prenatal sex selection and postnatal discriminatory behavior in nutrition and healthcare. This feature, in turn, leads to excess female deaths below five. This chapter aimed to update the knowledge on sex differentials in under-five mortality, focusing on geographical variation using recently available disaggregated data from the NFHS-5. The study findings suggest a clear downward trend in the excess mortality rate among girls from NFHS-2 to NFHS-5. The reduction in the gender gap in under-five mortality is sizable nationally in 2019–21. Female survival among children has

[4]Odds ratios measure the strength of the correlation with the outcome variable. Values above (below) one correspond to a positive (negative) association.

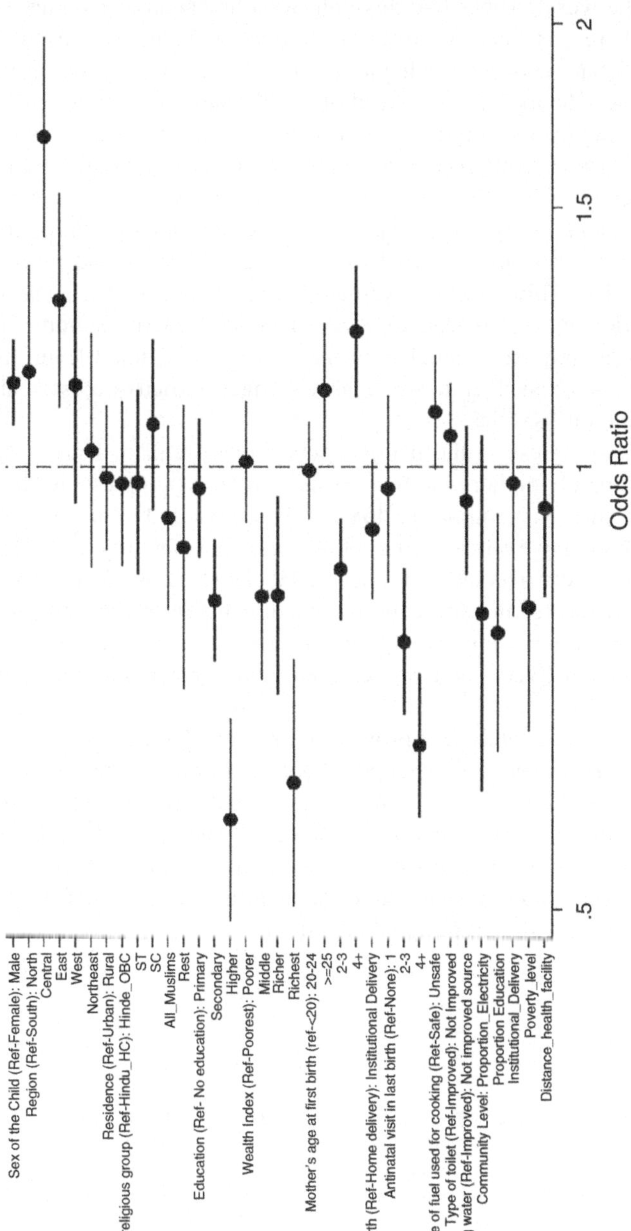

Fig. 6.3 Odds ratios of under-five deaths by selected background characteristics
Source: NFHS-5

finally become lower than male survival at the national and state levels, as observed elsewhere in the world. These findings indicate a few significant changes in recent times. First, there has been a substantial reduction in gender discrimination in nutrition, healthcare, and other behavioral variables at an early age in India in the most recent time. The most recent round of NFHS data shows an absence of gender disparity in immunization, nutrition, and treatment-seeking behaviors (Dixit et al. 2020). This may be a combined result of government efforts and civil society to increase awareness about the value of girl children. Second, a reduction in the fertility rate in India, implying a reduction in the proportion of high-parity children, might have been the source of improvements in healthcare and nutrition-related treatments for girls. Third, an improvement in the socioeconomic conditions of the Indian population may also lead to reduced gender discrimination. The various rounds of NFHS show substantial improvement in educational level, use of consumer durables, and basic facilities such as housing, electricity access, and improved water and sanitation facilities.

Despite such progress at the national level, there remain districts where girls experience marginally higher mortality levels than boys (not presented here). Out of 612 districts with robust estimates, 468 districts have under-five mortality higher than 25 per thousand live births, the target of under-five mortality of SDG 3. Approximately 25% of the districts record higher U5MR levels above 50 per 1000. Most of these districts are located in north-central India, notably in and around Uttar Pradesh. Maternal education, household wealth, higher age at childbirth, lower parity, ANC visit, institutional delivery, and higher caste status are associated with reduced under-five mortality.

Under-five mortality tends to improve faster for females than males at the national and state levels. However, higher female mortality is still present in a few districts. As SDG aims to eliminate "all forms of gender discrimination by 2030", it is essential to eradicate excess mortality among female children across all Indian regions and social groups. Because of substantial intrastate and interstate disparities, our study's findings recommend intensive intervention in selected geographical pockets and more investment in female children.

References

Bhattacharya, P. C. (2006). Economic development, gender inequality, and demographic outcomes: Evidence from India. *Population and Development Review, 32*(2), 263–292.

Bora, J. K., & Saikia, N. (2018). Neonatal and under-five mortality rate in Indian districts with reference to sustainable development goal 3: An analysis of the National Family Health Survey of India (NFHS), 2015–2016. *PLOS ONE, 13*(7), e0201125. https://doi.org/10.1371/journal.pone.0201125

Borooah, V. K. (2004). Gender bias among children in India in their diet and immunisation against disease. *Social Science and Medicine, 58*(9), 1719–1731.

Canudas-Romo, V., Saikia, N., & Diamond-Smith, N. (2015). The contribution of age-specific mortality towards male and female life expectancy differentials in India and selected states, 1970–2013. *Asia-Pacific Population Journal, 30*(2), 1–20.

Chen, L. C., Huq, E., & d'Souza, S. (1981). Sex bias in the family allocation of food and healthcare in rural Bangladesh. *Population and Development Review, 7*, 55–70.

Collaborators, M. D. S. (2010). Causes of neonatal and child mortality in India: A nationally representative mortality survey. *The Lancet, 376*(9755), 1853–1860.

Dixit, P., Cleland, J., & James, K. S. (2020). Sex differences in child health and health care: A reappraisal for India. *Population Studies, 74*(3), 379–398.

D'Souza, S., & Chen, L. C. (1980). Sex differentials in mortality in rural Bangladesh. *Population and development review*, 257–270.

Fledderjohann, J., Agrawal, S., Vellakkal, S., Basu, S., Campbell, O., Doyle, P., Ebrahim, S., & Stuckler, D. (2014). Do girls have a nutritional disadvantage compared with boys? Statistical models of breastfeeding and food consumption inequalities among Indian siblings. *PLOS ONE, 9*(9), e107172. https://doi.org/10.1371/journal.pone.0107172

Guilmoto, C. Z., Saikia, N., Tamrakar, V., & Bora, J. K. (2018). Excess under-5 female mortality across India: A spatial analysis using 2011 census data. *The lancet Global Health, 6*(6), e650–e658. https://doi.org/10.1016/S2214-109X(18)30184-0

Gupta, M. D. (1987). Selective discrimination against female children in rural Punjab, India. *Population and Development Review, 13*(1), 77–100.

Raman, T. R. (1998). Epidemiology of under-five malnutrition: Sex differential in healthcare and nutritional status (under-five malnutrition). *Medical Journal, Armed Forces India, 54*(4), 375–376. https://doi.org/10.1016/S0377-1237(17)30621-4

Rutstein, S. O., & Rojas, G. (2003). *Guide to DHS statistics*. ORC Macro.

Part II
Gender

Chapter 7
Women's Land Ownership and Patrilocality in India

Thomas Licart

On the eve of the release of her pioneering book on gender inequalities in properties in India (Agarwal, 1994a), Bina Agarwal argued that "the gender gap in the ownership and control of the property is the single most critical contributor to the gender gap in economic well-being, social status, and empowerment" (Agarwal, 1994b). Agricultural land was, and still is, the most critical asset in rural India. Land ownership is the primary source of income for many households and is also a marker of political power and social prestige. Agarwal highlighted three main benefits of women's land ownership. First is the welfare argument. Agricultural land is an essential asset for limiting the risk of poverty thanks to the direct source of income provided by its exploitation, as well as indirect (e.g., more accessible access to credit or valuable assets that can be sold). It positively impacts the welfare of women and children and reduces the risk of domestic violence (Batla et al., 2016; Panda & Agarwal, 2005). Second, women with land can improve their efficiency; they can feel more confident, willing, and able to invest in their land and improve productivity. Finally, land ownership is a significant source of empowerment. Women landowners enjoy greater autonomy, status, and respect within the community and increase their decision-making and bargaining power within the household (Valera et al., 2018).[1]

Nevertheless, women's access to the ownership and control of lands is limited in India. According to the last agricultural census (2015–2016),[2] the percentage share of female operational landholders is only 13.9%. In South Asia, India represents an

[1] See also Allendorf (2007) for an illustration of other benefits of women's land rights.

[2] Source: FAO Gender and Land Rights Database, Indian Agricultural Census (1995–1996; 2000–2001; 2005–2006; 2010–2011; 2015–2016); Agricultural Household Survey (Sri Lanka, 2016–2017); National Sample Census of Agriculture (Nepal, 2011–2012).

T. Licart (✉)
Université de Strasbourg, Strasbourg, France

C. Z. Guilmoto (ed.), *Atlas of Gender and Health Inequalities in India*, Demographic Transformation and Socio-Economic Development 16,
https://doi.org/10.1007/978-3-031-47847-5_7

average figure between Bangladesh (5% of women landowners in 2008) and Sri Lanka (23% in 2016–2017). Progress has been made over the past 20 years: from 9.5% in 1995–1996, the proportion of female landholders increased to 13.9% in 2015–2016. However, this growth appears to be particularly slow compared to some neighboring countries. From 2001 to 2011, the proportion increased only from 10.8% to 12.8%, while it has more than doubled in Nepal, from 8.6% to 19%. Surprisingly, this slow and steady increase does not appear to have been affected by the critical step taken by the Indian inheritance law in 2005.

On the fifth of September 2005, the Hindu Succession Act of 1956 was amended to reinforce gender equality in property inheritance and to remove the gender bias of the former law. While the law of 1956 was the first to introduce women's legal rights to inherit for Hindus, Sikhs, and Buddhists, the joint family's agricultural and ancestral properties were excluded from this provision. The reactions to this first attempt to improve gender equality on property rights depict customary regional practices and women's positions. While southern states, such as Kerala (1976), Andhra Pradesh (1986), and Tamil Nadu (1989), have amended the law to extend it to joint family property, other northern states, such as Haryana and Punjab, have tried, in vain, to abolish it (Chowdhry, 2009). Inheritance being India's primary land acquisition mode, the 2005 amendment should have been the final blow to gender inequality for Hindus, Sikh, and Buddhist communities. These gender inequalities enshrined in the law have long been less pronounced in other religions (Subramanian, 2008). For instance, the inheritance of Muslims has come under the Muslim Personal Law (Sharia) Application Act since 1937; it gives women the right to inherit ancestral properties, but only half the share of men. Most Christian communities are governed by the Indian Succession Act, which is older, dating from 1925, and more equalitarian, with equal property rights between sons and daughters. Thus, currently, most women have legal access to ancestral lands in each community. The low figure of women among landholders is due to two reasons. First, these laws concern only intestate succession and can be circumvented by testamentary succession. Second, there remains a significant gap between legislative and customary law.

Women face numerous obstacles to controlling and owning land; they must know their rights and be willing to exercise them. The gender gap in education remains the main barrier for the former. The latter has to deal with a traditional kinship system and social values that are hostile to these claims. While some matrilineal communities have long existed in south and northeast India, the country has long been governed by two patrilineal legal doctrines: The *Mitakshara* and the *Dayabhaga*. These schools of law can be considered the roots of the traditional joint family composed of coparceners of the ancestral properties (Shah, 1968). One of its main features is its patrilocality: married sons stay in the parental home and support them in old age, while married daughters leave their natal family to live with their in-laws.

In a pioneering study of the kinship system in India, the authors describe two kinship systems that coexist (Dyson & Moore, 1983). In the North Indian system, marriage is strictly patrilocality-cum-village exogamic. As noted by one author, "A girl child is allowed to remain a child only for short periods of life. It is always stressed that her relationship with her natal home is temporary" (Sonawat, 2001). Hence, after marriage, women tend to live far from their natal home, making it more difficult to claim their rights on parental land—and even more to exercise direct control over that land. This difficulty is reinforced by a social taboo on women claiming land. Women have already inherited through the dowry[3]; accordingly, they avoid asserting their rights to maintain peaceful relations with their natal family. In the South Indian kinship system, marriage within the family is more common, especially between uncle and niece or first cousins. Married women often stay close to their natal family and may live with their uncle and aunt. It is, therefore, more accessible for them to claim the inheritance from their parents' property. In addition, the presence of matrilineal communities in the past would reduce the patriarchal resistance to women's property. The patrilocal norm would also be more flexible; a return to her natal family in case of a marital or family crisis is less excluded. At the same time, some pseudo-matrilocal arrangements can be established when the daughter has inherited land, unlike her husband; however, this south/north dichotomy is now porous. The dowry system also prevails in South India. Although more common than in the north, consanguineous marriages are now a minority in South India: they represent 18% of marriages in Telangana and 28% in Tamil Nadu, according to NFHS-5. Kerala has only 4.4% of women aged 15–49 in consanguineous marriage.

Despite this well-established literature, few quantitative studies on the gender gap in agriculture ownership have focused on its overall spatial structure and correspondence to the different patrilocality norms. This chapter documented the women landowners' distribution across regions in India. After analyzing its main socioeconomic features, we aim at the geographical pattern of one of them: patrilocality.

Data and Measurement

The gender gap in land ownership has received greater attention in the fifth round of NFHS.[4] The issue has been addressed in two questions. First, the woman's questionnaire asks whether she owns land alone or jointly, regardless of its size or purpose, "Do you own any agricultural or non-agricultural land either alone or jointly with someone else?". However, this question has been asked only in the "State module" and is unsuitable for a district-level study. The second question is asked on the household questionnaire to each household owning agricultural land. It collects the gender of landowners as follows: "Male member," "Female member," or "Both." Agarwal (2003) underlines the greater virtues of individual ownership in comparison with the joint titles (more power over land, more independence from men...). However, for sample size reasons at the district level, the female land

[3] Even if girls often have limited access to the dowry for the benefit of the in-law family.

[4] The original NFHS dataset and the spatial analysis methodology are described in detail in Chap. 1.

ownership will correspond to both individual and joint ownership by women. Thus, the women's land ownership index corresponds to the share of female landowners (alone or together) among households' landowners. The other rich source on gender and land is the quinquennial agriculture census. However, the agriculture census focuses on operational holding, a distinct notion of ownership defined in NFHS. The holder will be responsible "for the operation of the agricultural holding and who exercises the technical initiative and is responsible for its operation," irrespective of the legal ownership status.

The index computed to study patrilocality is based on the sex of the children-in-law residing within joint families. In each district, we compute the proportion of daughters-in-law among children-in-law of the household head. A figure of 75% corresponds to a district where three-fourths of children-in-law living with their parents are daughters-in-law. The higher this proportion, the stronger the culturally prescribed norm of patrilocality among complex households. On the other hand, a lower index means a significant proportion of residing sons-in-law and a more frequent presence of married daughters in a joint family setup. We must stress that this indicator ignores the practice of neolocality since it only factors in households in which parents and a married couple coreside.[5] The proportion of daughters-in-law among children-in-law indicates the regional flexibility in the patrilocality norm and, more indirectly, the access of a married daughter to her natal place.

Findings and Discussion

The proportion of females among agricultural landowners was 10.8%, according to NFHS-5. This share of women landowners at the national level conceals the state-level heterogeneity. From less than 5.0% in Chandigarh and 6.0% in Jammu and Kashmir, this proportion exceeds one-fourth of landowners in Kerala (28.1%). However, about half of the landowners are women in Lakshadweep (48.4%) and Meghalaya (87.6%). These territories are well-known for their matrilineal societies, as for the Khasi, Jaintia, and Garo Tribes in Meghalaya.[6]

The district map of females' share among landowners shows more detailed sub-regional variations and national spatial patterns (Fig. 7.1). The South India/North India division is clear: almost half of the Indian districts record fewer than 10% of women among landowners, and they predominantly are located in North India, in a region ranging from Jammu and Kashmir to Gujarat, Odisha, and West

[5] Neolocal residence corresponds to situations in which newly married couples reside separately from the families of both the husband and the wife. As a matter of fact, the proportion of nuclear households (mostly based on neolocal residence) is only weakly correlated with the patrilocality index ($r = -0.26$).

[6] We must emphasize here that a matrilineal system differs from a matriarchal system. In a matrilineal system, property titles are traditionally in women's hands, but effective control and management are often masculine.

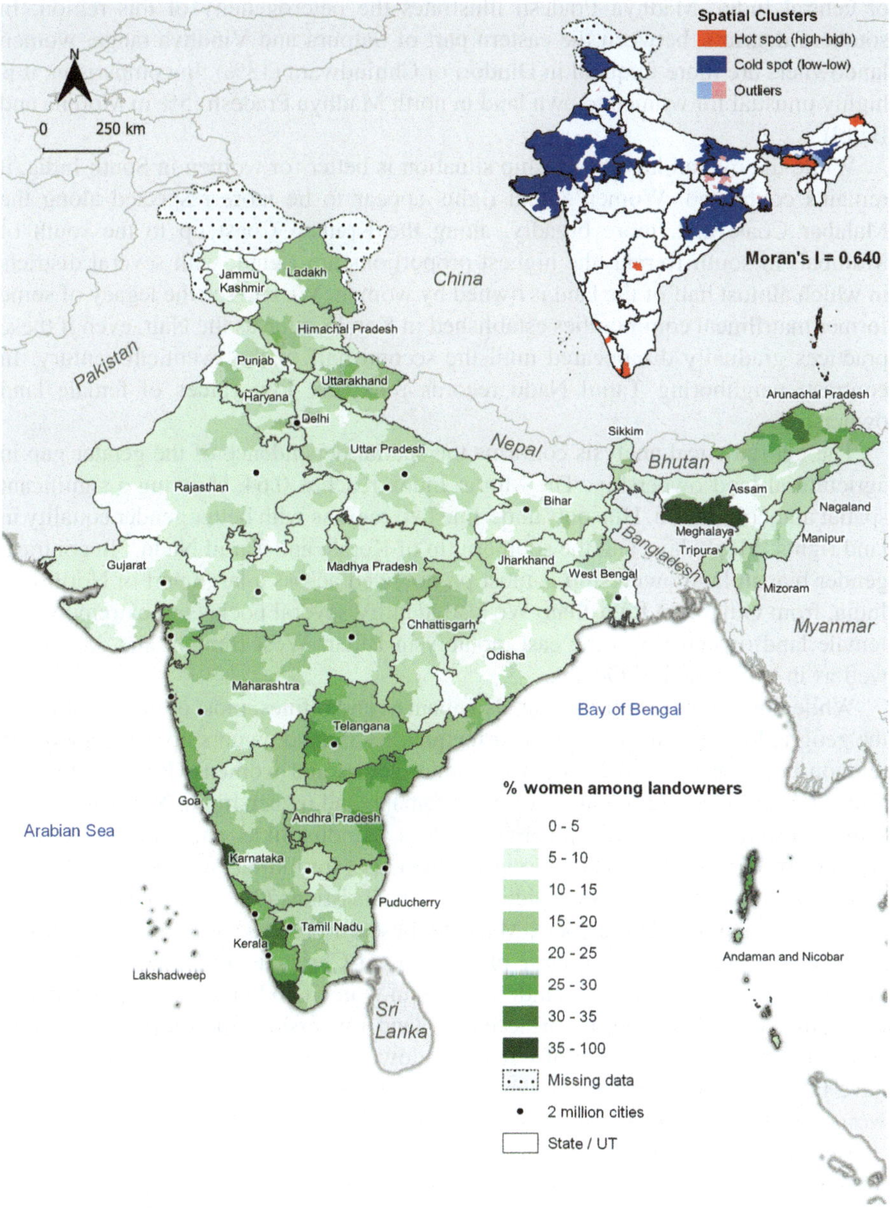

Fig. 7.1 Percentage of women aged 15–49 among the landowners
Source: NFHS-5, 2019–21
The map is for illustrative purposes and may not represent official boundaries

Bengal and encompassing the Indonesia-Gangetic Plains. Nevertheless, North India is not a homogenous territory of male landowners. The proportion of female landowners tends to rise in the western Himalayan (Himachal Pradesh, Uttarakhand) or central India. Madhya Pradesh illustrates the heterogeneity of this region. In southern districts, between the eastern part of Satpura and Vindhya range, women landowners are more frequent in Dindori or Chhindwara (18%). In comparison, it is highly unusual for women to own land in north Madhya Pradesh (5% in Morena and Betul).

While the overall land ownership situation is better for women in South India, it remains contrasted. Women's land rights appear to be more respected along the Malabar Coast and, more broadly, along the Konkan Coast up to the south of Mumbai. In south Kerala, the highest proportions are found, with several districts in which almost half of the land is owned by women. We can see the legacy of some former matrilineal communities established in Kerala, such as the Nair, even if these practices gradually disappeared until the second half of the twentieth century. In contrast, neighboring Tamil Nadu records relatively low values of female land ownership.

The geostatistical analysis confirms the spatial dependence of the gender gap in agricultural land ownership. The Moran Index reaches 0.64, showing a significant spatial autocorrelation. Hotspots underline two regions with better gender equality in land rights: Meghalaya and the southern tip of Kerala and Tamil Nadu.[7] In contrast, gender bias in land ownership is most pronounced across a large part of Northwest India, from Gujarat to Rajasthan. We also identify several pockets of extremely low female land ownership in the east, notably in Bihar, West Bengal, and Assam, as well as in tribal parts of Odisha.

While this chapter confirms, but also nuances and refines, most of the literature on the geographical disparities of gender inequalities in land ownership, what about the relation between the critical socioeconomic factors and women's land ownership? Table 7.1 provides additional statistics on female land ownership in North and South India. Despite the different inheritance laws, Hindus/Sikhs and Muslims have a similar proportion of women among landowners (around 8.3% to 10.3%). On the other hand, the difference is considerable with Christians (24%), who have twice as many women among landowners. Many of these differences stem from the regional religious distribution and the large proportions of Christians in Kerala and Meghalaya. If we focus only on North India, Christian women no longer have an advantage over other religions in terms of access to land ownership. In contrast, Christians record the highest proportion of female landowners in South India. Caste seems to have little effect in North India, while OBC households in South India have fewer women landowners than higher castes (15.9 vs. 21.1%).

Hence, historical differences in inheritance law seem to have a limited effect in this part of India compared to the cultural environment. To better examine individual variations in gender equity in land ownership, we present the result of a logistic model in which female land ownership is correlated with various background

[7]The Lakshadweep Islands are spatially isolated but would otherwise belong to the Southwestern hotspot due to their cultural proximity to Kerala.

Table 7.1 Females among agricultural landowners by socioeconomic characteristics

	North India	South India	Total
Woman's marital			
Married	7.1	14.6	8.4
No coresiding husband	10.5	23.6	11.7
Widow	35.7	41.5	37.0
Separated/divorced	9.3	17.3	10.5
Household type			
Nuclear	6.2	14.0	7.7
Joint with only married sons	10.1	17.7	11.0
Joint with only married daughters	16.2	28.1	20.8
Joint with both married sons and daughters	10.4	17.4	11.5
Other complex households	10.7	18.1	12.1
Religion			
Hindu	9.2	16.9	10.3
Muslim	7.9	17.3	8.3
Christian	9.2	21.3	24.0
Sikh	8.8	6.7	8.8
Other	12.5	7.1	13.2
Caste			
Scheduled caste	9.4	18.0	10.7
Scheduled tribe	9.6	16.9	11.6
Other backward class	8.5	15.9	9.9
None of them	9.7	21.1	10.7
Female educational level			
No school	9.6	17.5	10.9
Primary	8.7	16.2	9.9
Secondary	8.8	16.9	10.1
Higher	9.3	17.7	10.9
Do not know	13.1	17.2	13.5
Wealth index			
Poorest	9.0	17.7	9.5
Poorer	8.7	16.7	9.9
Middle	8.7	16.5	10.5
Richer	9.5	17.0	11.2
Richest	10.0	18.6	11.4
	9.1	**17.1**	**10.4**

Notes: All figures are in percentages; Northeastern states were excluded from the subnational comparison due to their high heterogeneity

individual and household variables (Fig. 7.2).[8] Once the essential demographic and socioeconomic variables are controlled, the women's religion remains associated

[8]Odds ratios measure the strength of the correlation with the outcome variable. Values above (below) one correspond to a positive (negative) association.

with land ownership, notably among Sikhs and Christians. Only the SC/ST (Dalit and Adivasi) women have slightly higher odds than other castes of owning land.

On the education level, a key variable in women's empowerment and awareness of legal rights, the evidence of its relationship with women's ownership is not strong at first sight. Both south and north Indian women who have continued their education after secondary school have almost similar land ownership levels. The effect of the age structure is modest, but women who own land are older than landless women. This difference is related to widowhood and divorce, critical correlates of female land ownership. As with age, we find a gradual increase in women's odds of owning land as their education level increases (Fig. 7.2). The association with wealth level is much more pronounced as female landownership appears significantly more frequent among the wealthiest households.

Socio-demographic factors may have some of the most substantial impacts on women's land ownership. Married women rarely own land; only 8.4% of land-owning households have women as owners, while the oldest woman lives with her husband. This proportion is higher for households with migrant husbands (no coresiding husband) and 4.4 times higher when the most senior woman in the home is a widow. The widowhood of the oldest woman in the household both marks the absence of the traditional patriarchal figure and a way for women to acquire land. Marital status explains much of the gender gap in land ownership between nuclear and complex households. The analysis by household type displays the expected

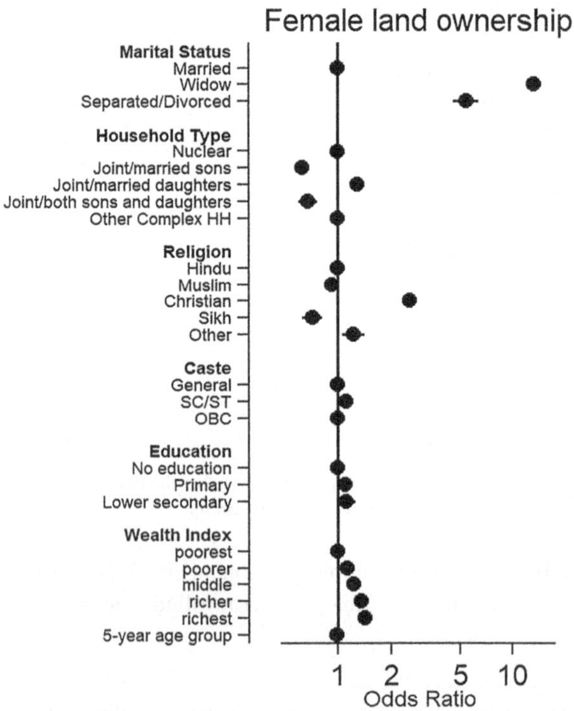

Fig. 7.2 Odds ratios of land ownership among the oldest ever-married women by selected socioeconomic characteristics

opposition between patrilocal and uxorilocal systems, with the former (respectively the latter) associated with lower (higher) proportions of female households. Women living in households with married sons have the lowest probability of owning any land.

These demographic factors alone remain insufficient to explain the geographical distribution of female land ownership described earlier. The proportion of women among landowners at the district level is not strongly correlated with the proportion of widows ($r = 0.28$) and nuclear households ($r = 0.21$).[9] It is not related to households with migrant husbands ($r = 0.05$). The only strong relationship observed is between the patrilocality index of the joint family and women's land ownership. At the district level, the proportion of daughters-in-law among children-in-law and the share of women among landowners appear to be strongly negatively correlated ($r = -0.82$). In other words, in a given district, the more married women who live with their in-laws, the lower women's access to land property compared to men's. On the contrary, districts that deviate most from the patrilocal norm will have more women among landowners.

Despite this strong relation between both gender dimensions, the spatial distribution of patrilocality displayed in Fig. 7.3 is not identical to that of land ownership. Overall, and not surprisingly, the Indian joint family is largely patrilocal: 96% of children-in-law are daughters-in-law. In other words, husbands live with their parents-in-law in only 4% of households with children-in-law. More than 99% of coresiding children-in-law are daughters-in-law in about one hundred districts.[10] Almost all of these districts are located in North India. The North India patrilocality pattern seems far less diversified than the land ownership pattern: Fig. 7.3 shows almost complete uniformity in patrilocal practices across North India. The vast majority of its districts have over 95% of daughters-in-law among children-in-law. We can, however, notice some pockets where patrilocality falls below 95%, notably in parts of east Madhya Pradesh and north Chhattisgarh or in Odisha and east Bihar. Tribal communities often inhabit these regions. The highest proportion of sons-in-law in North India is in Tapi (Gujarat), where 17% of coresiding children are sons rather than daughters-in-law. This territory is chiefly inhabited by Adivasis (84% of the total population in 2011), mainly from the Bhil and Gamit tribes.

While remaining predominantly patrilocal, South India is characterized by a slightly more prominent presence of sons-in-law in extended families than elsewhere, and a fair share of its districts have more than 10% of sons-in-law among children-in-law. Furthermore, intrastate variations are often considerable. In Karnataka, the North-South demarcation is evident, with stricter patrilocality in the Hyderabad Karnataka region but 27% of sons-in-law among coresiding children-in-law in Udupi, home of matrilineal Tuluvas. In Telugu-speaking areas, it is only along the Godavari valley that low levels of patrilocality are observed. On the

[9] Correlation coefficients are computed over NFHS-4 district values.

[10] Live-in sons-in-law are called *ghar jawai* in North India and a strong social stigma is attached to their presence in a family.

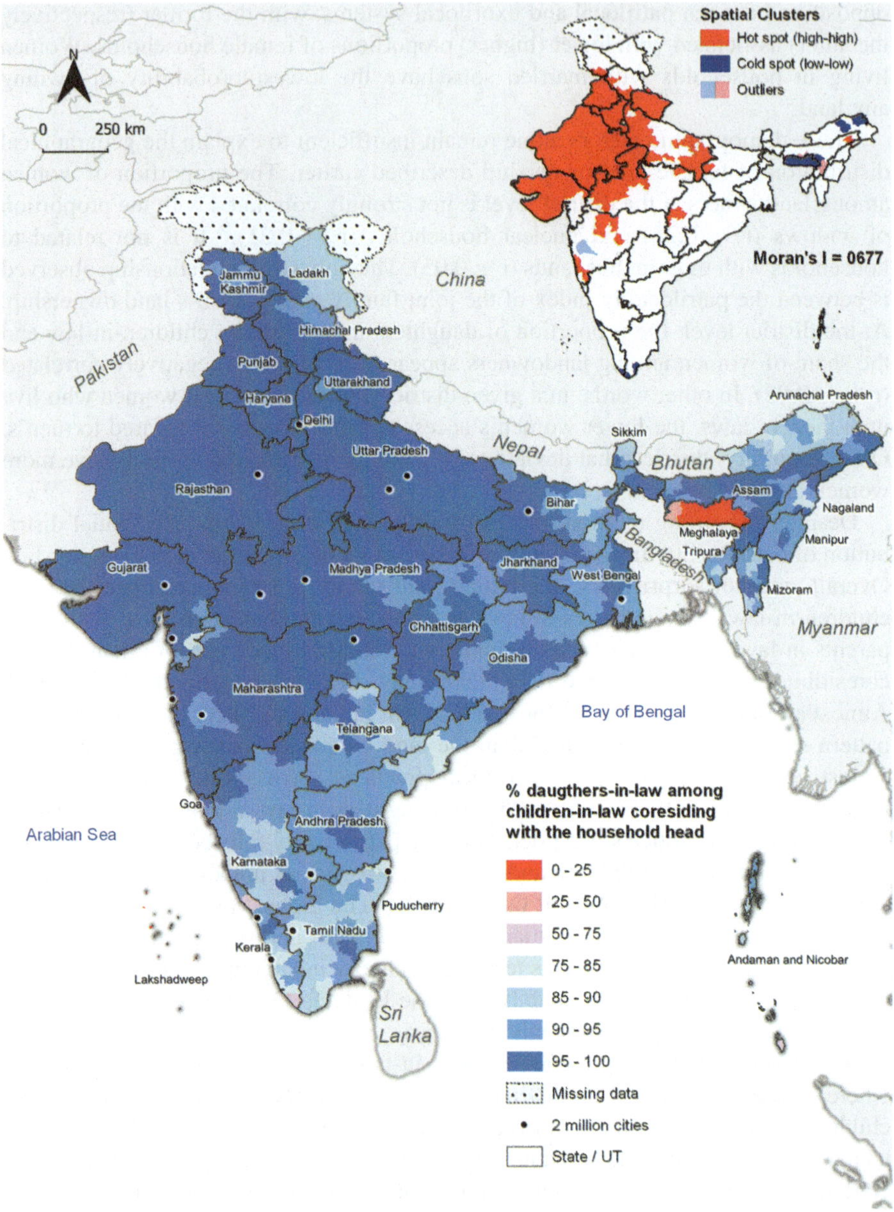

Fig. 7.3 Percentage of daughters-in-law among children-in-law coresiding with the household head
Source: NFHS-5, 2019–21
The map is for illustrative purposes and may not represent official boundaries

contrary, the Kaveri Delta and Chettinad in Tamil Nadu turn out to be much more patrilocal areas than the rest of the state. Kerala is itself highly composite. Staunchly patrilocal Malabar includes, for example, a more bilateral area like Kannur, where almost 30% of joint families include a son-in-law. Likewise, the proportion of sons-in-law among children-in-law living in complex families also jumps to 27% in Thiruvananthapuram (Travancore). Crossing the Arabian Sea to Lakshadweep, the share of sons-in-law surges further to 79% in an archipelago where matrilineality predominates.[11]

The Northeast is, as expected, showing a rather heterogeneous picture. Meghalaya stands as a perfect outlier because of its matrilocal communities. In one of its districts (East Jaintia Hills), more than 90% of married children residing with their parents are daughters living with their husbands. There are other areas of less strict patrilocality, such as Arunachal Pradesh or Mizoram, but the percentage of daughters-in-law never drops below 75%.

Moran's index of this indicator is 0.68, showing a spatial dependence slightly more pronounced than for women's land ownership. Besides Meghalaya and another area of low patrilocality centered on Kanyakumari, the LISA map highlights a broader high-patrilocality area extending from Punjab to Uttarakhand, western Madhya Pradesh (Malwa and Chambal), and Gujarat. This area represents the epicenter of patrilineal and patrilocal Indian society.

It should be emphasized that this region closely resembles other regions noted for their patriarchal traditions in this Atlas. Apart from its similitude with the map of female land ownership, the patrilocality map follows the contours of son preference displayed by the map of fertility preference (see Fig. 8.1) and girl-only families (see Fig. 9.2).

In addition, the spatial distribution of women's land ownership and the patrilocal index are linked to a demographic "supply effect." The norms of patrilocal residence and patrilineal inheritance can only persist if couples have sons to live with and to bequest to land later. Due to the ongoing fertility decline, many couples, particularly in South India, end up without a son (Chap. 9). The impact of fertility decline is partially slowed down in some regions by the masculinization of births (Allendorf, 2020; Chap. 8 in this Atlas). We may further observe that the proportion of sonless women aged 40–49 years is somewhat correlated at the district level with female landownership ($r = 0.33$) and the patrilocality index ($r = -0.34$)—even more so if we remove the matrilineal district from the analysis ($r = 0.47$ and $r = -0.46$, respectively).[12] Of course, the relationship between the spatial distribution of women among landowners and daughter-in-law among children-in-law goes beyond common demographic factors. It seems primarily rooted in an inherited kinship system typical of the patriarchal family in which unequal inheritance and land rights correspond to strict patrilocal norms (Agarwal, 1994b).

[11] Incidentally, Lakshadweep has been ruled for centuries by the Kingdom or Sultanate of Kannur, which stands today as Kerala's least patrilocal district.

[12] Correlation coefficients were computed on NFHS-4 district-level data.

Conclusion

Women's land ownership rates remain low in India despite recent marginal progress. Only 11% of landowners are women, while legal provisions exist to ensure equality in inheritance. While gender bias in favor of men is prevalent throughout most of the country, land deprivation for women reaches alarming levels in Northwest India and more rural areas of Bihar and Odisha. Religion, education, and the family situation appear to have an additional impact on women's land ownership. Moreover, the gender gap in land ownership is associated with kinship practice, especially patrilocality. The strictly patrilocal system in North India appears to act as a barrier to women's empowerment through land acquisition.

The frequency of patrilocal coresidence may slowly decrease in the future, notably due to the gradual nuclearization process (Licart, 2018). Nevertheless, the outcome of more common neolocal residence on gender land ownership remains uncertain. The gender gap can only be reduced if sex differentials in education diminish in rural India if the practice of dowry declines, and if legal awareness and sensitization on gender equality of inheritance become more widespread than in the past.

References

Agarwal, B. (1994a). *A field of one's own: Gender and land rights in South Asia*. Cambridge University Press.

Agarwal, B. (1994b). Gender and command over property: A critical gap in economic analysis and policy in South Asia. *World development, 22*(10), 1455–1478. https://doi.org/10.1016/0305-750X(94)90031-0

Agarwal, B. (2003). Gender and land rights revisited: Exploring new prospects via the state, family and market. *Journal of Agrarian Change, 3*(1), 184–224.

Allendorf, K. (2007). Do women's land rights promote empowerment and child health in Nepal? *World Development, 35*(11), 1975–1988.

Allendorf, K. (2020). Another gendered demographic dividend: Adjusting to a future without sons. *Population and Development Review, 46*(3), 471–499. https://doi.org/10.1111/padr.12337

Batla, N., Duvvury, N., & Chakraborty, S. (2016). Women's vulnerability, risk and social protection: An exploration of links between property ownership and domestic violence in South Asia. In S. Cook & N. Kabeer (Eds.), *Deficits and trajectories: Social protection as development policy in the Asia region* (pp. 219–244). Routledge.

Chowdhry, P. (2009). *Gender discrimination in land ownership*. SAGE Publications India.

Dyson, T., & Moore, M. (1983). On kinship structure, female autonomy, and demographic behavior in India. *Population and Development Review, 9*(1), 35–60. https://doi.org/10.2307/1972894

Licart, T. (2018). Étudier la structure des ménages en Inde à partir de l'enquête DLHS-3. *Working Papers Du CEPED, Paris, Ceped, 39*, 28.

Panda, P., & Agarwal, B. (2005). Marital violence, human development and women's property status in India. *World Development, 33*(5), 823–850. https://doi.org/10.1016/j.worlddev.2005.01.009

Shah, A. M. (1968). Changes in the Indian family: An examination of some assumptions. *Economic and Political Weekly, 3*(1/2), 127–134.

Sonawat, R. (2001). Understanding families in India: A reflection of societal changes. *Psicologia: Teoria e Pesquisa, 17*, 177–186. https://doi.org/10.1590/S0102-37722001000200010

Subramanian, N. (2008). Legal change and gender inequality: Changes in Muslim family law in India. *Law and Social Inquiry, 33*(3), 631–672. https://doi.org/10.1111/j.1747-4469.2008.00117.x

Valera, H. G. A., Yamano, T., Puskur, R., Veettil, P. C., Gupta, I., Ricarte, P., & Mohan, R. R. (2018). Women's land title ownership and empowerment: Evidence from India (working paper no. 559; issue 559). *ADB economics working paper series*. https://doi.org/10.22617/WPS189556-2.

Chapter 8
Spatial Patterns of Son Preference in India

Abhishek Singh and Ashish Kumar Upadhyay

Existing literature has documented marked son preference in several South and East Asian countries such as South Korea, China, Vietnam, India, Nepal, and Bangladesh (Arnold et al., 1998; Bhat & Zavier, 2003; Guilmoto, 2012; Gupta et al., 2003; Leone et al., 2003; Pandey & Astone, 2007). In India, son preference is associated with high fertility and low contraceptive use, girls' excess mortality, and sex ratio at birth in favor of males (Arnold et al., 1998; Arokiasamy, 2002; Bhat & Zavier, 2003; Clark, 2000; Singh et al., 2021). Son preference is also associated with discrimination against female children regarding food and nutrition, breastfeeding, immunization, or healthcare (Jayachandran & Kuziemko, 2011; Mishra et al., 2004; Pande, 2003). Although much research has been done on demographic manifestations of son preference in India, less research focuses on its spatial patterns across Indian districts. Some earlier studies examined state or broad geographic patterns (Arnold et al., 1998; Dyson & Moore, 1983; Yadav et al., 2020; Singh et al., 2022). These studies document higher son preference in the north compared with the south and the east.

Regarding states, these studies have highlighted higher son preference in Haryana, Punjab, Rajasthan, and Uttar Pradesh compared with Tamil Nadu, Kerala, and West Bengal. However, analyses at the state or broader regional levels often ignore vast spatial inequalities at the district level. Having identified this critical gap in the literature on son preference in India, the present study examines its spatial patterns with the Indian National Family Health Survey. Data from 707 districts of India in NFHS-5 provides us with a unique opportunity to examine spatial patterns of son preference in the districts of India.

A. Singh (✉) · A. K. Upadhyay
International Institute for Population Sciences, Mumbai, India
e-mail: abhishek@iipsindia.ac.in

C. Z. Guilmoto (ed.), *Atlas of Gender and Health Inequalities in India*, Demographic Transformation and Socio-Economic Development 16,
https://doi.org/10.1007/978-3-031-47847-5_8

Data and Measurements

In India, son preference can be studied based on three primary data sources: NFHS, District Level Household Surveys (DLHS), and India Human Development Surveys (IHDS). Of these, only the NFHS-4, NFHS-5, and DLHSs datasets can be used to understand patterns in son preference at the district level.[1] Unfortunately, the most recent round of DLHS was not conducted in Empowered Action Group (EAG)[2] states and Assam. The third round of the DLHS survey conducted in all the districts of India was performed in 2007–08. Therefore, NFHS-5 is the most recent data to provide a disaggregated picture of the spatial patterns of son preference in India.

In this study, we use differential fertility preference to identify gender bias. More precisely, we define son preference as the difference in the desire for additional children between women with sons and those without. The intention to have another child at different parity levels relates primarily to fertility levels (e.g., fertility decline in India is characterized by a rapid decline in the proportion of women desiring a third child). In the absence of gender bias, the presence of a son among previous births should have no impact on the desire for another birth, and the difference between women with or without previous male births should be zero. However, in the presence of son preference, sonless women will be more likely than other women to desire another child; the difference measured by our indicator will be sizable.

This difference was constructed using the following questions:

- For pregnant women: After the child you are expecting now, would you like to have another child, or would you prefer not to have any more children? (Have another child, no more, undecided/do not know); and
- Not pregnant or unsure: Would you like to have (a/another) child, or would you prefer not to have any (more) children? (Have (a/another) child, no more/none, says she cannot get pregnant, undecided/do not know).

Among pregnant women, those who responded as "no more" were coded as not desiring additional children, and the rest were coded as desiring additional children. Among non-pregnant women, those who responded as "no more/none" or "say she cannot get pregnant" were coded as not desiring additional children—the rest were coded as desiring additional children.

The magnitude of the difference in desired fertility between the two groups of women reflects the strength of the son preference. Population subgroups or areas having higher differences have higher son preferences. This indicator is easy to compute and may reveal attitudes that women may be less likely to articulate; it is also less likely to be affected by social desirability bias. Nevertheless, this indicator is expected to provide lower bounds to son preference estimates in populations marked by enormous sex-selective abortions or differential child mortality. Evidence

[1] The original NFHS dataset and the spatial analysis methodology are described in detail in Chap. 1.

[2] EAG states include Bihar, Jharkhand, Uttar Pradesh, Uttarakhand, Madhya Pradesh, Chhattisgarh, Odisha, and Rajasthan.

suggests this is not the case in most parts of India (Bhat & Zavier, 2007; IIPS and ICF, 2017; Registrar General of India, 2015).

We included a few district-level variables—percentages of women having five or more years of schooling, exposed to media (television, radio, or newspapers), employed, lowest wealth quintiles, and urbanization—to explain spatial patterns in son preference across the districts. In addition, the average number of children per woman among women aged 40–49, the percentage of children who are of birth order two or higher, the percentage of women from scheduled castes (SC) or scheduled tribes (ST), and the percentage of Muslim women were included as control variables in the regression models.

We prepared district-level maps and computed Moran's *I* and cluster maps based on the univariate local indicator of spatial autocorrelation (LISA). We finally estimated multivariable ordinary least squares (OLS) and multivariable spatial regression (SR) models to examine the adjusted associations between independent variables and son preference. We estimated the SR model to account for the spatial autocorrelations in the dependent and independent variables.

We used appropriate sampling weights in the estimations and adjusted our estimates for the complex survey design used in NFHS-5. We performed the statistical analyses with STATA 14.0.

Results

At the national level, the difference in not desiring additional children among women with son(s) and no son was 52%, which summarizes the intensity of son preference in India (Table 8.1). In other words, the proportion of women who do not want more children increases by 52 percentage points among women with sons.

Differences in not desiring additional children among women with son(s) and no son vary by potential covariates. For example, the difference in not desiring additional children declines from 57% in the lowest wealth decile to 47.7% in the highest wealth decile. Likewise, the difference in not desiring additional children differs by the level of women's schooling. Son preference initially rises with education but reduces again for women with more than 12 years of schooling. Son preference is also higher among non-working women compared with working women. The magnitude of son preference further declines with media exposure, from 56.5% (women not exposed to media) to 50.9% (exposed to media). Furthermore, son preference is higher in rural than urban areas (54.9% versus 46.4%).

Figure 8.1 allows us to focus on the regional differentials. The map shows the spatial distribution of our son preference indicator, viz., the difference in the percentage of women not desiring additional children among women who have and do not have sons. At the district level, the difference between desiring additional children ranges from a relatively low 17% in East Khasi Hills (Meghalaya) to an extreme 80% in Jind (Haryana). Overall, districts in North India show much higher son preference than districts in South India. In the north, the desire to have an

Table 8.1 Difference in the percentage of women not desiring additional children among women who have sons and who do not have sons by independent variables

Characteristics	Difference in the percentage of women not desiring additional children among women with and without sons
Wealth decile	
1	57.0
2	56.1
3	55.6
4	53.5
5	52.2
6	52.0
7	50.1
8	50.2
9	47.8
10	47.7
Schooling	
No schooling	48.7
Primary (1–5 years)	49.0
Secondary (6–12 years)	50.8
Higher (more than 12 years)	47.4
Currently working	
No	54.0
Yes	48.3
Media exposure	
No	56.5
Yes	50.9
Place of residence	
Urban	46.4
Rural	54.9
India	52.0

additional child among the sonless is generally higher by more than 50 percentage points. This difference rises to above 70% or even 80% in various parts of the Northwest. Son preference decreases as we move towards the east and the south. The level of son preference is significantly lower along the Indian littoral, from the Konkan Coast to the Sundarbans Delta. The absence of a son often results in less than a 30% difference in fertility desire in several areas, especially in Kerala, south Karnataka, south Tamil Nadu, and parts of Telangana and Andhra Pradesh.[3] Northeast India also shows considerably lower levels of son preference than the

[3]The Godavari Valley is also visible on the map of patrilocality (Fig. 7.3).

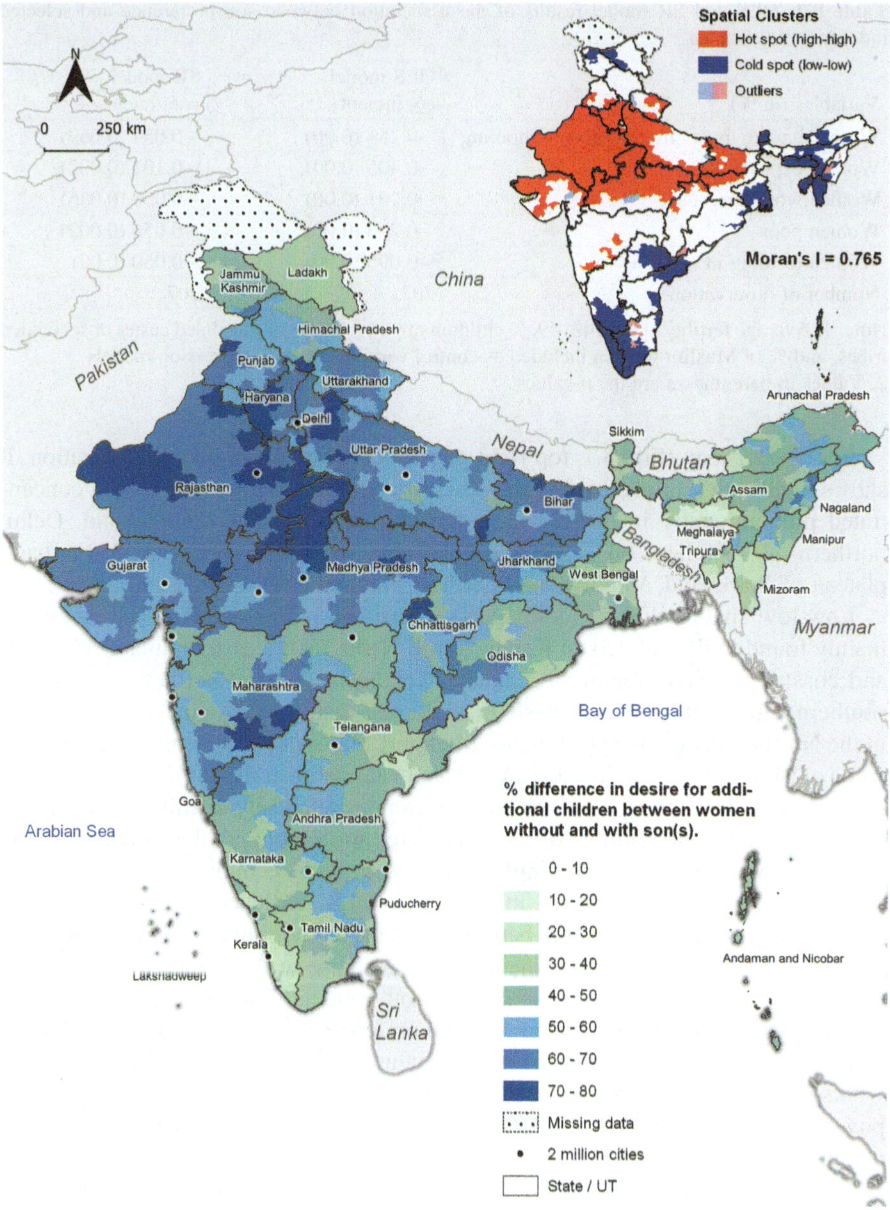

Fig. 8.1 Percentage difference in the desire for additional children between women without and with son(s)
Source: NFHS-5, 2019–21
The map is for illustrative purposes and may not represent official boundaries

north, with some of the lowest values of gender bias observed, particularly in Meghalaya, Mizoram, Manipur, or Tripura. Meghalaya especially stands out with an almost negligible level of son preference in fertility behavior.

Table 8.2 OLS and SR model results of the association between son preference and selected independent variables

Variables (in %)	OLS model coefficients	SR model coefficients
Women having five or more years of schooling	−0.259 (0.00)	−0.054 (0.069)
Women exposed to media	−0.405 (0.00)	−0.101 (0.002)
Women working	−0.161 (0.00)	−0.050 (0.035)
Women poor	−0.263 (0.00)	−0.056 (0.002)
Women residing in urban areas	−0.095 (0.00)	−0.060 (0.00)
Number of observation	707	707

Note: 1. Average fertility at ages 40–49, % children of parity 2+, % of scheduled castes or scheduled tribes, and % of Muslim women included as control variables in both regression models
2. Values in parentheses are the p-values

The cluster map (Fig. 8.1, top right panel) confirms this regional polarization. It shows high-high spatial clusters (hotspots) where extreme son preference is concentrated predominantly in the districts of Rajasthan, Haryana, Uttarakhand, Delhi, northern and southern upper Ganga plains regions of Uttar Pradesh, Hazaribagh plateau of Jharkhand, Vindhya, and north of Madhya Pradesh.

Low-low spatial clusters (cold spots) where son preference is at its lowest are mainly found in the districts of Kerala, Tamil Nadu, inland eastern, inland southern, and coastal and Ghat regions Karnataka, Telangana, coastal northern and coastal southern regions of Andhra Pradesh. In addition, a distinct cold spot can be identified in the Northeast (Meghalaya, Tripura, Manipur, Mizoram, Arunachal Pradesh). The value of Moran's *I* was 0.76; such an elevated value of overall spatial autocorrelation confirms that districts with similar son preference are closely distributed in space.

We conclude this examination with the regression analysis of the correlates of son preference at the district level using standard geographic, economic, and educational indicators. Results are displayed in Table 8.2. OLS (ordinary least square) model shows a significant association between son preference and women's schooling ($p < 0.05$). Son preference declined with an increase in the percentage of women having five or more years of schooling in both models. The percentage of women working was negatively associated with son preference in both models ($p < 0.05$). In contrast, the percentage of women residing in urban areas was negatively associated with son preference in both models. In the OLS and SR regression model, women's poverty was also negatively associated with son preference. Women's exposure to media was also associated with son preference in both the regression models.

Notice that the regression coefficients are lower in the SR model than in the OLS model. Introducing the spatial dimension in the regression explains why some characteristics, such as women's schooling, cease to be closely correlated with son preference. The strong spatial autocorrelation (see Moran's *I* value above) suggests that unobserved spatial-dependent variables affect son preference and confirm the SR model's fitness for studying the spatial association between son preference and independent variables.

Conclusion

Our analysis reveals widespread son preference in India, with a clear north/south divide. The northeastern states of India also behaved like the southern states regarding son preference. Clusters of entrenched son preference were predominantly located in Rajasthan, Haryana, southern Punjab, Uttarakhand, Delhi, northern and southern upper Ganga plains regions of Uttar Pradesh, Hazaribagh plateau region of Jharkhand, and Vindhya and northern regions of Madhya Pradesh. Low-low spatial clusters were seen mainly in Kerala, Tamil Nadu, inland eastern, inland southern, and coastal and Ghat regions of Karnataka, Telangana, coastal northern and coastal southern regions of Andhra Pradesh, Meghalaya, Tripura, Manipur, Mizoram, and Arunachal Pradesh. This geography closely resembles other forms of gender discrimination examined in this Atlas, such as that depicted on the maps of female landownership among women and girl-only families (see Chaps. 7 and 9).

Multivariable regressions illustrate some of the strongest associations between son preference and a set of variables. Son preference declined with an increase in the percentage of women exposed to media, currently working, poor, and living in urban areas. Women having five or more years of schooling was negatively and strongly associated with son preference in OLS regression only. However, ordinary regressions capture only a part of the country's diversity, and adding a spatial dimension in the SR significantly improves the modeling.

Our analysis offers a couple of important policy options. First, encouraging women of reproductive age to participate in the labor force is an essential policy option that India may consider for reducing son preference in general and in northern states in particular. We also found specific regions where son preference was substantial despite the high percentage of women having five or more years of schooling and currently working. Moreover, some regions in northwest India had high levels of son preference despite high media exposure and low poverty. Such findings emphasize the need to focus more on changing social norms that promote son preference in Indian society.

To conclude, we indeed find marked son preference in northern India. We also find crucial local spatial associations between son preference and select socioeconomic and residence-related variables. Moreover, our findings are robust to social desirability bias and reflect attitudes that women are less likely to articulate. Future research may examine the spatial patterns of son preference trends in India. Future research may also examine the spatial patterns in son preference using other indicators to check whether the spatial patterns based on fertility intentions are similar to those based on actual fertility behavior.

References

Arnold, F., Choe, M. K., & Roy, T. K. (1998). Son preference, the family-building process and child mortality in India. *Population Studies, 52*(3), 301–315. https://doi.org/10.1080/00324720310001150486

Arokiasamy, P. (2002). Gender preference, contraceptive use and fertility in India: Regional and development influences. *International Journal of Population Geography, 8*(1), 49–67. https://doi.org/10.1002/ijpg.236

Bhat, P. N. M., & Zavier, A. J. F. (2003). Fertility decline and gender bias in India. *Demography, 40*(4), 637–657. https://doi.org/10.2307/1515201

Bhat, P. N. M., & Zavier, A. J. F. (2007). Factors influencing the use of prenatal diagnostic techniques and the sex ratio at birth in India. *Economic and Political Weekly, 42*(24), 2292–2303.

Clark, S. (2000). Son preference and sex composition of children: Evidence from India. *Demography, 37*(1), 95–108. https://doi.org/10.2307/2648099

Dyson, T., & Moore, M. (1983). On kinship structure, female autonomy, and demographic behavior in India. *Population and Development Review, 9*(1), 35–60. https://doi.org/10.2307/1972894

Guilmoto, C. Z. (2012). Son preference, sex selection, and kinship in Vietnam. *Population and Development Review, 38*(1), 31–54. https://doi.org/10.1111/j.1728-4457.2012.00471.x

Gupta, M. D., et al. (2003). Why is son preference so persistent in East and South Asia? A cross-country study of China, India and the Republic of Korea. *The Journal of Development Studies, 40*(2), 153–187. https://doi.org/10.1080/00220380412331293807

IIPS and ICF. (2017). *National Family Health Survey (NFHS-4) 2015–16: India*. IIPS.

Jayachandran, S., & Kuziemko, I. (2011). Why do mothers breastfeed girls less than boys? Evidence and implications for child health in India*. *The Quarterly Journal of Economics, 126*(3), 1485–1538. https://doi.org/10.1093/qje/qjr029

Leone, T., Matthews, Z., & Zuanna, G. D. (2003). Impact and determinants of sex preference in Nepal. *International Family Planning Perspectives, 29*(2), 69–75. https://doi.org/10.2307/3181060

Mishra, V., Roy, T. K., & Retherford, R. D. (2004). Sex differentials in childhood feeding, healthcare, and nutritional status in India. *Population and Development Review, 30*(2), 269–295. https://doi.org/10.1111/j.1728-4457.2004.013_1.x

Pande, R. P. (2003). Selective gender differences in childhood nutrition and immunization in rural India: The role of siblings. *Demography, 40*(3), 395–418. https://doi.org/10.1353/dem.2003.0029

Pandey, R. P., & Astone, N. M. (2007). Explaining son preference in rural India: The independent role of structural versus individual factors. *Population Research and Policy Review, 26*(1), 1–29.

Registrar General of India. (2015). *Compendium of India's fertility and mortality indicators, 1971–2013*. Office of the Registrar General of India.

Singh, A., Kumar, K., Yadav, A. K., James, K. S., McDougal, L., Atmavilas, Y., & Raj, A. (2021). Factors influencing the sex ratio at birth in India: A new analysis based on births occurring between 2005 and 2016. *Studies in Family Planning, 52*(1), 41–58.

Singh, A., Upadhyay, A. K., Kumar, K., Singh, A., Johnson, F. A., & Padmadas, S. S. (2022). Spatial heterogeneity in son preference across India's 640 districts. *Demographic Research, 47*, 793–842. https://doi.org/10.4054/DemRes.2022.47.26

Yadav, A. K., Anand, A., Singh, R. A., & Jungari, S. (2020). Sex composition and son preference in India and major states: Evidence from the National Family Health Survey-4 (2015–16). *Clinical Epidemiology and Global Health, 8*(4), 1140–1146. https://doi.org/10.1016/j.cegh.2020.04.005

Chapter 9
Girl-Only Families in India

Mary E. John and Christophe Z. Guilmoto

India is well-known for its skewed sex ratio, pointing to an unexpected preponderance of males. Much has been written on this phenomenon since British officials in colonial India noted fewer women in certain provinces, such as Rajputana and Punjab, and among certain caste groups, such as the Jats, during the 1881 census. A century later, in the 1970s, demographers were shocked to discover a long-term secular decline in the proportion of women in India's population. Economists and anthropologists later highlighted practices of discrimination within households, leading to the more significant neglect of women and girls in terms of nutrition and healthcare, especially among the rural poor. A somewhat different phenomenon emerged in metropolitan India with newly introduced prenatal medical technologies to determine the sex of a fetus and the spread of sex-selective abortions (Jaising et al., 2007; John, 2014). Since the 1990s, gender discrimination, almost universal in some form or another, has had further consequences in India. The lack of value attached to women, and the obverse, the desire for a son in a largely patrilineal and patrilocal society, have led to a gender imbalance at the time of birth (masculinization of the sex ratio at birth) and in the life chances of women compared to men (female excess mortality).

The standard measure of the imbalance is the sex ratio at birth for a given age or for a particular population group. However, there is a limitation in using such a measure, regardless of how the ratio is computed. This ratio figure bears no direct relationship to the practice that has led to it, namely how families are "planning" their children's number and sex composition. When fertility patterns were still high (i.e., when families had over 4 or 5 children), biological probability told us that most

M. E. John
Formerly with the Centre for Women's Development Studies, New Delhi, India

C. Z. Guilmoto (✉)
Centre des Sciences Humaines/IRD (CEPED), New Delhi, India
e-mail: christophe.guilmoto@ird.fr

C. Z. Guilmoto (ed.), *Atlas of Gender and Health Inequalities in India*, Demographic Transformation and Socio-Economic Development 16,
https://doi.org/10.1007/978-3-031-47847-5_9

families would be mixed, with some combination of both boys and girls. Nevertheless, when fertility levels steadily decline, as in India, and more families realize their preferences for a smaller family, something new and exciting emerges due to the more significant risk of couples having only boys or only girls. Accordingly, son preference and daughter aversion manifest themselves in a new way in the era of fertility decline and the rise of the small family, where the ideal family includes only two children.

On the one hand, a growing proportion of families will, probabilistically, have one child of each gender, giving the impression of greater gender egalitarianism. On the other hand, there would also be significant families with only girls (sonless families) or only boys (families without daughters). Therefore, the suggestion is that in the era of the small family, we should not only speak about son preference or gender discrimination. We can focus more specifically on the fact that families must now—if they wish to remain small—anticipate the actual possibility of having only girls or decide to intervene almost immediately to change this undesirable situation through sex selection or additional births. Thus, this chapter proposes that the proportion of girl-only families—beyond considerations of the skewed sex ratio—can be turned into a valuable measure of the gender imbalance that better mirrors family building. The second advantage is that this is a positive measure. Rather than speak of "missing women," as done since Amartya Sen's computations (1990), why not speak of the emergence of girl-only families, whose presence could be an indicator of a positive change in gender systems (Sen, 1990)?

Without gender bias, the proportion of girl-only families would be determined only by biological hazards. For instance, if solely determined by the biological distribution, the proportion of sonless women with a single child should be 48.8% (using a standard sex ratio at birth of 105 male births per 100 female births). However, the observed proportion of girl-only families is much lower than expected in India: it represents only 35.3% of one-child families who want no more children, according to NFHS-5 data. This departure from the expected proportion represents a relative deficit of 28% of girl-only families (see below for explanations and computational procedures). Such a gap is caused by two specific dimensions of son preference: prenatal sex selection (sex-selective abortions) and gender bias in fertility behavior (fertility progression in the absence of a male birth). The prenatal sex selection of female fetuses artificially reduces the number of females born. It is common in families with only girls who want to ensure the next birth is a son. Bias in fertility behavior is a less detectable form of gender discrimination. Parents without a son are more likely to have additional children than parents who already have one (Chaudhuri, 2012). This bias notably results in a high proportion of sons among last births, as more parents stop having another child after having a boy than after having a girl. In a time of reductions in fertility when families wish to have just two or three children, this gender bias also means that families with more significant numbers of children tend to have more unwanted daughters in pursuit of the son they want.

Data and Measurements

Examining the gender composition of Indian families requires detailed demographic data, most notably the detailed birth history of women found only in large demographic surveys, such as the NFHS surveys.[1] Based on NFHS-5 data, we use the birth history of women who do not want or cannot have additional children because of infertility and sterilization. The lack of fertility data on women older than 49 prevents us from including them in our computation. The first indicator computed is the proportion of women with only daughters (or sonless women) among women with previous birth who either declare not to desire any more children or to be infertile (irrespective of age).

This indicator is not perfect. First, the size of district-wise samples of women who do not want more children varies from 216 in Jabalpur to 1600 in Barmer, and measurement is more fragile in areas with small populations. Second, we retained the total number of births rather than that of surviving children, which is often more relevant to understanding the reproductive strategies of parents. Third, the indicator reflects fertility behavior related to several decades before the survey. Finally, and more importantly, this indicator closely depends on the overall fertility level since the probability of remaining sonless decreases with increases in family size. In theory, the birth of an additional child divides the likelihood of remaining sonless by a factor of two. For this reason, the proportion of girl-only families is bound to be more prominent in low-fertility states, such as Kerala, than in high-fertility states, such as Madhya Pradesh.

To measure the extent to which a gender bias in reproductive behavior twists the proportion of girl-only families, we reclassified NFHS-5 mothers by parity. First, we computed the theoretical proportion of girl-only mothers among them based on the natural sex ratio at birth. For example, 24% of women with two children would be expected to have exactly two girls. Then, this expected proportion was compared at the district level with the observed proportion of mothers without sons after combining women by different parity levels. Our second indicator measures the gap between the expected and observed proportion of girl-only families and the relative deficit of girl-only families. For instance, the observed proportion of girl-only families in India has risen from 8.8% (NFHS-4) to 10.9% (NFHS-5).

This proportion remains significantly below the expected proportion of 18.9% based solely on parity distribution. This variation corresponds to a net deficit of 8% (=18.9−10.9%) of girl-only families. Therefore, our indicator is the relative deficit, measured as 42.3% (=8/18.9), i.e., the proportion of missing girl-only families among expected girl-only families. In other words, the combined effects of prenatal sex selection and gender bias in reproductive behavior have artificially reduced the risk of sonlessness by 42% in India. Nevertheless, wide disparities remain across India, and the apparent deficit of girl-only families can be almost non-existent in some areas or, on the contrary, become considerable.

[1]The original NFHS dataset and the spatial analysis methodology are described in detail in Chap. 1.

Results

Figure 9.1 gives the district picture of the proportion of girl-only families in India as per NFHS 5. Notice that just a handful of districts correspond to more than 20% of girl-only families. These districts are primarily located in Kerala (central and south Kerala) and adjacent districts of Tamil Nadu, one in Tamil Nadu (Perambalur), in seven Tripura and West Bengal districts, in the Andaman and Nicobar, and other isolated areas. More broadly, girl-only families appear on the map most frequently in South and East India as well as in Ladakh and east Himachal Pradesh. A much larger swath of districts is at the opposite end of the spectrum, where only a few percent of families have one or more daughters and no son. These are in the northwest—covering most of Rajasthan, Gujarat, Punjab, Haryana, Bihar, and West Madhya Pradesh (i.e., Malwa)—and some districts of Maharashtra, Uttar Pradesh, and Uttarakhand. A high level of spatial autocorrelation with Moran's *I* at 0.78 confirms the distinct spatial patterns of this map.

At this first level of analysis, girl-only families are more common within distinct clusters covering most of South India and Southwest Bengal, while we see high levels of avoidance of sonless families in northwest and northern India. However, this map closely resembles the contours of fertility differentials in India, with higher proportions of girl-only families in areas where women have, on average, the lowest number of children. It remains challenging to determine whether this gender composition is an unintended by-product of low fertility or signals greater acceptability of girl-only families in an otherwise patriarchal country (Sahoo & Nagarajan, 2020).

Differential fertility patterns across the country make it difficult to tell the difference between the involuntary and deliberate dimensions of the gender composition of offspring. This situation makes the patterns in Fig. 9.2 more significant, based on the computation of the deficit of girl-only families against the expected proportion, taking parity into account. Here, the lower the figure, the smaller the bias against being a girl-only family.

A small number of districts shown in pink, overlapping with the best girl-only districts from the previous map (Fig. 9.1), actually have slightly higher proportions of girl-only families than expected. Unsurprisingly, the most extreme proportion of girl-only families is found in the Khasi-dominated district of West Jaintia Hills in Meghalaya, where matrilineal practices are widespread. Such cases reflect some deliberate daughter preference and are also visible in several districts of Kerala. At the next level, many more districts are close to having the expected proportion of girl-only families. These districts are clustered in South India (Kerala, Tamil Nadu, South Karnataka, Andhra Pradesh, and Telangana). Other clusters of girl-only families are also discernable in the Northeast (chiefly in Meghalaya, but also in Assam, Mizoram, and Nagaland) and in West Bengal.

In contrast, the apparent deficit often exceeds 60% of expected girl-only families in the rest of India, with many specific districts where the deficit goes beyond 80%. These districts completely dominate the northwestern states and form a compact cluster that stretches from Gujarat in the west to Punjab in the north and

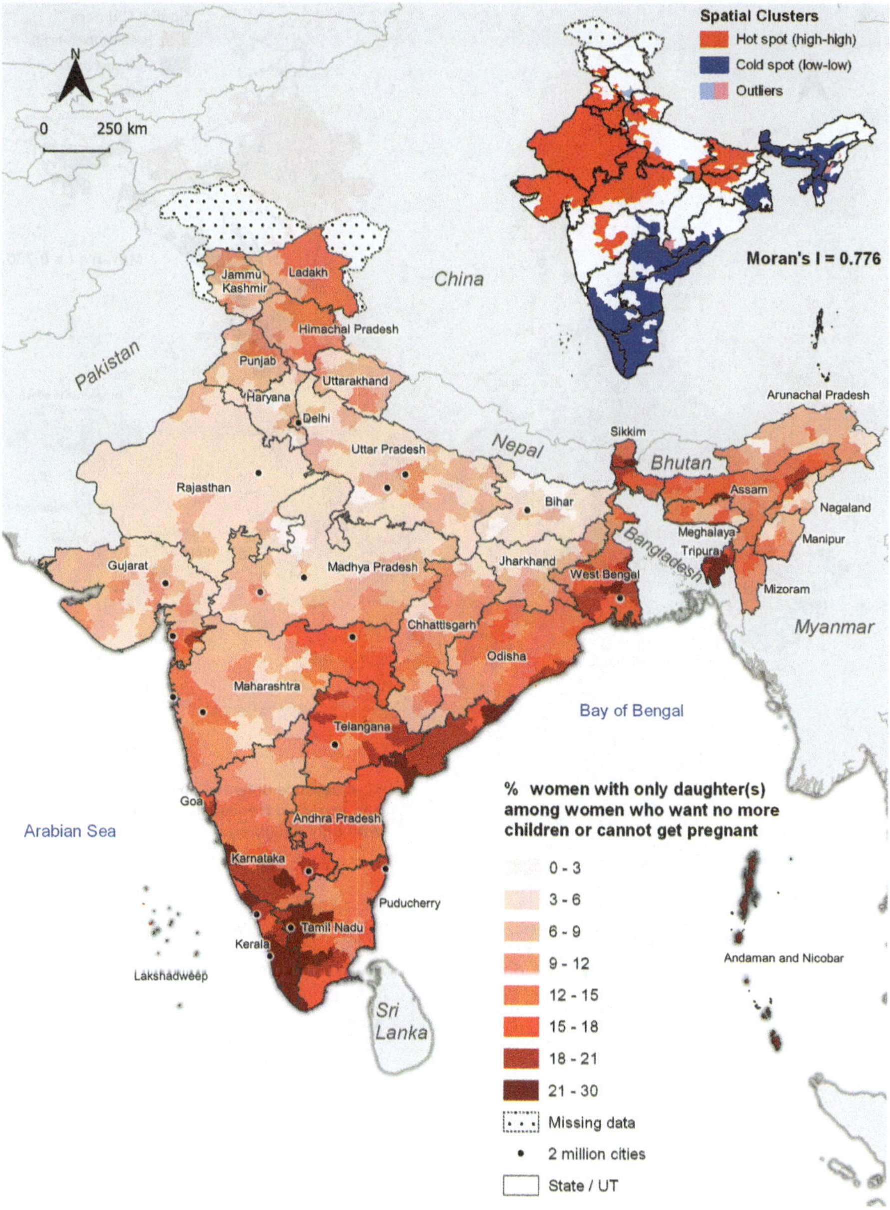

Fig. 9.1 Percentage of women of completed fertility with only daughters
Source: NFHS-5, 2019–21
The map is for illustrative purposes and may not represent official boundaries

Bundelkhand in the east. Bihar represents another hotspot of missing girl-only families, even if, in contrast with previously mentioned states to the west, Bihar is characterized by high fertility. Therefore, this more differentiated picture highlights

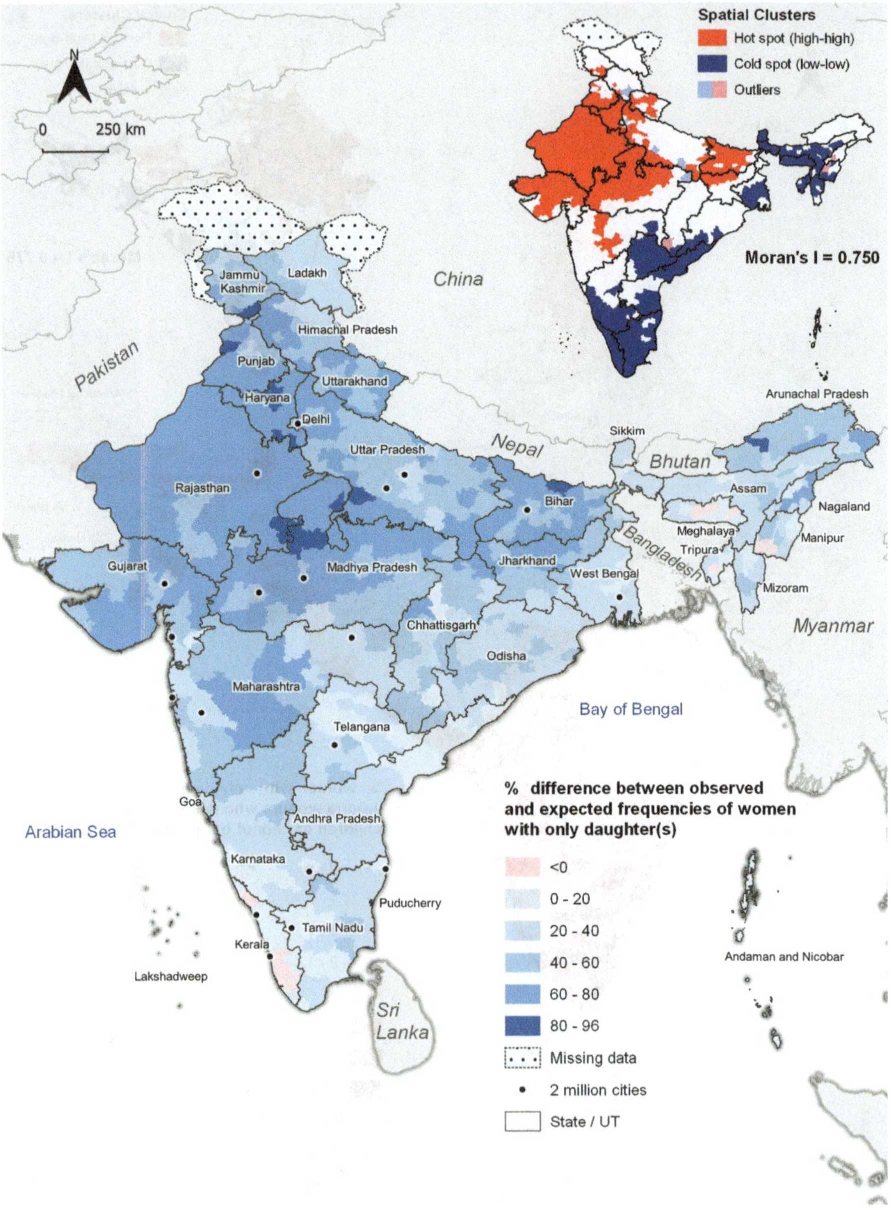

Fig. 9.2 Apparent relative deficit of girl-only families
Source: NFHS-5, 2019–21
The map is for illustrative purposes and may not represent official boundaries

the specificity of the girl-only family by netting out the effects of higher fertility levels. In Uttar Pradesh, where women have, on average, some of India's highest numbers of children, the threat of sonlessness is averted mainly by the sheer impact of high fertility. Nevertheless, our estimate of the net deficit of girl-only families, which factors in the effects of local fertility levels, suggests that the need for a son in this part of India remains strong but not as acute as in Northwest India or parts of Madhya Pradesh.

Figure 9.2 provides a much clearer picture of the regional avoidance of the girl-only family. The North-South divide typical of fertility levels has given way to the northwest-southeast gradient of son preference investigated in Chap. 8 of this Atlas. When mapped even more closely, the deficit of girl-only families resembles the percentage of vegetarian women displayed in Chap. 3. Again, the relatively high level of spatial autocorrelation (Moran's $I = 0.75$) points to the quality of the measurement based on women declaring not to want any more children or cannot get pregnant be willing or able to have more children.

It should be kept in mind that these specific figures correspond to the fertility behavior of older women at the end of their fertility cycle. Therefore, they reflect fertility decisions dating from the mid-1980s before the spread of gender-biased sex selection. However, more recent decades have seen a broader diffusion of the small family norm along with the geographical reach in sex selection. In other words, sex-selective practices among younger women may have changed the composition of their offspring to ensure the birth of a son over the last thirty years, with probably a sharper picture among younger women.

Discussion and Conclusion

How should we interpret the significance of girl-only families in India in the context of son preference and daughter aversion? The literature on the skewed sex ratio and "missing women" has emphasized that the dominant culture in India sees sons as a necessity (for carrying on the family line, for religious purposes, and for old age). Concurrently, daughters are a burden (since the family must find her a good marriage that will take her away to another family, attended by increasingly higher costs in the form of dowry). This bias translated into different types of discrimination in larger, mainly mixed families. However, in more recent years and with significant reductions in fertility, more and more families are explicitly planning to have only a few children.

A state like Kerala was among the first to undergo the demographic transition decades ago. It is also a state with its own version of gender discrimination: high levels of education go hand-in-hand with low work participation rates for women, marriages are characterized by large dowries, and reported levels of domestic violence and suicides are high. Even so, this is a state where half the districts have good proportions of girl-only families, as per our sample of women. Kerala represents a complex case that needs more careful analysis, where families are prepared to have only girls, and reported cases of sex selection are negligible—even while other patterns of gender discrimination are considerable. On the other hand, there are many districts in the northwest where families appear to be quite firmly set against being sonless, even when they want to keep their families small. These districts have some of the worst sex ratios; they seem to confirm the hypothesis that fertility decline would exacerbate sex selection under conditions where son preference and daughter aversion persist (Guilmoto, 2009; Gupta & Bhat, 1997).

The interesting question is whether the presence of girl-only families can make for positive change. Keera Allendorf has made some suggestions regarding the special place that girl-only families could occupy in transforming gender systems. She goes beyond existing discussions regarding the role of the demographic transition in facilitating more gender-equitable practices. We may indeed consider that parents are likely to treat sons and daughters more equally when the family is small and that mothers themselves would also be relieved of frequent childbearing and childcare to be able to take on other roles outside the home. Nevertheless, Allendorf argues that this gendered demographic dividend is taken to a different level when a family is sonless. In such families, daughters can become more like sons, including caring for their parents in old age. (Allendorf, 2015, 2020). Her analysis uses IHDS data and is based on state-level analysis. She sees mothers adjusting their expectations when faced with the reality of having only daughters and looks to a future where the growing presence of such families would be more fully gender transformative.

A micro-level study undertaken in 2018 in urban locations in two states—Haryana and Maharashtra—has examined the phenomenon of the acceptability of girl-only families more closely (John, 2018). The analysis undertaken in Rohtak and Jhajjar in Haryana confirms the active avoidance of sonless families illustrated by our maps. Among the minimal numbers of girl-only families, some were considering still trying for a son, and others were more or less resigned to the fate "that God willed." The picture was more mixed with Beed and Pune in Maharashtra, where the proportion of girl-only families was more prominent than elsewhere. Still, within these, some mothers did not believe that a son was necessary for the family's future.

It is too soon to conclude on the gender transformative potential of the growing presence of girl-only families. The slide in the sex ratio imbalance has yet to change direction. However, we strongly suggest that, beyond discussing son preference or skewed sex ratios, the emergence of girl-only families should be critical in considering family-building strategies in twenty-first-century India's economic and social context.

References

Allendorf, K. (2015). Fertility decline, gender composition of families, and expectations of old age support. *Population Research and Policy Review, 34*(4), 511–539. https://doi.org/10.1007/s11113-014-9354-5

Allendorf, K. (2020). Another gendered demographic dividend: Adjusting to a future without sons. *Population and Development Review, 46*(3), 471–499. https://doi.org/10.1111/padr.12337

Chaudhuri, S. (2012). The desire for sons and excess fertility: A household-level analysis of parity progression in India. *International Perspectives on Sexual and Reproductive Health, 38*(4), 178–186.

Guilmoto, C. Z. (2009). The sex ratio transition in Asia. *Population and Development Review, 35*(3), 519–549. https://doi.org/10.1111/j.1728-4457.2009.00295.x

Gupta, M. D., & Bhat, P. N. M. (1997). Fertility decline and increased manifestation of sex bias in India. *Population Studies, 51*(3), 307–315. https://doi.org/10.1080/0032472031000150076

Jaising, I., Sathyamala, C., & Basu, A. (2007). *From the abnormal to the normal: Preventing sex-selective abortions through the law*. Lawyers Collective (Women's Rights Initiative).

John, M. E. (2014). *Sex Ratios and Gender Biased Sex Selection: History, Debates, and Future Directions*. UNFPA/UN Women.

John, M. E. (2018). *The Political Economy of Sex Selection: Exploring Family Development Linkages*. UNFPA.

Sahoo, H., & Nagarajan, R. (2020). "Daughter-only" families in selected high and low son preference states in India: A comparative analysis. *Indian Journal of Human Development, 14*(2), 234–256.

Sen, A. (1990). More than one hundred million women are missing. *New York Review of Books, 37*(20), 61–66.

Chapter 10
Migration of Husbands of Indian Women

Kirti Gaur and Kunal Keshri

Migration is one of the crucial components of demographic change, along with fertility and mortality. It uniquely transforms the national population's size, distribution, and composition (Charles-Edwards et al., 2019). In the post-globalization era, the volume of international and internal migrants has increased, to a large extent, because of the enhancement of transport and communication facilities. Interestingly, the volume of internal migrants remains four times that of international migrants (UNDP, 2009). Still, this realm of internal migration has received less attention from policymakers until recently (Srivastava, 2020). Of late, migration has taken center stage and has grasped the attention of policymakers, notably to the plight of migrants highlighted during the COVID-19 outbreak.

There have been arguments that the Indian population is less mobile than in other countries (Davis, 1951). Recent studies also support this contention as the Aggregate Crude Migration Intensity (ACMI) of India is the lowest (5.2%) among Asian countries (Charles-Edwards et al., 2019), of which South Korea is the highest (52.8%). The authors found a slight ascent to 6.6% in ACMI using Census 2011 data (Bhagat & Keshri, 2020). There has been an increase of 10% in migration rate (as per the place of last residence information) in the previous three censuses, as shown in Table 10.1. However, it is to be noted that the census data are deficient in capturing temporary labor migration, which consists of a more significant proportion of labor migrants in India. For instance, a study based on National Sample Survey data found that annual temporary labor migration is seven times larger than

K. Gaur
Salaam Bombay Foundation, Mumbai, India

K. Keshri (✉)
International Institute for Population Sciences, Mumbai, India
e-mail: kunal.keshri@iipsindia.ac.in

C. Z. Guilmoto (ed.), *Atlas of Gender and Health Inequalities in India*, Demographic Transformation and Socio-Economic Development 16,
https://doi.org/10.1007/978-3-031-47847-5_10

Table 10.1 Trends of internal migration in India, census 1991–2011

	Population	Internal migrants		Intercensal migrants	
Year	millions	millions	%	millions	%
1991	838.5	225.8	26.9	8.1	9.7
2001	1018.5 (1028.6)	307.6 (309.4)	30.2 (30.1)	9.7 (9.7)	9.5 (9.5)
2011	1198.3 (1210.8)	447.1 (449.9)	37.3 (37.2)	13.9 (14.1)	11.7 (11.6)

Source: Authors' calculation using D-Series Census tables for 1991, 2001, and 2011
Note: Figures in the parentheses show numbers and percentages, including Jammu and Kashmir for 2001 and 2011. There was no census in 1991 in Jammu and Kashmir

permanent labor migration (Keshri & Bhagat, 2013). Arguments about lower mobility rates in India may be accordingly deceptive (Bhagat & Keshri, 2020).

While the level and volume of migration may be difficult to estimate, mobility profoundly affects all the spheres of life, including health, aging, and gender roles. Migration in India is often characterized by a typical pattern of men migrating alone and leaving their wives and children behind. This male-centered phenomenon is most prevalent in long-distance migration (Desai & Banerji, 2008).

Despite its significance, this feature of Indian migration remains sparingly studied. Two recent case studies from North India have found that the migration of men improves the autonomy of left-behind women (Choithani, 2020; Singh, 2018). These micro-level studies do not qualify to be generalized to the country. A previous study also tried to compare the autonomy of wives of migrant and non-migrant husbands in rural India, employing National Family Health Survey data (2005–2006). It concluded that women not living with their husbands have more autonomy than their counterparts (Ganguly & Negi, 2010). However, to our knowledge, there have been no studies on the spatial dimensions of migrant husbands in India. This chapter tries to fill the gap in the literature by studying the migration status of husbands of women aged 15–49 years (hereafter referred to as "migrant husbands") utilizing the data from the National Family Health Survey (2019–21). Unlike other data sources, this survey provides a unique opportunity to explore the migration rate at the district level. In addition, the spatial analysis of the migrant husbands has also been conducted to underline the geographical clustering of out-migrating districts across the country.

Data and Measurement

Though migration is not the focus of the National Family Health Survey (NFHS), some of the earlier studies have used the earlier rounds of NFHS data to establish an association between migration and different domains of maternal and child health (Keshri & Bhagat, 2013; Singh et al., 2012; Prusty & Keshri, 2015). Furthermore, NFHS-5 includes information about the change in the usual place of residence (UPR) of migrant husbands.[1] However, we do not know the type of mobility

[1] The original NFHS dataset and the spatial analysis methodology are described in detail in Chap. 1.

involved, i.e., whether it is a local migration within the district or an inter-district or interstate migration. Despite this shortcoming, the NFHS-5 remains the only source to provide district-level estimates of husbands' migration.

All the currently married women aged 15–49 have been asked the same question: "Is your husband living with you, or is he staying elsewhere?" The response has been categorized into (a) living with her and (b) living elsewhere. Women whose husbands were living elsewhere were asked an additional question: "For how long (years/month) have you and your husband not been living together (IIPS and ICF, 2022)?" There might be chances that absent husbands may reside elsewhere with another woman and, hence, are not staying with their wives. We restricted the analysis to currently married women whose husbands have no other spouses to exclude them. These three questions have been used to determine the migration status of women's husbands aged 15–49. The migration status of the husband is categorized into two categories: "non-migrant husband" refers to women whose husbands are living with their wives or are absent for less than a month, while "migrant husband" refers to women whose husbands are away for more than a month.[2]

Findings and Discussion

Table 10.2 shows that the proportion of migrant husbands in India was 8.5%, according to the NFHS-5. The figure is twice as high in rural (10.2%) as in urban (4.8%) areas. The table also emphasizes different characteristics associated with migration. As age increases, the percentage of women whose husband is migrant decreases. Migration of husbands is also more frequent among Muslims and OBC castes than in the rest of the population. We find an inverse relationship between the frequency of husbands' migration and the wealth index of the household. Migration probability declines from 12.9% among the first poorest decile to 5.1% among the tenth richest decile, suggesting that poverty may be a significant driver of migration. In contrast, the migration-education relationship follows a U-shape. In addition, non-nuclear (extended) families have a higher percentage of migrant husbands than nuclear families (Table 10.2).

The map (Fig. 10.1) is based on district-level averages and illustrates the regional variation in husbands' migration in greater detail. It highlights the highly skewed regional distribution of migration over the country. Around 162 districts exhibit a percentage of migrants greater than 10% than the national average of 7.5%. In the rest of India, migration among married men appears far more infrequent, with over 150 districts reporting migration rates below 2%.

Starting our regional examination from the north, we find some pockets in the middle and lower Himalayas, comprising districts from two hill states of

[2]Husbands with more than one wife are excluded from the analysis.

Table 10.2 Percentage of migrant husbands among women aged 15–49 years by different background characteristics

Background characteristics	Migrant husband	Background characteristics	Migrant husband
Age group		**Place of residence**	
15–19	15.7	Urban	4.8
20–24	12.9	Rural	10.2
25–29	10.0	**Education**	
30–34	8.4	No education	9.3
35–39	7.1	Incomplete primary	7.8
40–44	6.0	Complete primary	7.9
45–49	4.9	Incomplete secondary	7.7
Caste		Complete secondary	9.5
Scheduled caste	8.6	**Wealth deciles**	12.9
Scheduled tribe	5.3	1st	12.3
OBCs	9.9	2nd	10.9
None of them	7.5	3rd	9.7
Religion		4th	8.2
Hindu	8.3	5th	7.2
Muslim	10.9	6th	6.8
Others	5.89	7th	6.3
Household structure		8th	5.7
Nuclear	6.8	9th	5.1
Non-nuclear	10.1	10th	8.5
Household headship			
Male	4.5		
Female	36.9	**Total**	**8.5**

Source: Computed from NFHS-5 data

Uttarakhand and Himachal Pradesh, where husband migration is a relatively frequent phenomenon. For instance, the eastern parts of Uttarakhand (Kumaon), which has been well-known for its male outmigration for decades (Tumbe, 2018), is characterized by a remarkably high prevalence (more than 30%) of husbands' migration in Almora and Rudraprayag. In western parts of Himachal Pradesh, the leading out-migrating districts are Hamirpur and Kangra.

Moving towards the east, we find an extremely high prevalence of migrant husbands in the Terai region near the Nepal border and the middle and lower Ganga Plain. This region corresponds to northeast Uttar Pradesh and most of Bihar, including bordering districts of Jharkhand. These regions have a distinctly higher prevalence of migrants than the rest of the country.

The recurrent floods may explain the migration drive, making these regions some of India's poorest regions in terms of economic development. Less developed districts of eastern Uttar Pradesh (Keshri, 2019), such as Azamgarh, Basti, and Deoria, report a higher outmigration (more than 30%) of husbands. Likewise,

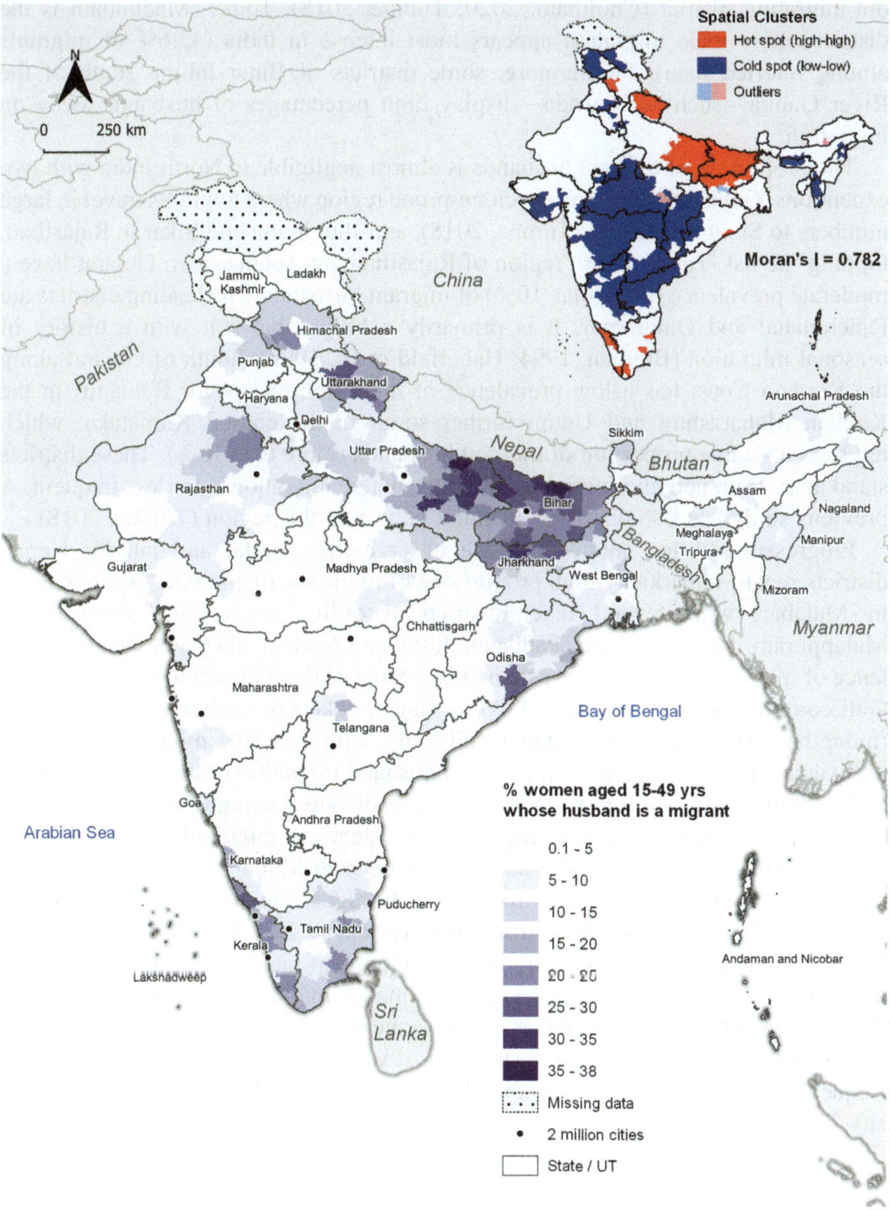

Fig. 10.1 Percentage of women aged 15–49 years whose husband is a migrant
Source: NFHS-5, 2019–21
The map is for illustrative purposes and may not represent official boundaries

districts in the Terai and those on the northern bank of the Ganges River—Madhubani, Sheohar, Madhepura, Siwan, and Saran—also have a remarkably high percentage of migrant husbands. For decades, Saran has been dubbed a male out-migrating district (Choithani, 2020; Tumbe, 2018). Today, Madhubani is the district where male migration appears most intense in India (43.6% of migrants among married men). Furthermore, some districts of Bihar falling south of the River Ganga—such as Nawada—display high percentages of husbands away on migration.

The proportion of migrant husbands is almost negligible in North India with two exceptions: Ganjam in Odisha, a cyclone-prone region where migrants travel in large numbers to Surat or Kolkata (Tumbe, 2018), and Jhunjhunu and Sikar in Rajasthan, topping the list. The southern region of Rajasthan and southeastern Gujarat have a moderate prevalence (more than 10%) of migrant husbands. The leading districts are Panchmahal and Dungarpur. It is primarily a hilly tribal belt with a history of seasonal migration (Breman, 1994; Haberfeld et al., 1999). South of Gujarat along the Konkan Coast has a low prevalence of migration except for Ratnagiri in the Konkan Maharashtra and Udupi further south in the coastal Karnataka, which registers a sizable proportion of migrant husbands (more than 10%). These districts stand apart from neighboring inland districts, where migration is far less frequent. A previous study has also observed a similar pattern in this region (Tumbe, 2018).

Progressing further southwards, we observe that coastal and interior Kerala districts record remarkably high proportions of migrants, topping at 27% in Kannur in Malabar, with several other districts recording proportions above 20%: Malappuram, Mahe, Thrissur, Pathanamthitta, and Kollam. have a moderate prevalence of migrant husbands (more than 10%). Most of these absent husbands work in Gulf countries. In the Coromandel Coast, some pockets of medium-level migration (more than 10%) were observed in Tamil Nadu, with over 20% migrating husbands in Sivaganga and Perambalur. In contrast, husband migration is almost non-existent in Andhra Pradesh and limited in Telangana to the areas around Nizamabad.

The spatial analysis of the district-wise prevalence of migrant husbands in India shows a remarkably high spatial autocorrelation with Moran's I value at 0.78. We find an apparent clustering of districts with higher migration of husbands in Uttarakhand and Bihar and the surrounding districts in Uttar Pradesh and Jharkhand. These regions are characterized by poor development indicators, which may cause the distress-driven migration of husbands. Smaller migration pockets are found in the south, most notably in Malabar and Travancore regions.

While low income acts as a push factor, it would be misleading to attribute the frequency of male migration in these clusters to the sole effect of economic adversity. The spatial analysis highlights many other less-developed districts in North and Central India where poverty could also lead to labor migration but where male migration, as measured by the absence of husbands, appears modest or almost nonexistent. In contrast, outmigration appears to be clustered in specific, well-circumscribed migration pockets, as attested by the high spatial autocorrelation measured and exemplified by the large clusters found in Bihar, Uttarakhand, or more isolated pockets such as Ratnagiri in coastal Maharashtra. The history of intense mobility in the past has created a local culture of migration in these areas, with solid networks that allow prospective migrants to find specific jobs in selective destination areas.[3] Young men are encouraged early on to become migrants, while women are not hesitant to marry men who may spend months or years away from home later in life.

Conclusion

The present chapter explored the spatial variation of migrant husbands of women aged 15–49 and offered significant findings. As measured by NFHS-5 wealth deciles, household socioeconomic status negatively affects the husband's migration. However, this relationship is not linear with the social status of women. Women living in non-nuclear households are more likely to have migrant husbands. It is considered unusual for women to live alone, and husbands' migration may be feasible only if they live with other family members (De Haan, 2006). Compared to rural women, the husbands of women living in urban areas tend to be less mobile, probably due to better local job opportunities.

The spatial analysis of district averages leads to a unique clustered map with no strong correlation with other demographic or health indicators examined in this Atlas. Most northern and eastern states have a higher prevalence of out-migrating husbands, but intrastate variations are significant. The middle and lower Ganga Plain, the Terai regions of Himalaya, followed by the southern Konkan coastal region, record many migrant husbands. The highly significant spatial autocorrelation confirms the strong regional clustering of male outmigration. To conclude, most out-migrating regions are mostly economically backward, leading to the departure of married men towards the urban growth centers of the economically developed regions. Nevertheless, many other poor regions, notably in central India, do not benefit from such well-established migration networks.

References

Bhagat, R. B., & Keshri, K. (2020). Internal migration in India. In M. Bell, A. Bernard, E. Charles-Edwards, & Y. Zhu (Eds.), *Internal migration in the countries of Asia: A cross-national comparison* (pp. 207–228). Springer. https://doi.org/10.1007/978-3-030-44010-7_11

Breman, J. (1994). *Wage hunters and gatherers: Search for work in the urban and rural economy of South Gujarat*. Oxford University Press.

[3]Tumbe (2018) notably described the contemporary labor connection between Ganjam in Odisha and Surat in Gujarat, where many migrants from Ganjam work in the powerloom sector.

Charles-Edwards, E., Bell, M., Bernard, A., & Zhu, Y. (2019). Internal migration in the countries of Asia: Levels, ages and spatial impacts. *Asian Population Studies, 15*(2), 150–171. https://doi.org/10.1080/17441730.2019.1619256

Choithani, C. (2020). Gendered livelihoods: Migrating men, left-behind women and household food security in India. *Gender, Place and Culture, 27*(10), 1373–1394. https://doi.org/10.1080/0966369X.2019.1681366

Davis, K. (1951). *The population of India and Pakistan*. Princeton University Press.

De Haan, A. (2006). Migration, gender, poverty: Family as the missing link. In *Poverty, gender and migration* (pp. 107–128). Sage India.

Desai, S., & Banerji, M. (2008). Negotiated identities: Male migration and left-behind wives in India. *Journal of Population Research, 25*(3), 337–355.

Ganguly, S., & Negi, N. S. (2010). *The extent of association between husbands' outmigration and decision-making power among left behind wives in rural India* (SSRN Scholarly Paper ID 1,743,932; Issue ID 1,743,932). Social Science Research Network. https://doi.org/10.2139/ssrn.1743932

Haberfeld, Y., Menaria, R. K., Sahoo, B. B., & Vyas, R. N. (1999). Seasonal migration of rural labor in India. *Population Research and Policy Review, 18*(5), 471–487.

IIPS and ICF. (2022). *National Family Health Survey 2019–21, India*. International Institute for Population Sciences (IIPS).

Keshri, K. (2019). Temporary labour migration. In S. Irudaya Rajan & M. Sumeetha (Eds.), *Handbook of internal migration in India*. Sage India.

Keshri, K., & Bhagat, R. B. (2013). Socio-economic determinants of temporary labour migration in India: A regional analysis. *Asian Population Studies, 9*(2), 175–195.

Prusty, R. K., & Keshri, K. (2015). Differentials in child nutrition and immunization among migrants and non-migrants in urban India. *International Journal of Migration, Health and Social Care, 11*(3), 194–205.

Singh, R. (2018). Impact of male out-migration on women left behind: A study of two villages in Uttar Pradesh. *Remittances Review, 3*(1), 75–92.

Singh, P. K., Rai, R. K., & Singh, L. (2012). Examining the effect of household wealth and migration status on safe delivery care in urban India, 1992–2006. *PLoS One, 7*, e44901.

Srivastava, R. (2020). *Understanding circular migration in India: Its nature and dimensions, the crisis under lockdown and the response of the state* (Centre for Employment Studies Working Paper Series-WP, 4, 2020). Institute for Human Development.

Tumbe, C. (2018). *India moving: A history of migration*. Penguin Random House India Private Limited.

UNDP. (2009). *Human development report 2009: Overcoming barriers: Human mobility and development.* http: //hdr.undp.org/en/content/human-development-report-2009

Chapter 11
Age at Marriage of Indian Women

Aparajita Chattopadhyay and Akancha Singh

Marriage has classically been ubiquitous and remains so, particularly in South Asia. For example, according to NFHS-5, only 1.3% of Indian women remain unmarried when they reach 40. While there is slow progress in raising the age of marriage, child marriage among girls is still a concern in South Asia. Around 285 million girls are married under 18 in South Asia, constituting about 44% of the global burden of child marriage (UNICEF, 2018). Despite a decline of nearly 30% in the rate of child marriage in the last 25 years (UNICEF, 2018), the rates are still considerably high in most South Asian countries. Bangladesh has the highest rate of child marriage among South Asian countries (59% 2014), followed by Nepal (40% 2016), Afghanistan (35%, 2015), India (27%, 2015–16), and Pakistan (21%, 2012–13) (UNICEF, 2018).

Estimates suggest that India is home to the most significant number of child brides in the world (UNFPA, 2012). Child marriage is defined as when girls and boys are under 18 and 21 years of age at marriage, respectively. By this definition, over 41% of Indian women aged 20–49 were married off below the legal age, according to NFHS-5. Nearly 36% of women aged 20–24 married before attaining 18 years of age. However, NFHS data shows that the prevalence of female child marriage has declined by 20% in the last ten years. Deep-rooted patriarchal socio-cultural practices, control over women's sexuality, poor socioeconomic conditions, low literacy rates, and lack of awareness of family planning methods are the main factors for adolescent marriage and teenage pregnancies (Caldwell, 2005; Roest, 2016).

Child marriage has a significant deleterious impact on the health and well-being of both women and children. It not only leads to early childbearing, closed-spaced pregnancies, unwanted pregnancy, and pregnancy termination but is also strongly

A. Chattopadhyay (✉) · A. Singh
International Institute for Population Sciences, Mumbai, India
e-mail: aparajita@iipsindia.ac.in

C. Z. Guilmoto (ed.), *Atlas of Gender and Health Inequalities in India*, Demographic Transformation and Socio-Economic Development 16,
https://doi.org/10.1007/978-3-031-47847-5_11

associated with maternal morbidity and mortality (Kamal, 2012; Paul, 2018). Early marriage also places women at an escalated risk of intimate partner violence (Kidman, 2017; Raj et al., 2012; Yount et al., 2016), further exacerbating sexually transmitted diseases, including HIV (Campbell, 2002; Nour, 2009). Child marriage and early pregnancies are also linked to an increased risk of children's physical growth, lower educational attainment, and higher mortality (Bates et al., 2007; Chari et al., 2017). Child brides are usually trapped in a poverty circle linked to a lower level of education or limited economic opportunities. The time between marriage and parenthood is short in India. Data from the 2011 Census confirm that approximately 30% of females aged 15–19 years who are married are already mothers, and 10% have had at least two children (ORGI, 2011).

The average age at marriage in India is increasing at a snail's pace. The major hurdles are the traditional practices and social norms, poor socioeconomic status of the parents, and poor enforcement of laws that induce parents to arrange a daughter's marriage at an early age. India also displays a substantial regional diversity in age at marriage. This geographical diversity in marriage timing corresponds to well-recognized regional features affecting different dimensions of family and gender (Dyson & Moore, 1983), thus providing an outstanding opportunity to examine how the gendered background might be linked to age at marriage. It is commonly acknowledged that patriarchy is less stringent in southern societies than in northern societies. Women in South India, in general, enjoy more significant levels of autonomy and freedom than their northern counterparts in many aspects of their lives (Dyson & Moore, 1983). There has been sufficient evidence to believe that, even within states, the prevalence of child marriage may differ. Even in a state with an overall high rate of child marriage, it is probable that certain districts would have a lower prevalence of child marriage because of specific cultural, social, or administrative characteristics that make these districts stand out from the rest of the state.

After the Child Marriage Restraint Act in 1929 (also popularly known as the Sarda Act), the government took nearly five decades to increase women's age at marriage from 16 to 18 years in 1978. The central government established a task force following the Budget speech of the finance minister in 2020. With emerging opportunities in education and employment, India needs to encourage its women to pursue higher studies and engage in productive activities, thus automatically lowering the health risks of early marriage. This chapter analyzes the National Family Health Survey (NFHS-5) data on age at marriage and discusses its policy implications.[1]

[1] The original NFHS dataset and the spatial analysis methodology are described in detail in Chap. 1.

Methods and Materials

We initially calculated the mean and median age at marriage but limited our analysis to the median age because of a negligible difference between the two indicators. We also calculated the median age at marriage by the wealth quintile of the households. The tables and figures presented in the chapter are based on the NFHS-5 data.

The district-level maps are plotted for all women of childbearing age (18–29 years). Moran's *I*, a measure of the degree of spatial autocorrelation, has been calculated and is used to identify local clusters of high and low proportions of child marriage.

We conducted logistic regressions to establish the relationship between selected covariates and child marriage. A dichotomous variable for child marriage is used as a dependent variable. We used socioeconomic indicators such as education (no education, primary, secondary, and higher), wealth quintile (poorest, poorer, middle, richer, and richest), religion (Hindu, Muslim, and others), and caste (scheduled castes, scheduled tribes, other backward classes, and others), mass media exposure (newspaper, radio, and television) and husband's education as the predictors in the regression model.

Findings

A fall in early marriage over time is evident from the different cohorts of NFHS-5 conducted in 2019–21. NFHS-5 reveals that marriage before the legal age of 18 is 26.6% for women aged 20–29, compared with 45% for women aged 45–49. Also, nearly 15.4% of women under 25 years of age in 2019–21 got married before the legal age. There has been an increase over the years in the age at marriage among women aged 20–49, but this increase has been quite small. It rose from 16.7 years in 1998–99 to 17.2 in 2005–06, 18.6 years in 2015–16, and then to 18.8 in 2019–21.

Interestingly, there is clear evidence of age heaping in the reporting of age at marriage in India. This phenomenon corresponds to a tendency to report the age near the legal age at marriage to avoid the supposed flouting of government norms related to age at marriage. The average ages reported here may entail a slight underestimation of the proportion of female marriages below age 18.

To understand the prevalence of child marriage within India, we prepared a map showing the proportion of females marrying below the legal age of 18 across Indian districts (Fig. 11.1). This map summarizes the extreme variations in female marriage schedules across the country, ranging from a negligible proportion of child marriage in Lakshadweep (4%) to almost half in West Bengal (42%). At the district level, the disparities are even wider between Kohima, the capital of Nagaland (1% of females married before 18), and Purba Medinipur (40.5%), a West Bengal rural district lying 20 km south of Kolkata.

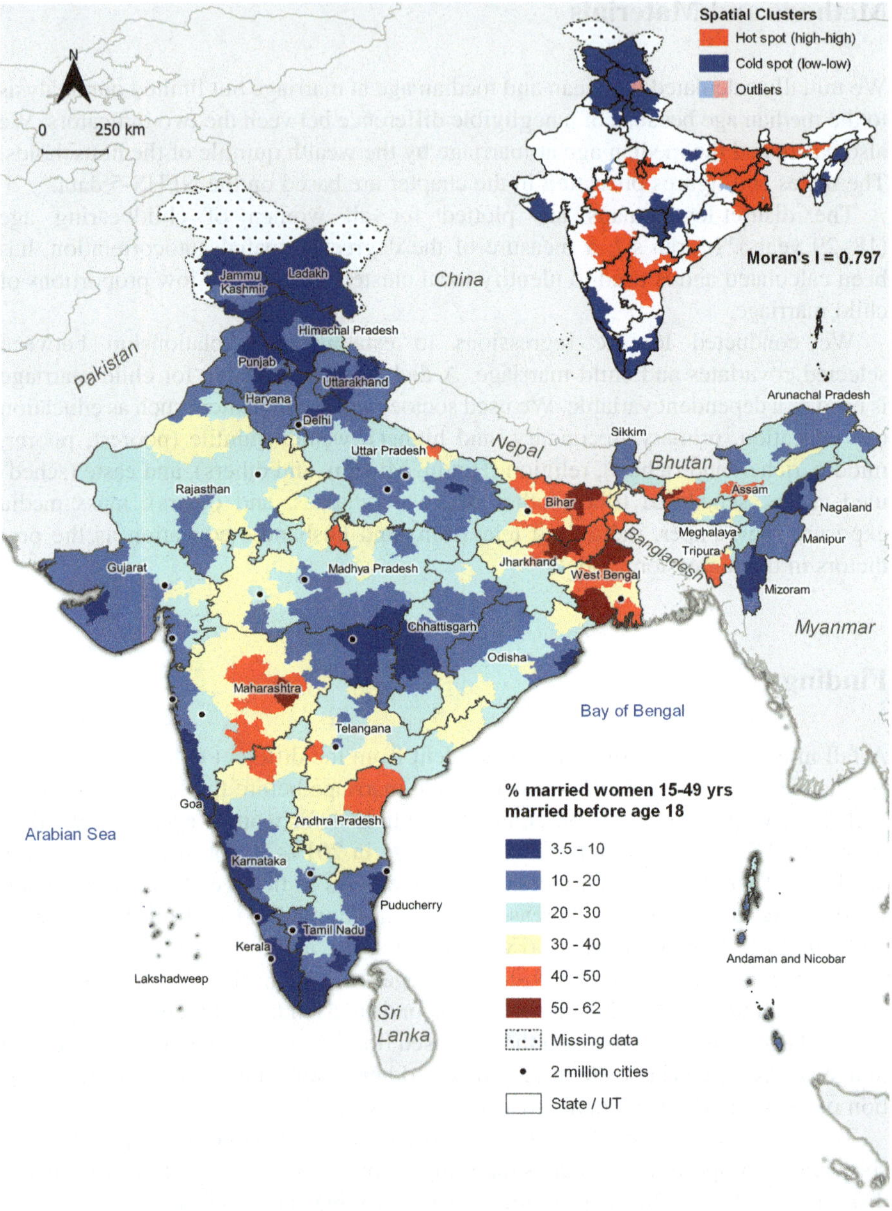

Fig. 11.1 Percentage of women aged 15–49 years married before the age of 18
Source: NFHS-5, 2019–21
The map is for illustrative purposes and may not represent official boundaries

Female child marriage is widespread in East India. In several dozen districts of Bihar, Jharkhand, and West Bengal, over 40% of women have married before 18. Child marriage can also be identified along a strip of land extending from Rajasthan to Madhya Pradesh, Maharashtra (50% in Parbhani), and finally, Andhra Pradesh, where child marriage reaches record levels (above 40% in the Krishna Delta).

In contrast, child marriage has become extremely rare (less than 10%) along the Konkan coast, from Goa to Kerala, and the Coromandel coast. Another distinct cluster of low frequency of child marriage emerges in North India, encompassing Jammu and Kashmir, Ladakh, Himachal Pradesh, and Punjab, along with bordering areas in Haryana, Delhi, western Uttar Pradesh, and Uttarakhand. Finally, a third and smaller cluster covers three adjacent states of the Northeast, viz. Mizoram, Manipur, and Nagaland. Interestingly, we can distinguish smaller areas where child marriage appears relatively uncommon (concerning less than 20% of women), including one centered on Nagpur in Vidharba and neighboring Chhattisgarh.

The geostatistical analysis of the distribution of child marriage across the country yields a high spatial autocorrelation (Moran's $I = 0.80$). The cluster map confirms high spatial autocorrelation among the districts. The hotspot of child marriage emerges in north-central India in opposition to the late-marriage clusters found in Northwest and Southwest India. We may also note that this map resembles the fertility map (see Chap. 18 in this Atlas) since child marriage is associated with a larger family size. However, early marriage also presents alarming similarities with the distribution of underweight women in India (Chap. 2 in this Atlas).

Understanding the differences in ascribed and attained character on age at marriage is essential. Marriage is often said to be deeply affected by customs and traditions. Nevertheless, socioeconomic determinants are also prominent. Figure 11.2 shows, for instance, the female age at marriage computed over the wealth quintiles. The data point to a clear positive curvilinear relationship ($r^2 = 0.99$), with the median age at marriage rising from 17 years among the poorest quintile to almost 20 among the richest. Age at marriage fails to change from the first

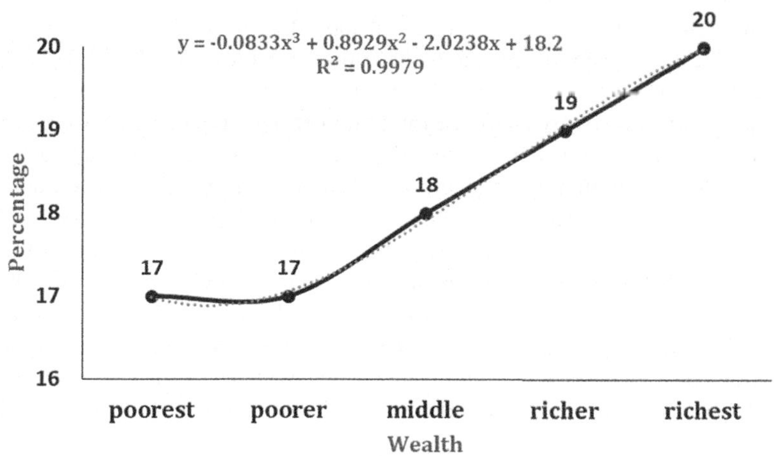

Fig. 11.2 Age at marriage by wealth level

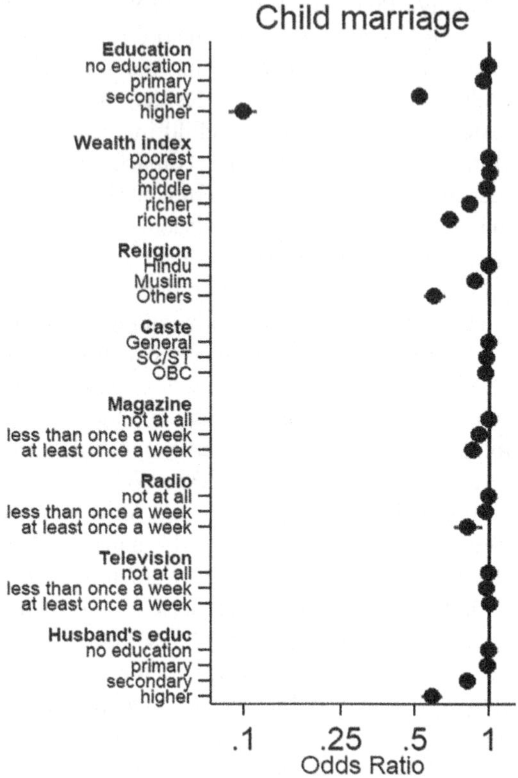

Fig. 11.3 Odds ratios of female child marriage by selected background characteristics
Source: NFHS 5

to the second wealth quintile but records a regular increase for the wealthier quintiles.

A comprehensive regression analysis of the odds of child marriage provides a better idea of the respective influence of various variables (Fig. 11.3). This logistic analysis demonstrates, in particular, that women's years of schooling correspond to the variable most positively associated with higher age at marriage.[2] Moreover, the coefficients have a clear negative gradient as women's educational attainment increases. Women with higher levels of education marry much later than those with relatively lower years of schooling, and the odds ratio associated with the highest educational attainment shrinks to 0.1. As for the wealth indicator examined earlier, the results remained the same even after controlling the role of other background variables, but the regression analysis shows that higher education has a more substantial impact on child marriage than wealth. We also found a significant association between caste and religious minorities, with age at marriage at its highest among Christians and Sikhs. In addition, child marriage occurs less often among

[2]Odds ratios measure the strength of the correlation with the outcome variable. Values above (below) one correspond to a positive (negative) association.

women with a higher level of mass media (television, radio, and magazine reading) exposure.

To sum up, both education and wealth play a distinctive role in raising women's median age at marriage. In comparison, important ascribed characteristics related to marriage, such as religion and caste, play a more modest role, as the odds ratio plotted in Fig. 11.3 indicates. In comparison, low education and poverty remain foremost in explaining the frequency of child marriage.

Discussion

Nuptiality is one of the essential components of population growth. The median age at marriage is a critical summary measure for describing the timing of nuptiality. The notion of marriage varies—it can be formal or informal, governed by various laws, or simply a customary practice in various parts of India. Blake hypothesized that the age at marriage would be significantly lower in societies where parents arrange marriages than in those with a relatively free choice of partners (Blake, 1965). Daughters are frequently seen as burdens in India because of gender inequality (e.g., dowry) and the low market demand for female labor. Impoverished parents often consider that marriage will secure a daughter's future since a husband or his family will be responsible for her care. When parents face economic adversities or in humanitarian crises/unsafe societies, marriage is a way to safeguard daughters from violence.

This chapter highlights the trends and patterns of median age at marriage and its change over time, identifying districts performing poorly. Further, it underscores the role of education and wealth in enhancing age at marriage by employing the latest NFHS-5 data that details age at marriage across Indian states. Our findings reveal that girls' marriage under the legal age of 18 is still rampant across Indian states. From Rajasthan in the west to Tripura in the east and parts of Maharashtra, Karnataka, Andhra Pradesh, and Telangana, many girls marry under 18. Early marriages persist in India even after the legal age was increased to 18 in 1979. Past evidence suggests that poverty is one of the significant drivers of early marriage among females in developing countries (UNFPA, 2012; UNICEF, 2018), and our analysis confirms that girls from poorer households are more likely to be married off at younger ages than more prosperous families. Poverty forces parents to marry off their daughters early, in part because the demand for dowry is low for younger girls. Girls are also married early to avoid the cost of education and release the financial burden of girls (IRCW and Plan Asia, 2013).

Our multivariate analysis provides suggestive evidence that the wealth index is strongly associated with the median age at marriage. This result explains, to some extent, the regional variations measured across districts. The lowest proportions of child marriage characterize more affluent areas, such as Punjab or Kerala. While the literature suggests that most women expressed favorable attitudes towards higher age at marriage, poorer and less educated families continue to resort to child marriage because they cannot afford to keep young daughters at home for long with no education or employment. In India, parental control over the decision to marry may be compatible with the postponement of marriage to a higher age only when families accept and can afford to educate their daughters, which will, in turn, allow young women to make independent and better-informed decisions on their future.

Beyond education and socioeconomic status considerations, child marriage has been known to depend on economic uncertainty and fear of violence. For instance, in societies where parents directly influence the decision to marry, maintaining premarital chastity may be a social obligation. When daughters are considered a liability, fulfilling this responsibility may be a source of satisfaction to the parents. Furthermore, when parents systematically arrange marriages, parental decisions may favor low age at marriage. Religion and caste impact age at marriage, as supported by the regression analysis in the current study. The entrenched spatial patterns of child marriage illustrated by our map confirm the persisting role of local gender and family traditions that favor early female marriage. Child marriage is still common among certain religious and caste groups, so there is an urgent need to address various cultural practices and religious dogmatism that encourage parents to ignore the law. In places where child marriage persists, the practice remains often well-accepted by community leaders and parents. However, prohibitions are not always sufficient, and any further rise in the age of marriage will depend upon the people's socioeconomic conditions, young women's education, local social mobilization, and adequate legislation.

References

Bates, L. M., Maselko, J., & Schuler, S. R. (2007). Women's education and the timing of marriage and childbearing in the next generation: Evidence from rural Bangladesh. *Studies in Family Planning, 38*(2), 101–112. https://doi.org/10.1111/j.1728-4465.2007.00121.x

Blake, J. (1965). *Parental control, delayed marriage, and population policy.* International Population and Urban Research, Institute of International Studies and Department of Demography, College of Letters and Science, University of California.

Caldwell, B. K. (2005). Factors affecting female age at marriage in South Asia. *Asian Population Studies, 1*(3), 283–301. https://doi.org/10.1080/17441730500441160

Campbell, J. C. (2002). Health consequences of intimate partner violence. *The Lancet, 359*(9314), 1331–1336. https://doi.org/10.1016/S0140-6736(02)08336-8

Chari, A. V., Heath, R., Maertens, A., & Fatima, F. (2017). The causal effect of maternal age at marriage on child well-being: Evidence from India. *Journal of Development Economics, 127*, 42–55. https://doi.org/10.1016/j.jdeveco.2017.02.002

Dyson, T., & Moore, M. (1983). On kinship structure, female autonomy, and demographic behavior in India. *Population and Development Review, 9*(1), 35–60. https://doi.org/10.2307/1972894

IRCW and Plan Asia. (2013). *Asia child marriage initiative: Summary of research in Bangladesh, India and Nepal.*

Kamal, S. M. M. (2012). Decline in child marriage and changes in its effect on reproductive outcomes in Bangladesh. *Journal of Health, Population, and Nutrition, 30*(3), 317–330.

Kidman, R. (2017). Child marriage and intimate partner violence: A comparative study of 34 countries. *International Journal of Epidemiology, 46*(2), 662–675. https://academic.oup.com/ije/article/46/2/662/2417355?login=true

Nour, N. M. (2009). Child marriage: A silent health and human rights issue. *Reviews in Obstetrics and Gynecology, 2*(1), 51–56.

ORGI. (2011). *Office Register General of India. 2011. Size, growth rate and distribution of population*. Registrar General of India. http://censusindia.gov.in/2011-prov-results/prov_results_paper1_india.html

Paul, P. (2018). Maternal age at marriage and adverse pregnancy outcomes: Findings from the India Human Development Survey, 2011–2012. *Journal of Pediatric and Adolescent Gynecology, 31*(6), 620–624. https://doi.org/10.1016/j.jpag.2018.08.004

Raj, A., Saggurti, N., Lawrence, D., Balalah, D., & Silverman, J. G. (2012). Association between adolescent marriage and marital violence among young adult women in India. *International Journal of Gynecology & Obstetrics, 110*(1), 35–39.

Roest, J. (2016). Child marriage and early child-bearing in India: Risk factors and policy implications. *Young Lives Policy Paper, 10*, 12–34.

UNFPA. (2012). *Marrying too young: End child marriage*. United Nations Population Fund.

UNICEF. (2018). *Global databases*. United Nations Children Fund. https://data.unicef.org/topic/childprotection/child-marriage/

Yount, K. M., Crandall, A., Cheong, Y. F., Osypuk, T. L., Bates, L. M., Naved, R. T., & Schuler, S. R. (2016). Child marriage and intimate partner violence in rural Bangladesh: A longitudinal multilevel analysis. *Demography, 53*(6), 1821–1852. https://doi.org/10.1007/s13524-016-0520-8

Part III
Reproductive Health

Chapter 12
Menstrual Hygiene Practices Among Indian Women

M. Sivakami

Menstrual health and hygiene management (MHM) are central to girls' and women's health and well-being because of their strong interaction with sexual and reproductive health, psychosocial health, education, and gender equality (Sommer et al., 2019; Babbar & Sivakami, 2023). The inability to maintain proper menstrual hygiene leads to reproductive tract infections (Das et al., 2015; Sivakami & Rai, 2019), affecting women's quality of life and dignity (Anand et al., 2015; Van Eijk et al., 2016). Improving menstrual health and hygiene has recently acquired attention in most low- and middle-income countries as a significant public health priority requiring multiple interventions to achieve desired outcomes.

The menstrual health of girls and women is marred with issues related to accurate information and support, as well as several structural problems that stem from cultural taboos and inadequate "Water, Sanitation, and Hygiene" (WASH) infrastructure (MacRae et al., 2019). The challenges to information and awareness regarding menstruation and menstrual hygiene management are immense. Adolescent girls lack knowledge or are misinformed regarding menstruation and receive minimal support to manage it (Phillips-Howard et al., 2016; Sivakami & Rai, 2019; Sommer et al., 2015). The knowledge of appropriate materials for menstrual hygiene is limited in many sections of society, including in India. Furthermore, women rarely have the autonomy to opt for the most appropriate solution.

The structural issues about cultural taboos and infrastructure for menstrual hygiene management represent significant barriers. The stigma around menstrual hygiene related to notions of "purity" and "pollution" and the ensuing discrimination against girls and women during their periods are severe. Women are considered impure during their period of menstruation and may not enter the kitchen or places of worship, must avoid certain food items and bathing, and, in severe cases, are not

M. Sivakami (✉)
Tata Institute of Social Sciences, Mumbai, India
e-mail: sivakami@tiss.edu

C. Z. Guilmoto (ed.), *Atlas of Gender and Health Inequalities in India*, Demographic Transformation and Socio-Economic Development 16,
https://doi.org/10.1007/978-3-031-47847-5_12

allowed to touch other members of their family (Garg et al., 2001; Narayan et al., 2001). The infrastructure available at school is inadequate for proper menstrual hygiene management, resulting in reduced participation and absenteeism of girls in schools (Sivakami & Rai, 2019) and higher dropout rates among adolescent girls from schools (Sommer et al., 2016; UNICEF, 2012). In workplaces, women have limited privacy to manage WASH needs (Taylor, 2011), and the menstrual hygiene needs of women are not perceived as a priority (Sommer et al., 2016). Recent media reports highlight the deplorable situation of menstruating women in India who get their uterus removed to avoid wage loss because of the lack of facilities available at the workplace (see Chap. 16 of this Atlas).

Menstrual hygiene is a gendered issue, and differential gender roles in Indian society pose a significant challenge to menstrual hygiene management (Khanna & Das, 2016). However, the nature of patriarchy and the gender roles assigned to men and women vary across the geography of the Indian subcontinent based on their existing customs and traditions. The current inequities due to socioeconomic status, educational status, caste, tribe, age, marital status, and others intersect with gender. Gender acts through multiple pathways across multiple marginalizations amplify women's lack of autonomy over their menstrual health and hygiene practices and call for a better understanding of menstrual hygiene practices across India. The chapter explored geographical inequality in menstrual hygiene practices in India's districts, employing cross-sectional data from the National Family Health Survey-5.

Data and Measurements

Unlike other demographic and health indicators, information on menstruation was not available until recently from any nationally representative surveys in India. For the first time, District Level Household Survey-3 (DLHS-3, 2007–2008) provided information on menstrual practices among married women aged 15–49 and unmarried girls (IIPS, 2010).

The district-level unit data from the recent NFHS-5 provided information on different protection methods during menstruation for women aged 15–24 in India.[1] NFHS-5 obtained information on women's use of various methods to prevent blood stains from becoming evident, such as cloth, locally prepared napkins, sanitary napkins, tampons, menstrual cups, others, and nothing to protect during their menstrual period. Women may use any of the above or a combination of different protection methods during their menstrual cycle. From the above information, NFHS-5 categorizes women who use locally prepared napkins, sanitary napkins, tampons, and menstrual cups during their menstruation as women using "hygienic methods"; those using cloths and others as "unhygienic methods" and those who are

[1] The original NFHS dataset and the spatial analysis methodology are described in detail in Chap. 1.

Table 12.1 Percentage of women aged 15–24 who have ever menstruated by type of protection used during their menstrual period

Type of protection	DLHS-3	NFHS-4	NFHS-5
	2007–2008	2015–2016	2019–2021
Cloths	92.2	62.1	49.61
Locally prepared Napkin	3.1	16.3	14.97
Sanitary Napkin	9.5	41.8	64.37
Tampon	NA	2.4	1.67
Menstrual cup	NA	NA	0.3
Nothing	0.9	0.5	0.21
Other	0.2	0.1	0.23
Use of any hygienic method	12.6	57.6	77.61

Note: *NA* not available

not using anything as "nothing." Following the exact definition, "Use of any hygienic methods" is computed for 241,112 women who use or used them at some point during their menstruation. This information is tabulated by district and social groups to assess inequity in menstrual hygiene practices in India and its districts. Although the exclusive hygienic method would be a better indicator, as it would reveal the extent of women who use only clean methods, it was felt after the initial analysis that the samples at the district level posed challenges, which reinforced us to stick to the NFHS-5 definition.

Findings and Discussion

Table 12.1 presents information on the percentage of women aged 15–24 who menstruate by type of protection used during their menstrual cycle. The proportion of women using hygienic methods has significantly increased in the last decade, between DLHS-3 (2007–2008) and NFHS (2019–21). Apart from changing life-styles and economic progress, such sizable improvement may also be attributed to state and central government schemes to provide low-cost napkins for girls (especially schoolgirls) and women in the last decade. Despite this overall increase, according to NFHS-5, most women in the 15–24 age group still used cloth (49.6%) for protection during their menstrual period. The second most commonly used material was sanitary napkins (64.4%), followed by locally prepared napkins (15.0%). Tampons were used by 1.7% of women, menstrual cups were used by 0.3%, and 0.2% did not use any material for protection during the menstrual period.

As expected, women in rural areas are less likely to use hygienic methods than women in urban areas. Over 89.6% of the women in urban areas (72.6% in rural areas) use hygienic methods during menstruation. Figure 12.1 presents the proportion of women using hygienic methods by socioeconomic deciles computed from the

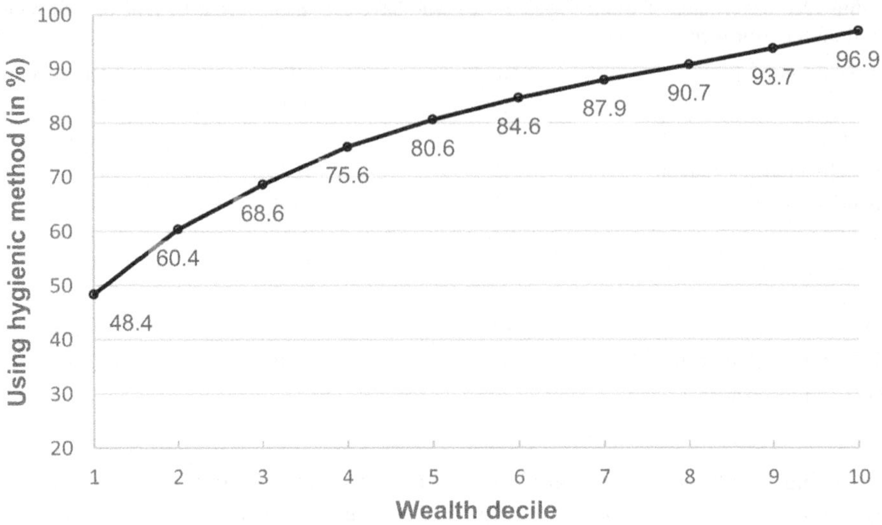

Fig. 12.1 Percentage of women aged 15–24 using hygienic methods during their menstrual period by wealth decile

NFHS-5 wealth index. This figure reveals that only 48.4% of women use any hygienic material in the lowest decile compared to the highest decile, where the proportion rises to 96.9%. The proportion of women using hygienic methods during menstruation systematically increases with socioeconomic status ($r^2 = 0.99$). The same is true with education, which is also strongly associated with menstrual hygiene. These results suggest that income and awareness about hygiene, access, and affordability of menstruation products play crucial roles in the uptake of hygienic material during menstruation (MacRae et al., 2019; Sommer et al., 2015).

The state-wise variation in hygiene materials among women aged 15–24 years during their menstrual cycle reveals considerable variation, with southern and northernmost regions showing the highest proportion of women using hygienic materials during their menstruation. However, in the entire east-central belt of India, Gujarat, Assam, Meghalaya, and Tripura from the Northeast, women report the lowest use of hygienic methods. Such a low proportion of hygienic materials in these regions primarily highlights issues, such as a lack of awareness regarding hygienic materials, no access to protective materials, higher cultural stigma, and lower levels of women's autonomy.[2]

While Puducherry (99.1%) is at the top, followed by Andaman and Nicobar (98.9%) and Tamil Nadu (98.4%), women in Bihar and Madhya Pradesh rank the

[2]An analysis based on earlier NFHS-4 data highlights some of statistical correlates of better menstrual hygiene: women's education and household socioeconomic status, as well as women's autonomy and exposure to mass media, and urban residence (see Roy et al., 2021).

lowest (with only 59.2% and 60.9%, respectively) among hygienic material use during their menstruation. Assam, Meghalaya, and Tripura do not fare well compared to other northeastern states. Among the union territories (UTs), women using hygienic material is above the national average (77.6%) in all UTs (except Jammu and Kashmir), with Puducherry and Lakshadweep over 98%. Although 26 states and all UTs (except one) show proportions above the national average, 20 states and UTs exhibit proportions below 90%, indicating that the use of sanitary methods remains a severe issue in India (Van Eijk et al., 2016). From this analysis, one can safely assume that the practice of hygienic methods during the menstrual cycle is likely to be worse for older women, as menstrual hygiene programs primarily target young adolescent girls.

The district map (Fig. 12.2) shows in greater detail the vast disparities across the districts of India, ranging from a low 32.8% in West Jaintia Hills (Meghalaya) to 100% in several districts such as Chennai or Karaikal. The proportion of women who use any hygienic materials is high among all the districts in South India (except Hyderabad Karnatak) and Goa, as well as in the Punjab-Himachal Pradesh-Uttarakhand region. Proportions are also high in several states of the Northeast (Sikkim, Mizoram, and Manipur). However, figures are, on the contrary, low in almost all districts of Central India, in a broad region encompassing Gujarat, Madhya Pradesh, Bihar, Chhattisgarh, Bihar, and adjoining districts. Low proportions are also observed in Assam, Tripura, and parts of Rajasthan. Most districts with low usage come under Empowered Action Group (EAG) states, regions with the least advanced health and development indicators. One of the most disconcerting results comes from Meghalaya. Better women's status characterizes this state, but less than half of young women use hygienic menstrual methods in some districts.

Some intriguing regional variations are also observed. For example, disparities within Maharashtra are pronounced, with coastal districts or in Vidarbha recording proportions of women using hygienic methods that are significantly higher than in Marathwada. Similarly, despite the impressive picture in Arunachal Pradesh, Mizoram, Manipur, or Nagaland, the immediate neighboring districts in Assam and Tripura have far fewer women using hygienic materials.

The geostatistical analysis of the distribution of hygienic methods across India leads to a high spatial autocorrelation with Moran's *I* at 0.72. The cluster analysis confirms that the largest concentration of high values (usually above 80%) lies in Tamil Nadu, Kerala, and parts of Karnataka, Andhra Pradesh, and Telangana. The next hotspot where more women use hygienic materials during their menstruation is centered in Punjab and covers Haryana, Himachal Pradesh, Uttarakhand, and north Rajasthan.

The broad region with the lowest estimates of the use of hygienic material ranges from north Gujarat and encompasses most of Madhya Pradesh and Bihar, as well as many districts of Uttar Pradesh, Chhattisgarh, and Odisha. These districts represent the poorest areas of the country. Interestingly, urban areas such as Kanpur,

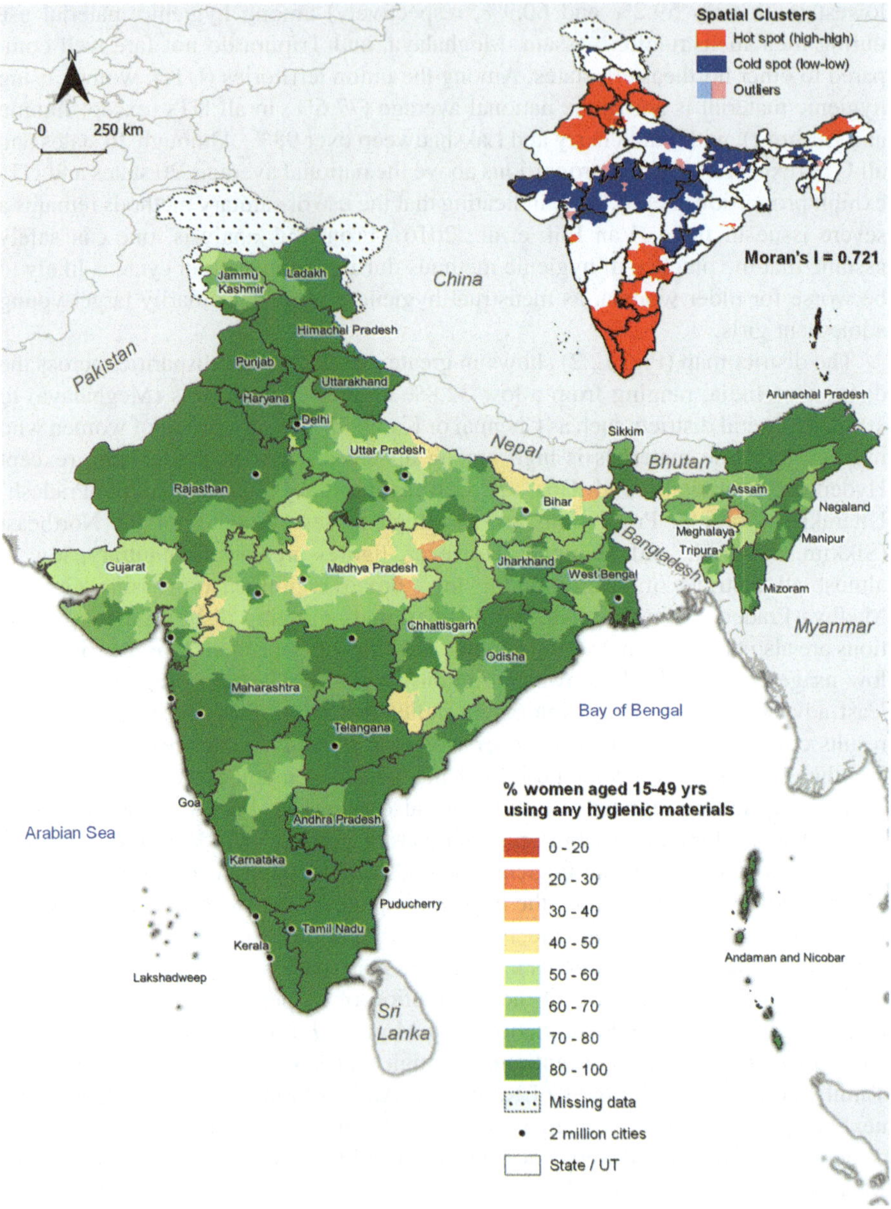

Fig. 12.2 Percentage of women aged 15–49 years using hygienic materials during their periods
Source: NFHS-5, 2019–21
The map is for illustrative purposes and may not represent official boundaries

Lucknow, Indore, or Bhopal do not belong to this regional cluster as they record proportions of use of hygienic methods distinctly higher than rural districts around them.

Conclusion

In summary, although women's use of hygienic methods during menstruation has improved in the last ten years (between DLHS-3 and NFHS-5), India still has a long way to go, as only a few states with near-universal use of hygienic methods by menstruating women. At the national level, about 22.4% of women are not using hygienic methods. While about half of the women still use clothes, only about 64.8% use sanitary napkins. Our analysis also shows substantial inequality in using hygienic methods by place of residence (90% in urban areas vs. 73% in rural areas), but the range of variations is far more comprehensive by household wealth (48% among the poorest decile vs. 97% among the richest). Thus, using sanitary methods is primarily associated with the socioeconomic status of women.

The state-level use of hygienic methods emphasizes massive inequality across Indian states, where hygienic methods during menstruation seem to be a significant issue in many forms. Among the northeastern states, the EAG states and Assam show deplorable conditions that call for immediate action from the policy and program managers. It indirectly indicates a lower level of awareness and lesser supply of hygienic methods in these states, along with the poor socioeconomic status of women. The district-level maps show the vast disparity and hotspots even within the state with better hygienic methods. This anomaly needs further investigation as context; geographic-specific cultural factors may play a significant role in education and access to menstrual hygiene materials.

Recently, the government has placed greater emphasis on providing sanitary pads for menstruating girls, especially schoolgirls. Nevertheless, we must recognize that ensuring good menstrual hygiene management requires a multifaceted approach. The issue does not concern only young girls; efforts should also focus on adult women and address sociocultural and behavioral issues and WASH facilities. A massive awareness at the grassroots level and the supply of low-cost yet effective sanitation pads are needed to improve menstrual hygiene in India.

Acknowledgments Thanks to Mr. Gulsan Kumar and Dr. Harihar Sahoo's for preparing the preliminary maps for the study at a short request, which was instrumental in shaping the chapter.

References

Anand, E., Singh, J., & Unisa, S. (2015). Menstrual hygiene practices and their association with reproductive tract infections and abnormal vaginal discharge among women in India. *Sexual and Reproductive Healthcare: Official Journal of the Swedish Association of Midwives, 6*(4), 249–254. https://doi.org/10.1016/j.srhc.2015.06.001

Babbar, K., & Sivakami, M. (2023). *Promoting menstrual health: Towards sexual and reproductive health for all* (ORF Issue Brief, 613). Observer Research Foundation. https://www.orfonline.org/research/promoting-menstrual-health/

Das, P., Baker, K. K., Dutta, A., Swain, T., Sahoo, S., Das, B. S., Panda, B., Nayak, A., Bara, M., Bilung, B., Mishra, P. R., Panigrahi, P., Cairncross, S., & Torondel, B. (2015). Menstrual hygiene practices, WASH access and the risk of urogenital infection in women from Odisha, India. *PLoS One, 10*(6), e0130777. https://doi.org/10.1371/journal.pone.0130777

Garg, S., Sharma, N., & Sahay, R. (2001). Socio-cultural aspects of menstruation in an urban slum in Delhi, India. *Reproductive Health Matters, 9*(17), 16–25. https://doi.org/10.1016/s0968-8080(01)90004-7

IIPS. (2010). *District level household and facility survey (DLHS-3), 2007–08: India*. IIPS.

Khanna, T., & Das, M. (2016). Why gender matters in the solution towards safe sanitation? Reflections from rural India. *Global Public Health, 11*(10), 1185–1201. https://doi.org/10.1080/17441692.2015.1062905

MacRae, E. R., Clasen, T., Dasmohapatra, M., & Caruso, B. A. (2019). "It's like a burden on the head": Redefining adequate menstrual hygiene management throughout women's varied life stages in Odisha, India. *PLoS One, 14*(8), e0220114. https://doi.org/10.1371/journal.pone.0220114

Narayan, K. A., Srinivasa, D. K., Pelto, P. J., & Veerammal, S. (2001). Puberty rituals, reproductive knowledge and health of adolescent schoolgirls in South India. *Asia-Pacific Population Journal, 16*(2), 225–238. https://doi.org/10.18356/65d467c6-en

Phillips-Howard, P. A., Caruso, B., Torondel, B., Zulaika, G., Sahin, M., & Sommer, M. (2016). Menstrual hygiene management among adolescent schoolgirls in low- and middle-income countries: Research priorities. *Global Health Action, 9*. https://doi.org/10.3402/gha.v9.33032

Roy, A., Paul, P., Saha, J., Barman, B., Kapasia, N., & Chouhan, P. (2021). Prevalence and correlates of menstrual hygiene practices among young currently married women aged 15–24 years: An analysis from a nationally representative survey of India. *The European Journal of Contraception and Reproductive Health Care, 26*(1), 1–10.

Sivakami, M., & Rai, S. (2019). What do we know about sexual and reproductive health of adolescents and youth in India: A synthesis of literature. In *Health and well being of India's young people* (pp. 121–156). https://doi.org/10.1007/978-981-13-6593-5_5

Sommer, M., Sutherland, C., & Chandra-Mouli, V. (2015). Putting menarche and girls into the global population health agenda. *Reproductive Health, 12*, 24. https://doi.org/10.1186/s12978-015-0009-8

Sommer, M., Chandraratna, S., Cavill, S., Mahon, T., & Phillips-Howard, P. (2016). Managing menstruation in the workplace: An overlooked issue in low- and middle-income countries. *International Journal for Equity in Health, 15*(1), 86. https://doi.org/10.1186/s12939-016-0379-8

Sommer, M., Zulaika, G., Schmitt, M., & Gruer. (2019). *Monitoring menstrual health and hygiene measuring progress for girls related to menstruation*. Columbia University/WSSCC.

Taylor, A. (2011). *Women and the city: Examining the gender impact of violence and urbanisation: A comparative study of Brazil, Cambodia, Ethiopia, Liberia and Nepal*. ActionAid.

UNICEF. (2012). *Girls today, women tomorrow: Research highlights on knowledge, practice, attitude and norms on menstrual hygiene, India*. UNICEF.

Van Eijk, A. M., Sivakami, M., Thakkar, M. B., Bauman, A., Laserson, K. F., Coates, S., & Phillips-Howard, P. A. (2016). Menstrual hygiene management among adolescent girls in India: A systematic review and meta-analysis. *BMJ Open, 6*(3), e010290. https://doi.org/10.1136/bmjopen-2015-010290

Chapter 13
Utilization of Antenatal Care Services Among Indian Women

Junaid Khan

The utilization of antenatal care (ANC) services during pregnancy plays a significant role in ensuring maternal health, timely pregnancy monitoring, maternal nutritional health, and newborn care (Lincetto et al., 2006; Murphy et al., 2020). ANC utilization plays a crucial role in determining maternal and perinatal mortality since it provides essential healthcare support to pregnant mothers and promotes newborn care (Hall et al., 1980; McCarthy & Maine, 1992; WHO, 2015). Along with family planning, safe delivery, and obstetric care, ANC is one of the four most crucial pillars; it is the gateway to safe motherhood to identify threats to pregnancy and provides important nutrition counseling to the mother for better progression of the pregnancy (McDonagh, 1996). As per the WHO guidelines and recommendation, a pregnant mother is expected to complete four ANC check-ups, initiating the first check-up during the first trimester and the last at around the 37th week of the pregnancy (Lincetto et al., 2006). Though India has experienced a gradual and consistent decrease in maternal mortality from 437 to 178 per 100,000 live births from 1990 to 2012, India could not achieve Goal 5-A of the Millennium Development Goals (MDGs) by 2015. The maternal mortality ratio (MMR) in 2014–16 by the Office of the Registrar General's Sample Registration System (SRS) is 130 deaths per 100,000 live births. Target 3.1 of Sustainable Development Goals (SDG) set by the United Nations aims to reduce the global maternal mortality ratio to less than 70 per 1,00,000 live births.

When SDGs target the countries to reduce the maternal mortality ratio by two-thirds from the 2010 level by 2030, maternal healthcare utilization is still an ongoing challenge in India (Awasthi et al., 2016). The National Rural Health Mission (NRHM), launched in 2005, aimed at improving maternal healthcare utilization among Indian women, as well as child and adolescent health. During

J. Khan (✉)
Vivekananda College, Kolkata, India
e-mail: statjun@gmail.com

C. Z. Guilmoto (ed.), *Atlas of Gender and Health Inequalities in India*, Demographic Transformation and Socio-Economic Development 16,
https://doi.org/10.1007/978-3-031-47847-5_13

the last decade, NRHM played a crucial role in improving maternal healthcare utilization and strengthening the healthcare infrastructure and accessibility. Taking care of a sizable rural population and its economic well-being through NRHM has been strategized to integrate the public healthcare centers to make maternal healthcare more accessible. Routine antenatal care service has been promoted at the public healthcare system's lowest level (sub-centers). Beyond the basic pregnancy monitoring and management service, such sub-centers are connected to referral centers (e.g., community health centers or district hospitals) to provide advanced care.

Despite improved ANC coverage during the NRHM period, socioeconomic and geographic variations in ANC service utilization remain wide in India. Disparities in access to healthcare utilization within a country play a determining role in the low uptake of antenatal care service, one of the most crucial maternal healthcare components (Say & Raine, 2007). In addition, state-level estimates on MCH care service utilization conceal significant variations across districts within states. These district-level maternal healthcare indicators are essential to improve existing policies and to target future interventions on ANC utilization.

Data and Measurement

The NFHS-5 produced many health indicators at the district level. Although the different rounds of the District Level Household Survey (DLHS) provide the estimates of maternal care components at the district level, NFHS-5 delivers the most recent estimates for all 707 districts of India, and it represents the most suitable source for this study of antenatal care.[1] The data utilized in this study come from the fourth round of NFHS and refer to the most recent birth during the last five years of birth history. This study focuses on two different ANC components:

- ANC visits: percentage of women who completed at least four ANC visits during their nine-month pregnancy.
- Neonatal tetanus protection: percentage of the women whose last birth was protected against tetanus.

Findings and Discussion

According to NFHS-5, about 6.1% of women did not go to ANC during their last pregnancy. There has been a continuous decline of such women over the last decades, thanks to increased accessibility and awareness. Table 13.1 shows the

[1] The original NFHS dataset and the spatial analysis methodology are described in detail in Chap. 1.

Table 13.1 Utilization of ANC services in India, 1992–2021

Percentage of women in India	1992–93	1998–99	2005–06	2015–16	2019–21
No ANC	36.8	34	22.8	16.4	6.1
ANC visit in the first trimester	24	33	43.9	58.6	58.5

gradual decline in the proportion of women with no ANC visit, while the number of ANC during the first trimester of pregnancy has improved since the 1990s. Women who did not utilize ANC dropped from 37% in 1992 to 6.1% in 2019–21. The ANC visit in the first trimester has increased from 24% in 1992–93 to 58.5% in 2019–21.

We now use the percentage of women who have had at least four ANC visits during their last pregnancy for the district-level analysis—with an average of 58.5% in India, according to NFHS-5 figures. The data plotted in Fig. 13.1 illustrate the wide disparities observed in India, with rates ranging from 25% or less in Nagaland and Bihar to more than 90% in Goa and Lakshadweep. At the district level, ANC rates stretch from 4% in Tuensang (Nagaland) to 99% in Theni (Tamil Nadu) and Wayanad (Kerala). In 76 districts, less than one-third of pregnant had at least four antennal care visits. Most of these districts are in Nagaland, Uttar Pradesh, Bihar, and Jharkhand. In contrast, the highest rates of at least four ANC visits (above 80%) are observed in the north (Jammu and Kashmir, Ladakh, Himachal Pradesh, as well as Chandigarh and New Delhi), in the east (West Bengal and Odisha) and more prominently in South India from Maharashtra to Andhra Pradesh and Kerala.

A broader look at the map underlines the pronounced difference between north-central India and the rest of the country, i.e., South, Northwest, and Northeast India. We distinguish in particular an almost continuous line separating a compact block made of Madhya Pradesh, Uttar Pradesh, Bihar, and Jharkhand from their southern, northern, and eastern neighbors, with ANC rates jumping by 10–50 percentage points when we cross this invisible border. Jharkhand and Bihar are, for instance, surrounded to the south and the east by districts (in West Bengal and Odisha) that record ANC rates that are two to three times higher. As suggested by the regional patterning, ANC rates show substantial spatial autocorrelation when measured in terms of Moran's I (0.71).

The sharp variations observed between adjoining states also point to the crucial role of regional health policies in the diffusion of proper antenatal care. Some states fail to ensure that pregnant women have the same quality of care as their neighbors. To some extent, the frequency of ANC visits epitomizes the progress of reproductive health in India, and its map is closely related to those of institutional deliveries, cesarean sections, menstrual hygiene as well as low fertility (see Chaps. 12, 14, and 18 in this Atlas).

Tetanus vaccination indicates progress in eradicating maternal and neonatal tetanus (Roper et al., 2007; Singh et al., 2012). Yet, despite their importance, numerous women in India do not take these vaccinations. Lakshadweep remains the only union territory where women have systematically received tetanus

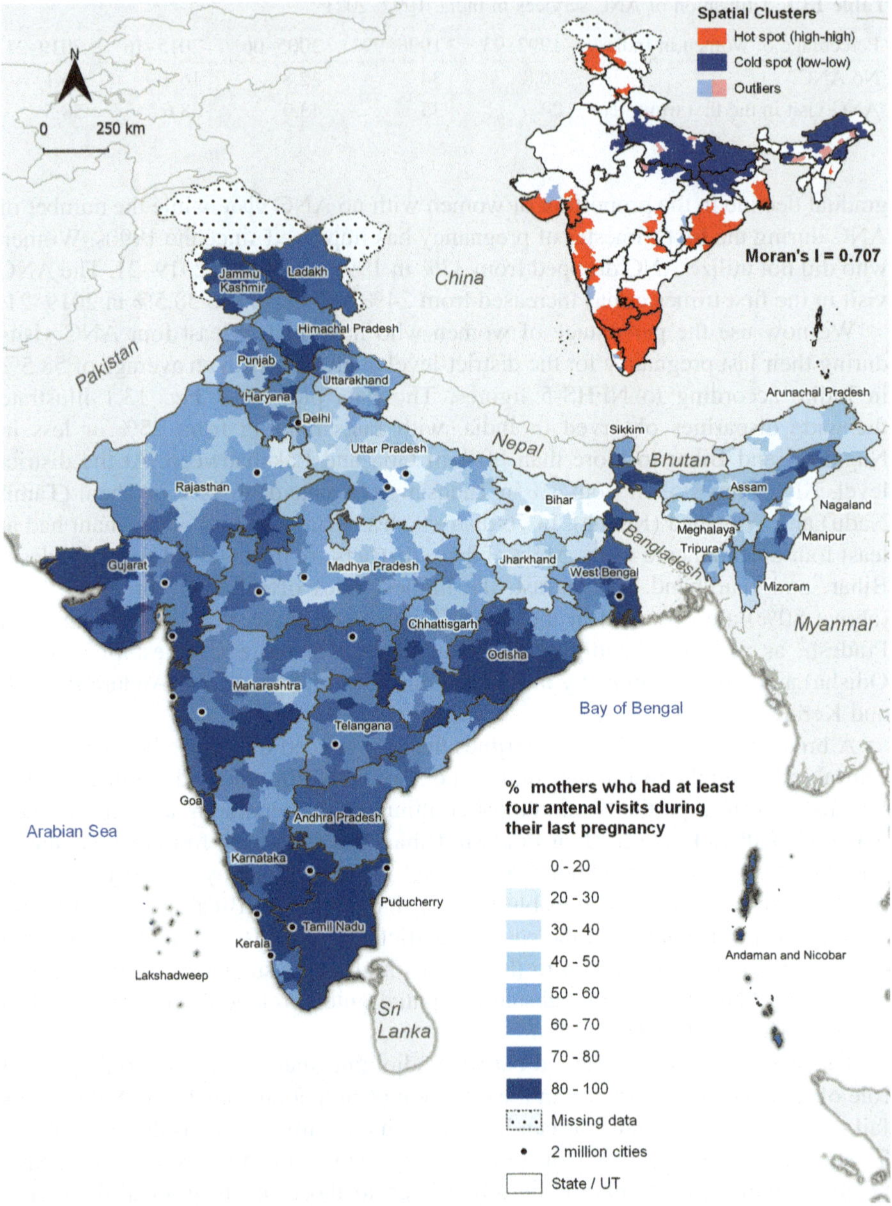

Fig. 13.1 Percentage of women who had four antenatal visits
Source: NFHS-5, 2019–21
The map is for illustrative purposes and may not represent official boundaries

vaccination for their last live birth. Nevertheless, several states are getting close to this achievement, notably Odisha, Madhya Pradesh, Goa, and Tamil Nadu, where ANC rates exceed 95%.

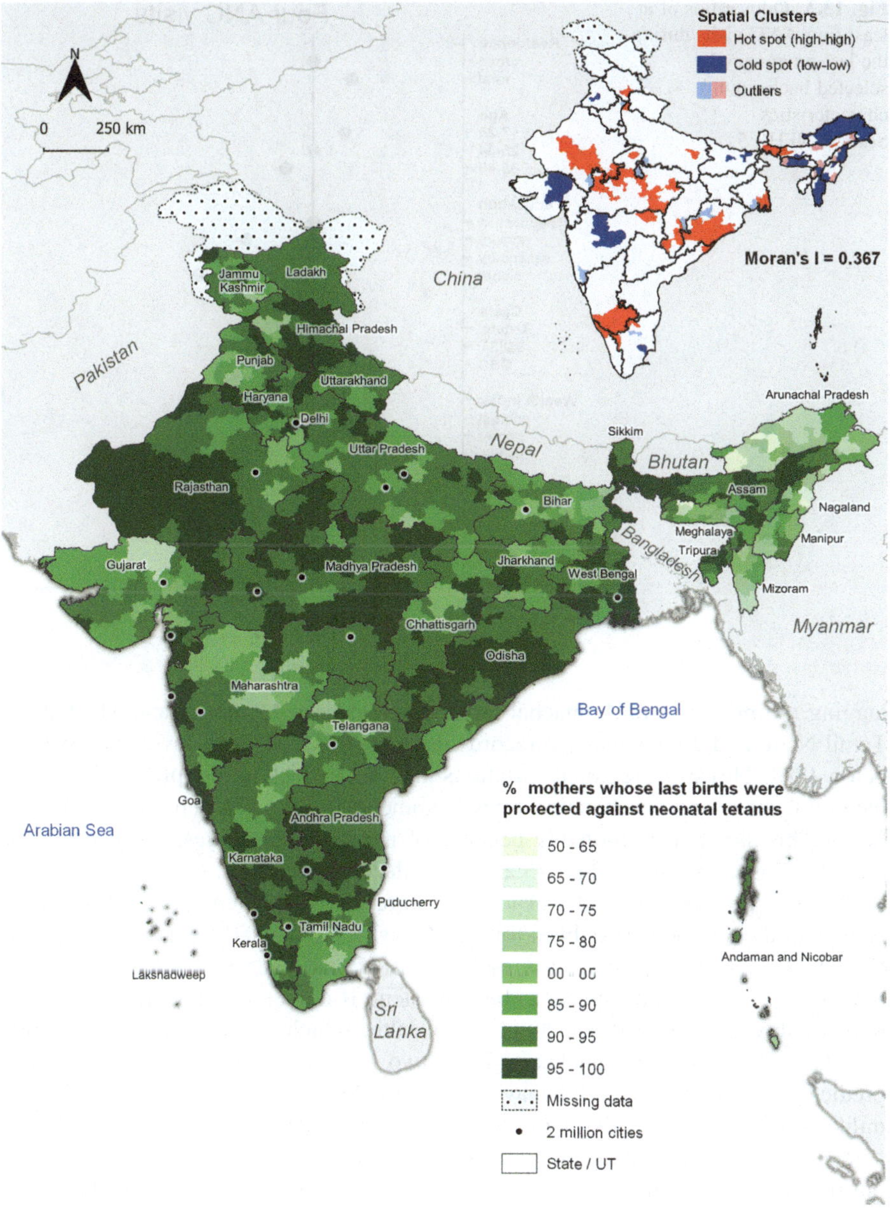

Fig. 13.2 Percentage of women whose last births were protected against neonatal tetanus
Source: NFHS-5, 2019–21
The map is for illustrative purposes and may not represent official boundaries

District-level rates of neonatal tetanus protection for the most recent live births show good coverage across India, as 494 districts exhibit a coverage above 90% (Fig. 13.2). All other districts now record vaccination rates above 50%. States

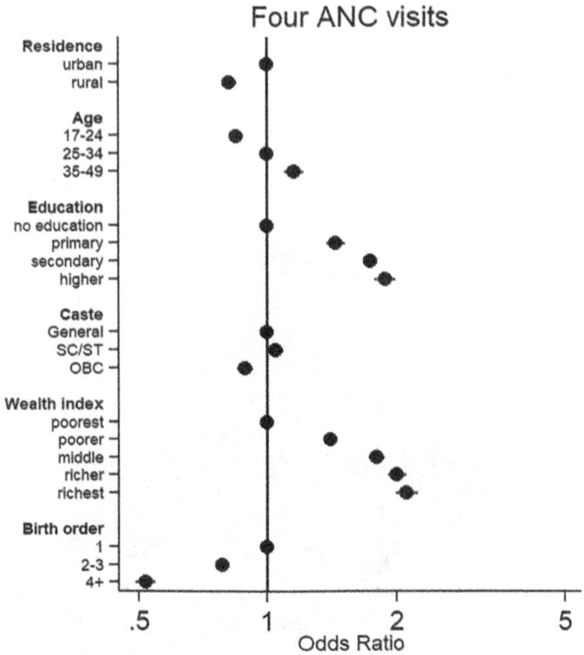

Fig. 13.3 Odds ratios of at least four ANC visits during the last pregnancy by selected background characteristics
Source: NFHS 5

lagging are primarily in Arunachal Pradesh, Nagaland, Mizoram, and Meghalaya. Tamil Nadu and Telangana also record somewhat disappointing levels of coverage below 90%. However, regional variations may be difficult to interpret as the spatial patterning of tetanus vaccination rates is somewhat weak (Moran's *I* is as low as 0.37). This situation is probably because of measurement issues. As a result, the regional clusters shown in Fig. 13.2 may be deceptive.

We also present the results of logistic regressions of antenatal health behavior using two dichotomous variables: four ANC visits and neonatal tetanus vaccination. Figures 13.3 and 13.4 show the odds ratios of various variables for these two models.[2] Overall, results appear to be consistent, if not similar, for the two models. It is notably the case for education and wealth, which are, as expected, strongly correlated with better antenatal care. These two variables are usually the most potent predictors of antenatal health behavior. Nevertheless, it may also be observed that, unlike for health or gender indicators, wealth has a more significant impact on antenatal health than education. This result provides suggestive evidence that out-of-pocket costs (including access to facilities) may act as a greater barrier to antenatal care than a lack of information or awareness.

[2]Odds ratios measure the strength of the correlation with the outcome variable. Values above (below) one correspond to a positive (negative) association.

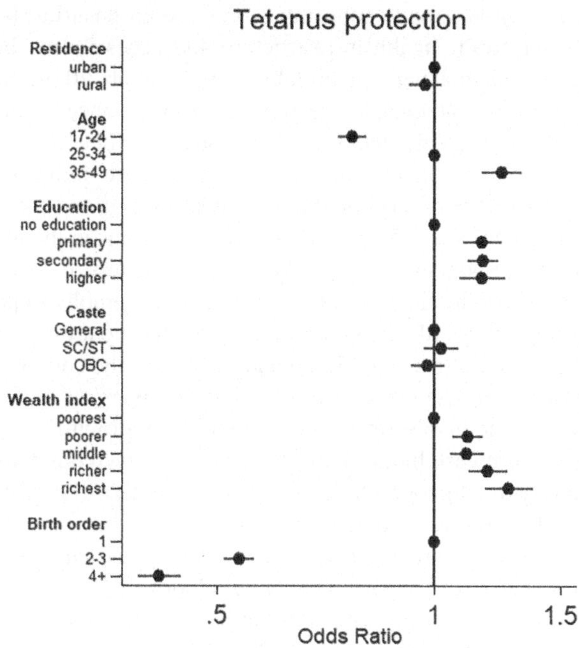

Fig. 13.4 Odds ratios of neonatal tetanus protection among last births by selected background characteristics
Source: NFHS 5

On the contrary, birth order is negatively associated with antenatal care indicators, which explains to some extent the higher vulnerability of these births for both mothers and children. The rural residence also tends to depress ANC and neonatal tetanus indicators. Young mothers aged 17–24 across districts are less likely to complete four ANC visits or to start them during the first trimester (results not shown here), which suggests that young mothers in India may be reluctant or unaware of the benefits of antenatal care. Older mothers aged 35–49 also have a lower chance of starting ANC in the first trimester. Similarly, protection against tetanus appears less common among young mothers. The effect of age is not identical across indicators. Caste differences are modest, except for Adivasi mothers with insufficient neonatal tetanus protection.

Conclusion

The importance of antenatal care utilization on mother and child health is well established (Lincetto et al., 2006; Ogbo et al., 2019). ANC provides health support and pregnancy monitoring and promotes and educates women about the next level of maternal and healthcare services, like institutional delivery and child immunization.

India has made substantial progress in ensuring better maternal health through better public health infrastructure and accessibility, but antenatal care services are still inadequate and inequitable (Kumar et al., 2019). Still, there remain women who do not use antenatal care services. For instance, women's last birth was often not protected against tetanus. This study provides an understanding of the significant components of antenatal care. The selected indicators were disaggregated at the district level to document in finer detail variations in antenatal care utilization among Indian women. The maps show the variations in the utilization of different antenatal care components and identify compact clusters of districts where maternal healthcare utilization is still particularly low. This geography of poor antenatal care is relatively straightforward when measured by the frequency of ANC visits, with a strong divide between north-central India and the rest of the country. But the mapping of neonatal tetanus protection also leads to the discovery of more unusual regional patterns, in which the higher rates do not coincide at all with more developed districts of South or Northwest India. This observation may require more research to confirm this unexpected geography and explore its potential explanations.

This study also identifies the main social and demographic determinants of antenatal behavior. It shows, in particular, that uneducated and poor mothers go for fewer ANC visits. The same relationship is valid for the frequency of neonatal tetanus protection. These findings are consistent with the previous studies (Mihret et al., 2018; Nandi et al., 2020). Like a recent study (Fulpagare et al., 2019), this study also presents evidence that the utilization of antenatal care services among young women aged 15–24 is substantially lower. It appears thus that ANC coverage is lower among women who need it the most: poor, less educated, socially backward mothers, and among those mothers of higher parity and living in rural areas.

References

Awasthi, A., Pandey, C. M., Chauhan, R. K., & Singh, U. (2016). Disparity in maternal, newborn and child health services in high focus states in India: A district-level cross-sectional analysis. *BMJ Open, 6*(8), e009885. https://doi.org/10.1136/bmjopen-2015-009885

Fulpagare, P. H., Saraswat, A., Dinachandra, K., Surani, N., Parhi, R. N., Bhattacharjee, S. S. S., Purty, A., Mohapatra, B., Kejrewal, N., Agrawal, N., Bhatia, V., Ruikar, M., Gope, R. K., Murira, Z., De Wagt, A., & Sethi, V. (2019). Antenatal care service utilization among adolescent pregnant women—Evidence from Swabhimaan Programme in India. *Frontiers in Public Health, 7*. https://doi.org/10.3389/fpubh.2019.00369

Hall, M., Chng, P. K., & Macgillivray, I. (1980). Is routine antenatal care worthwhile? *The Lancet, 316*(8185), 78–80. https://doi.org/10.1016/S0140-6736(80)92950-5

Kumar, G., Choudhary, T. S., Srivastava, A., Upadhyay, R. P., Taneja, S., Bahl, R., Martines, J., Bhan, M. K., Bhandari, N., & Mazumder, S. (2019). Utilisation, equity and determinants of full antenatal care in India: Analysis from the National Family Health Survey 4. *BMC Pregnancy and Childbirth, 19*(1), 1–9.

Lincetto, O., Mothebesoane-Anoh, S., Gomez, P., & Munjanja, S. (2006). Antenatal care. In *Opportunities for Africa's newborns: Practical data, policy and programmatic support for newborn care in Africa* (pp. 55–62). Partnership for Maternal, Newborn & Child Health.

McCarthy, J., & Maine, D. (1992). A framework for analyzing the determinants of maternal mortality. *Studies in Family Planning, 23*(1), 23–33. https://doi.org/10.2307/1966825

McDonagh, M. (1996). Is antenatal care effective in reducing maternal morbidity and mortality? *Health Policy and Planning, 11*(1), 1–15. https://doi.org/10.1093/heapol/11.1.1

Mihret, M. S., Limenih, M. A., & Gudayu, T. W. (2018). The role of timely initiation of antenatal care on protective dose tetanus toxoid immunization: The case of northern Ethiopia postnatal mothers. *BMC Pregnancy and Childbirth, 18*(1), 235. https://doi.org/10.1186/s12884-018-1878-y

Murphy, M., McHugh, S., O'Keeffe, L. M., Greene, R. A., Corcoran, P., & Kearney, P. M. (2020). Preventive health counselling during antenatal care using the pregnancy risk assessment monitoring system (PRAMS) in Ireland. *BMC Pregnancy and Childbirth, 20*(1), 98. https://doi.org/10.1186/s12884-020-2756-y

Nandi, A., Kumar, S., Shet, A., Bloom, D. E., & Laxminarayan, R. (2020). Childhood vaccinations and adult schooling attainment: Long-term evidence from India's Universal Immunization Programme. *Social Science and Medicine (1982), 250*. https://doi.org/10.1016/j.socscimed.2020.112885

Ogbo, F. A., Dhami, M. V., Ude, E. M., Senanayake, P., Osuagwu, U. L., Awosemo, A. O., Ogeleka, P., Akombi, B. J., Ezeh, O. K., & Agho, K. E. (2019). Enablers and barriers to the utilization of antenatal Care Services in India. *International Journal of Environmental Research and Public Health, 16*(17), 3152. https://doi.org/10.3390/ijerph16173152

Roper, M. H., Vandelaer, J. H., & Gasse, F. L. (2007). Maternal and neonatal tetanus. *The Lancet, 370*(9603), 1947–1959. https://doi.org/10.1016/S0140-6736(07)61261-6

Say, L., & Raine, R. (2007). A systematic review of inequalities in the use of maternal healthcare in developing countries: Examining the scale of the problem and the importance of context. *Bulletin of the World Health Organization, 85*, 812–819. https://doi.org/10.1590/S0042-96862007001000019

Singh, A., Pallikadavath, S., Ogollah, R., & Stones, W. (2012). Maternal tetanus toxoid vaccination and neonatal mortality in rural North India. *PLoS One, 7*(11), e48891. https://doi.org/10.1371/journal.pone.0048891

World Health Organization. (2015). *World health statistics 2015*. World Health Organization.

Chapter 14
Institutional Delivery and Cesarean Births in India

Christophe Z. Guilmoto

From the standpoint of global reproduction, trends in childbirth observed in India are of utmost importance. According to the United Nations population forecasts, the country will record the most significant number of births during the twenty-first century. Beyond their sheer volume, however, Indian deliveries are also of great relevance to understanding the profound transformations in childbirth practices in an era characterized by rising middle classes, public health policy efforts, and the rapid expansion of the private healthcare sector.

Giving birth in rural areas has long been a frightening experience for both mothers and children, as illustrated by the persistence of high maternal and infant mortality rates associated with maternal facilities and services (Griffiths & Stephenson, 2001). The lack of proper delivery conditions represented a typical form of passive gender discrimination, in which maternal and child health was considered a low priority. As a result, the proportion of home deliveries had only declined from 73.7% in 1992–93 to 61.3% in 2005–06 during a post-reform period otherwise characterized by sustained economic development and the lessons drawn from Cairo's International Conference on Population and Development in 1994. The slow progression of institutional births until the early 2000s set India in a league of countries with distinctly lower GDPs and higher fertility. The recourse to cesarean in case of delivery complications was also severely constrained in India by the lack of access to institutional facilities.

This chapter will describe, on the contrary, the revolution that followed the introduction of new schemes to ensure access to safe hospital deliveries for the most vulnerable women. The advances in several health outcomes since the mid-2000s seem remarkable in numerous fields. The most impressive transformation is reflected in the surge in the proportion of institutional births recorded between the

C. Z. Guilmoto (✉)
Centre des Sciences Humaines/IRD (CEPED), New Delhi, India
e-mail: Christophe.Guilmoto@ird.fr

C. Z. Guilmoto (ed.), *Atlas of Gender and Health Inequalities in India*, Demographic Transformation and Socio-Economic Development 16,
https://doi.org/10.1007/978-3-031-47847-5_14

last three rounds of the NFHS surveys, when it more than doubled from 38.7% to 88.6%. This continuous progress has indeed taken India to rates above 95%, according to the 2021–22 figures from the HMIS (Health Management Information System), and the same period also witnessed a parallel jump in cesarean rates, from 8.5% to 17.2% in the fourth NFHS round and finally to 21.5% in the fifth round. In this chapter, we will document the gradual progression of institutional deliveries across regions and classes and chart the contours of the uneven map of C-sections in India.

Data and Measurement

Data on childbirth practices have been collected since the first NFHS rounds in India, with information on the place and type of deliveries.[1] The definition of possible places of birth has only marginally changed over survey rounds, but more information is now available on C-sections. Other sources on childbirth practices include the rounds of the District-Level Household Surveys (DLHS) and the Indian Human Development Surveys (IHDS). More recently, the series from the HMIS also provided some estimates of institutional and cesarean births by district and year.

The data on institutional and cesarean births from the latest NFHS-5 round have been computed for individual districts and social groups. Cesarean rates are calculated here only over institutional births (since there cannot be surgical deliveries in the case of home births). NFHS-5 figures are based on the last three births during 2019–21.

Data on childbirth are expected to be of excellent quality, as birth and mode of delivery represent information easy to collect during the survey. The only statistical limitation is the sample size, with an average sample of 329 births at the district level during the last three years. In some 18 districts, fewer than 150 births were recorded; however, a previous study confirmed the quality of NFHS-4 estimates (Guilmoto & Dumont, 2019), which should also hold for the following NFHS round.

Findings and Discussion

The proportion of births delivered in hospitals and clinics has recorded an impressive rise during the last fifteen years, even if the lack of annual estimates prevents us from drawing a more precise picture of what has happened since 2000. For example, in 2001–06 (NFHS-3), institutional births still accounted for only 38.7% of all deliveries (Table 14.1). Within a few years, this proportion had already increased to 46.9% in 2004–08 (DLHS-3), but the most spectacular change occurred in the

[1] The original NFHS dataset and the spatial analysis methodology are described in detail in Chap. 1.

Table 14.1 Percentage of institutional and cesarean births in 1993–2021

Survey	NFHS-1	NFHS-2	NFHS-3	NFHS-4	NFHS-5
Institutional births	26.30	34.00	38.70	78.90	88.6
Cesarean births[a]	11.00	20.90	22.00	21.80	24.3

[a]Rates computed on institutional births

subsequent years, with a sudden jump to 78.9% in 2010–16 and a further progression to 88.6% five years later (NFHS-5). This recent increase is primarily linked to the Janani Suraksha Yojana, a scheme that promotes institutional births among underprivileged women (Randive et al., 2013).

Significant variations, however, persist between states. Many advanced areas from Chandigarh to Karnataka record institutional rates above 95%, with Kerala, Tamil Nadu, and Puducherry topping the list with almost universal institutional deliveries (above 99%). Conversely, more than a fifth of all deliveries still occur at home in Bihar or Jharkhand. The highest rates of deliveries outside health facilities are otherwise primarily found in the Northeast, with rates in Nagaland as high as 46%.

The map of district-level differentials (Fig. 14.1) illustrates in greater detail the variations still characterizing access to safe births at the time of the NFHS-5. It also shows that spatial patterning often cuts across state boundaries. While the national average stands at 89% (87% and 94% for rural and urban areas, respectively), more than a third of Indian districts exhibit rates above 95%. The map reveals that these areas cover most of South India and significant portions of Western India and Maharashtra, except for Khandesh and Marathwada. The rates closest to universal institutional deliveries (i.e., above 99%) are observed along the Konkan coast from Goa to Kerala but also cover south Karnataka and almost all Tamil districts. Incidentally, South India is on par with neighboring Sri Lanka, where nearly all births today are attended by skilled practitioners.

North Central and East India do not fare as well in comparison. For instance, rates in the middle Ganga River Valley, from Uttar Pradesh to Bihar and Jharkhand, are distinctly lower. Peripheral districts along the Pakistani border in Rajasthan or the Nepalese border in Uttar Pradesh and Bihar record the lowest rates (often below 80%), suggesting the somewhat centripetal nature of India's infrastructural development and political mobilization. Districts with rates below 80% are also found in some predominantly tribal areas of Central India, such as in Jharkhand or among Bhils inhabiting the borders of Madhya Pradesh and Maharashtra. As an illustration of pronounced subregional heterogeneity, we can also highlight the noticeable dip in the proportion of institutional deliveries observed in south Haryana: the less advanced districts of Palwal and Mewat may lie less than 50 km from the National Capital Region and yet register relatively low rates of institutional deliveries. The same is true of the adjacent district of Mathura in Uttar Pradesh, located between Agra and Delhi metropolises.

Somewhat more surprising is the deplorable situation in several northeastern states. While measurement issues may stem from the small sample of births in less

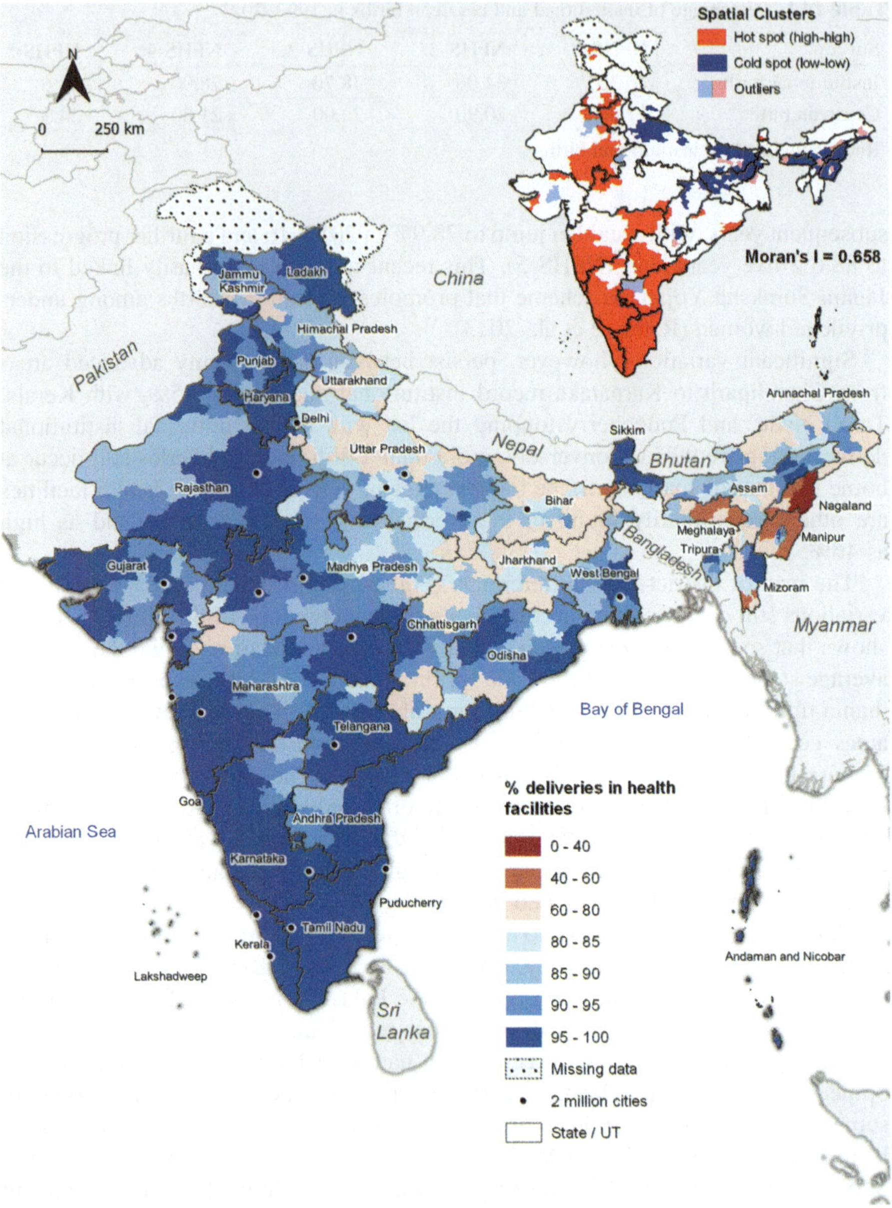

Fig. 14.1 Percentage of births delivered in health facilities
Source: NFHS-5, 2019–21
The map is for illustrative purposes and may not represent official boundaries

populated districts, the regional analysis emphasizes the concentration of the worst delivery conditions of the country in the states of Meghalaya, Manipur, and Nagaland, where the proportion of institutional deliveries often lies below 50% at the district level. Six districts register rates of institutional births below 40%, with India's lowest level of 22% found in Mon, a relatively isolated district of Nagaland lying next to Myanmar. These low values seem particularly at odds with this region's relatively favorable educational levels. Female literacy rates in several northeastern states tend, for the most part, to be higher than in the rest of the country. Nagaland presents the most unlikely combination of high literacy and poor delivery facilities. These maternal health inequalities observed in Northeast or Central India are mainly related to the poor health infrastructures in peripheral regions and the limited impact of government efforts to provide accessible, safe deliveries to local women.

The geostatistical analysis of institutional delivery rates across India confirms this indicator's relatively strong spatial autocorrelation, with Moran's *I* at 0.66. This spatial dependence level stems from the geographical concentration of modern and poor maternal health services in different regions of India. Following my previous observations, this analysis points to a cluster of almost universal institutional delivery extending from southwest Maharashtra to South India. Other hotspots of high institutional delivery rates are found in Haryana, east Rajasthan, and Telangana. The cold spots lie along the border with Nepal in Uttar Pradesh and Bihar, as well as in Jharkhand. The Northeast constitutes another distinct cluster of low institutional births, especially south of the Brahmaputra Valley. This geography resembles that of low fertility and adequate antenatal care (see Chaps. 13 and 18 in this Atlas) and points to parallel trends in the main components of improved reproductive health.

Since the highest rates are observed in the most developed regions, such as the six states and territories of South India, it is worthwhile contrasting the regional variations with differentials across economic groups. The chart presented here (Fig. 14.2) demonstrates the weight of wealth inequalities in the choice of the delivery place. Institutional rates steadily increase with socioeconomic status, rising

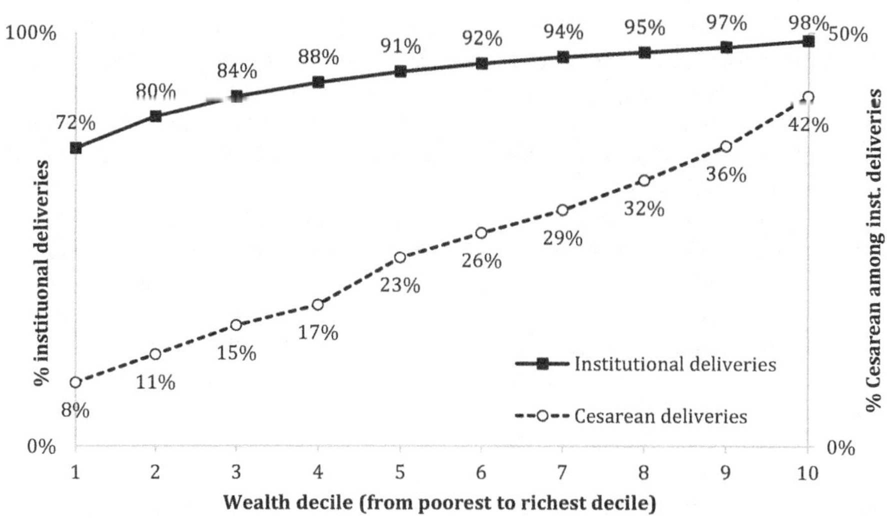

Fig. 14.2 Wealth decile and childbirth practices, 2020–21

from 72% among the poorest decile to 98% among the most prosperous ones. These differentials across wealth deciles are more modest but still visible when analyzed in more advanced regions of South India (data not shown here). In this regard, comparing data from the previous NFHS-3 round of 2005–06 is illuminating (data not shown). Such a comparison shows that the recent reduction in home deliveries did not impact all socioeconomic classes similarly. Among the wealthiest decile, rates of institutional births were already extremely high and close to or above 90%. However, among poorer deciles, the progression within fifteen years (i.e., between NFHS-3 and NFHS-5) was considerable as the proportion of institutional births soared from 11% to 72% in fifteen years. This jump demonstrates that most of the progression in institutional delivery chronicled here occurred among underprivileged communities that had long been excluded from hospital access. This transformation also serves as an indirect testimony of the effectiveness of the policy interventions mentioned above. Current rates below 80% suggest that health inequalities affecting the poorest communities were still pronounced in most of North India at the time of the NFHS-5. Continuous progress in providing safe deliveries to women from vulnerable groups and regions should close this gap shortly.

According to NFHS-5, 21.5% of all births were delivered by cesarean in India (17.6% and 32.3% for rural and urban areas, respectively). When restricted to births delivered in health facilities, India's net (or institutional) cesarean rate rises to 24.3%. It should be noted that these rates are already distinctly above the 10–15% proportion of cesarean deliveries recommended by the WHO (2015). The WHO considers that cesarean deliveries should represent around 10–15% of all births. Women in countries with rates below 10% are at risk of being unable to access surgical deliveries in case of complications. Otherwise, cesarean rates above 15% are indeed excessive. Most West European nations have rates close to 15–25% today, but various countries, notably in Latin America, have recorded much higher rates (Boerma et al., 2018).

NFHS-5 data show that the net cesarean rate in India is never below 10% in any state. The net cesarean rate increases from 20.3% in rural areas to 34.3% in towns and cities. The urban rate is, therefore, more than twice as high as the recommended 15% threshold. In several states such as Punjab, Jammu and Kashmir, Tamil Nadu, Andhra Pradesh, and Telangana, the cesarean rates among births delivered in health institutions are well above 40%.

The district map of net cesarean rates (Fig. 14.3) displays thought-provoking features. First, rates below 10% remain unfortunately frequent, found in over 100 districts, primarily in North and Central India. Northeastern states also stand out, with a conspicuous deficit of surgical deliveries reported in Mizoram, Nagaland, and Meghalaya. In a few isolated districts, spread from Rajasthan to Nagaland, even less than 5% of institutional births are delivered by cesarean. For instance, in Tuensang (Nagaland), only 35% of women deliver in an institution; among them, only 4% reported a cesarean delivery.

We can identify distinct spatial patterns from the cluster map, with a broader region with low cesarean rates extending from Rajasthan to Bihar. This cluster corresponds to inadequate health institutions across North India, where local

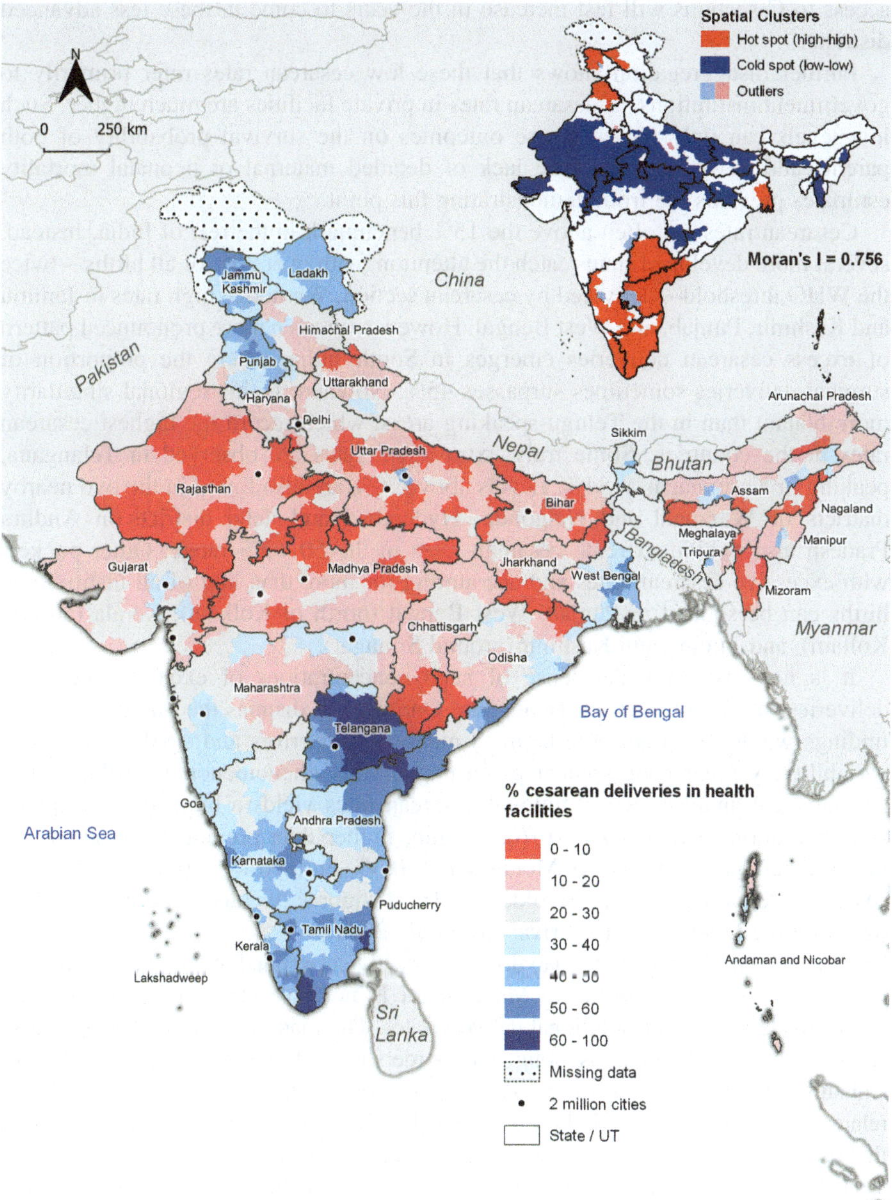

Fig. 14.3 Percentage of institutional births delivered by cesarean section
Source: NFHS-5, 2019–21
The map is for illustrative purposes and may not represent official boundaries

maternity homes lack adequate facilities to perform C-sections in cases of need. The map of districts with cesarean rates lower than 10% appears, however, extremely patchy; this regional segmentation suggests that things are changing rapidly and that access to C-sections will fast increase in the years to come in these less advanced districts.

Further disaggregation shows that these low cesarean rates refer primarily to government institutions, as cesarean rates in private facilities are much higher. Such low levels can only have adverse outcomes on the survival probability of both parents and newborns. Still, the lack of detailed maternal or neonatal mortality estimates prevents me from demonstrating this point.

Cesarean rates are often above the 15% benchmark in the rest of India. Instead, several more developed states catch the attention, with over 30% of all births—twice the WHO threshold—delivered by cesarean section. We notice high rates in Jammu and Kashmir, Punjab, and West Bengal. However, an even more pronounced pattern of excess cesarean deliveries emerges in South India, where the proportion of surgical deliveries sometimes surpasses 45%. Nowhere is this regional singularity more blatant than in the Telugu-speaking areas, which record the highest cesarean rates in the countries. Some truly extravagant rates are observed in Telangana, peaking in Karimnagar at 84%. Levels above 70% are also found in the two nearby districts of Warangal and Nalgonda. Hyderabad and delta districts in Andhra Pradesh also exhibit extreme cesarean rates in the 50–65% range. Other pockets with excessive cesarean rates and accounting for more than half of all institutional births can be spotted in Punjab, West Bengal (north of Kolkata), Kerala (around Kollam), and Jammu and Kashmir (around Srinagar).

It is not easy to make sense of such concentrations of excessive cesarean deliveries in regions such as Telangana. One way to dismiss the validity of these findings would be to attribute them to measurement errors and small sample size variability, yet the geographical patterning of this phenomenon is striking. The geostatistical analysis of institutional cesarean rates yields a high level of spatial autocorrelation (Moran's I is 0.76), a figure higher than previously observed for institutional births for which Moran's I is 0.66. Furthermore, prior mapping of cesarean deliveries based on older NFHS-4 figures yielded a similar picture (Guilmoto & Dumont, 2019; Srivastava et al., 2020).

It is also intriguing that the map does not exactly correspond to the previous map of institutional births; for instance, Maharashtra is not characterized by unnecessary cesareans despite high institutional delivery rates. The map of cesarean deliveries also shows well-marked variations along state borders (e.g., Telangana vs. Maharashtra or Chhattisgarh; Punjab vs. Haryana). This feature would suggest that regional legislation related to hospitals—particularly private hospitals and clinics that are primarily behind the rise in cesarean rates in India—directly affects these rates. The high rates in Telangana may be due to a broader spread of a new "culture of cesarean deliveries" among practitioners and patients lying at the root of this undue enthusiasm for surgical deliveries that are often unnecessary as dangerous for the parturient. The closest correlate of C-sections that we can find in this Atlas is the map of overweight (see Chap. 2), another indirect indicator of the impact of changing lifestyles among the Indian middle class.

Nevertheless, institutional delivery and cesarean rates are not identical. There are many districts in India where institutional delivery rates have crossed 95% while the cesarean rates still lie within the 10–20% range.[2] This observation is reassuring as it shows that cesarean rates need not increase everywhere to extreme levels as they did in Telangana.

Apart from the pronounced regional variations, the likelihood of cesarean delivery is also closely related to a host of social and health factors. We have already hinted at the role of private health facilities, where the proportion of cesarean deliveries has risen to 35.8% (Lee et al., 2021; Bhatia et al., 2020). However, investigations based on NFHS-4 data (Mohanty et al., 2019; Srivastava et al., 2020) have already documented several other correlates of cesarean births, starting with specific health conditions (BMI of the mother, parity, multiple births, diabetes). Moreover, low fertility is also a strong correlate, suggesting that parents of smaller families invest more in children and maternal care and delivery conditions. Finally, cesarean delivery correlates with better socioeconomic status, measured by urbanization, education, or household wealth. The cesarean rate among the highest decile group is already above 40% (see Fig. 14.2); however, these health, institutional, and socioeconomic variables do not explain away the unusual situation of Telangana, where the institutional cesarean rate is at an extreme 63%. Unique regional factors likely explain the spike in cesarean deliveries in Telugu-speaking districts, even if this trend is also part of a broader epidemic of cesareans observed worldwide (Boerma et al., 2018).

Conclusion

In retrospect, it is probably no exaggeration to say that India has recently undergone a revolution in childbirth. The advances in several health outcomes since the mid-2000s seem remarkable in many fields, and the jump in the proportion of institutional births between the last two rounds of the NFHS surveys heralds a profound transformation in India's reproductive landscape—placing the country well ahead of Bangladesh, Pakistan, or Nepal. The recent increase in institutional delivery rates corresponds to a progression of several percentage points per year. If this progression continues simultaneously, almost all Indian women should deliver in hospitals and clinics in the late 2020s. Nevertheless, the benefits of institutional deliveries are not automatic, and recent research (Lee et al., 2022) shows institutional delivery had no impact on newborn mortality in areas with poor-quality health systems.

Our maps point to persisting inequalities in access to institutional delivery, even if recent trends suggest that regional variations are shrinking. However, the singularity of the rise in cesarean rates exemplified by South India requires more investigations to understand the source of this fixation for surgical deliveries. It is no idle question.

[2] One of the many examples could be Porbandar (Gujarat), where more than 99% of births are delivered in health facilities, but no more than 19% of them via a cesarean procedure.

While all pregnant women will soon gain access to hospitals, they also need to be ensured of adequate and competent care and be free of the various forms of mistreatment and obstetric violence recently reported in India (Chattopadhyay et al., 2018; Diamond-Smith et al., 2016). It means preventing medically unjustified C-sections, operations far more expensive than vaginal deliveries—and potentially detrimental to both mothers and children (Sandall et al., 2018). With 1.8 million unnecessary cesareans already occurring every year in India at the time of the NFHS-4 (Guilmoto & Dumont, 2019), the issue is mounting; it will soon call for a fully-fledged policy response to check the overuse of C-sections.

References

Bhatia, M., Banerjee, K., Dixit, P., & Dwivedi, L. K. (2020). Assessment of variation in cesarean delivery rates between public and private health facilities in India from 2005 to 2016. *JAMA Network Open, 3*(8), e2015022–e2015022.

Boerma, T., Ronsmans, C., Melesse, D. Y., Barros, A. J. D., Barros, F. C., Juan, L., Moller, A.-B., Say, L., Hosseinpoor, A. R., Yi, M., de Lyra Rabello Neto, D., & Temmerman, M. (2018). Global epidemiology of use of and disparities in cesarean sections. *The Lancet, 392*(10,155), 1341–1348. https://doi.org/10.1016/S0140-6736(18)31928-7

Chattopadhyay, S., Mishra, A., & Jacob, S. (2018). "Safe", yet violent? Women's experiences with obstetric violence during hospital births in rural North-east India. *Culture, Health and Sexuality, 20*(7), 815–829. https://doi.org/10.1080/13691058.2017.1384572

Diamond-Smith, N., Sudhinaraset, M., Melo, J., & Murthy, N. (2016). The relationship between women's experiences of mistreatment at facilities during childbirth, types of support received and person providing the support in Lucknow, India. *Midwifery, 40*, 114–123.

Griffiths, P., & Stephenson, R. (2001). Understanding users' perspectives of barriers to maternal healthcare use in Maharashtra, India. *Journal of Biosocial Science, 33*(3), 339–359.

Guilmoto, C. Z., & Dumont, A. (2019). Trends, regional variations, and socioeconomic disparities in cesarean births in India, 2010–2016. *JAMA Network Open, 2*(3), e190526.

Lee, H.-Y., Kim, R., Oh, J., & Subramanian, S. V. (2021). Association between the type of provider and cesarean section delivery in India: A socioeconomic analysis of the National Family Health Surveys 1999, 2006, 2016. *PLoS One, 16*(3), e0248283. https://doi.org/10.1371/journal.pone.0248283

Lee, H. Y., Leslie, H. H., Oh, J., Kim, R., Kumar, A., Subramanian, S. V., & Kruk, M. E. (2022). The association between institutional delivery and neonatal mortality based on the quality of maternal and newborn health system in India. *Scientific Reports, 12*(1), 1–10.

Mohanty, S. K., Panda, B. K., Khan, P. K., & Behera, P. (2019). Out-of-pocket expenditure and correlates of cesarean births in public and private health centres in India. *Social Science and Medicine, 224*, 45–57. https://doi.org/10.1016/j.socscimed.2019.01.048

Randive, B., Diwan, V., & Costa, A. D. (2013). India's conditional cash transfer Programme (the JSY) to promote institutional birth: Is there an association between institutional birth proportion and maternal mortality? *PLoS One, 8*(6), e67452. https://doi.org/10.1371/journal.pone.0067452

Sandall, J., Tribe, R. M., Avery, L., Mola, G., Visser, G. H., Homer, C. S., Gibbons, D., Kelly, N. M., Kennedy, H. P., Kidanto, H., Taylor, P., & Temmerman, M. (2018). Short-term and long-term effects of cesarean section on the health of women and children. *The Lancet, 392*(10,155), 1349–1357. https://doi.org/10.1016/S0140-6736(18)31930-5

Srivastava, S., Chaurasia, H., Kumar Singh, K. J., & Chaudhary, P. (2020). Exploring the spatial patterns of cesarean section delivery in India: Evidence from National Family Health Survey-4. *Clinical Epidemiology and Global Health, 8*(2), 414–422. https://doi.org/10.1016/j.cegh.2019.09.012

World Health Organization. (2015). *WHO Statement on Cesarean Section Rates*. WHO. https://apps.who.int/iris/bitstream/handle/10665/161442/WHO_RHR_15.02_eng.pdf

Chapter 15
Immunization Coverage Among Indian Children

Basant Kumar Panda and Gulshan Kumar

Immunization is regarded as the most cost-effective intervention to protect children from life-threatening diseases such as tuberculosis, diphtheria, polio, tetanus, and other infectious diseases, which have short and long-term consequences (Andre et al., 2008). Childhood immunization is directly associated with many SDGs, such as good health and well-being, gender equality, and education. In addition, immunization in childhood played a significant role in substantially reducing child mortality globally. However, each year, millions of children, particularly from low- and middle-income countries, fail to receive the necessary vaccines for survival and good health. In most low-income countries, childhood immunization has been provided free of cost since 1974 through the Expanded Program on Immunization (EPI), Universal Childhood Immunization, and, since 2000, through Gavi, the Vaccine Alliance (Hinman & McKinlay, 2015; Lim et al., 2008). Between 1980 and 2018, relatively lower-income regions (most of which started from deficient levels of coverage) showed better progress than higher-income regions. Despite their relatively better progress, the immunization coverage rates of most countries in the Africa and Southeast Asia WHO regions still fall short of the ≥90% national target recommended by the Global Vaccine Action Plan (GVAP) (Wariri et al., 2021; VanderEnde et al., 2018). For example, a recent study on fifteen West African countries reveals that although measles-containing-vaccine coverage (MCV) has increased from 45% in 2001 to 66% in 2019, an estimated 4.5 million children (aged 12–23 months) did not receive the first dose of MCV in 2019 (Wariri et al., 2021).

B. K. Panda (✉)
Population Council Consulting, New Delhi, India

G. Kumar
Kashi Sahu College, Seraikela, India

C. Z. Guilmoto (ed.), *Atlas of Gender and Health Inequalities in India*, Demographic Transformation and Socio-Economic Development 16,
https://doi.org/10.1007/978-3-031-47847-5_15

Various governmental efforts have been made to achieve universal immunization in India in the last two decades. They have been associated with a dramatic increase in full-immunization coverage, including each vaccination dose. Evidence shows steady progress in full immunization coverage, rising from 34% in 1992 to 44% in 2005–06 and from 62% in 2015–16 (IIPS and ICF, 2017) to 77% in 2019–21 (IIPS and ICF, 2021). However, about one-fourth of the children still cannot receive complete vaccination in India. Further, there remain substantial regional and socio-economic disparities in healthcare access in India. As the national estimate masks the considerable variation across the subgroup, exploring the spatial patterning of immunization, including within states, is noteworthy.

This study has a primary objective: to understand the regional variations of the full-immunization coverage among children aged 12–23 months in India. The district-level map prepared for the chapter underlines space as a specific determinant of disparity in immunization coverage in India. The study findings can help to uplift the focus to the disadvantaged geographical areas and the populations carrying the maximum burden (Panda et al., 2020). Identifying areas of need is the first step in discovering and addressing the causes of inequity. We also examine the extent of sex differentials in immunization, as previous evidence suggested a gender disparity in full immunization coverage in favor of males (Pande, 2003).

Data and Measurement

Data on immunization in India have been collected regularly through national health surveys (National Family Health Surveys) since 1992. This study is based on the data from the latest round of the NFHS conducted during 2019–21.[1] The survey collected immunization information based on the reporting on the vaccination card. This information was collected through the mother's reference in case of the unavailability of vaccination cards. The reference group for the information is children aged 12–23 months, which is the ideal practice of several DHS surveys. Our sample size consists of 43,247 children of this age. The unweighted average number of children per district is about 61. This relatively modest sample size may account for some measurement imprecision at the district level.

Findings and Discussion

The coverage of full immunization by sex of the child at the national level in India is presented in Fig. 15.1. The trends over the last three decades point to a slow improvement till the 2000 decade, followed by a sudden jump in 2015–16 as the

[1] The original NFHS dataset and the spatial analysis methodology are described in detail in Chap. 1.

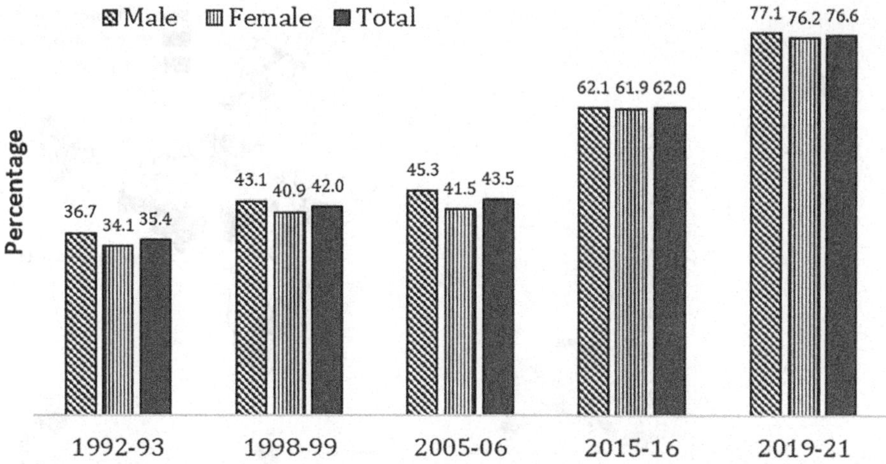

Fig. 15.1 Percentage of full immunization among children aged 12–23 months by sex in 1991–2021

proportion of fully immunized children increased by almost half within ten years. It further increased to 77.2% in 2019–21. Interestingly, female immunization rates until NFHS-3 were systematically lower than male immunization rates by 1–2 percentage points. In contrast, the latest NFHS-4 and NFHS-5 results showed a complete reduction of the sex differentials in immunization. Presently, immunization rates are identical for girls and boys.

Despite such recent improvement in vaccination coverage, about one-fourth of the children (23.4%) in India remain either not immunized or partially immunized in 2019–21. This situation is still far from the ideal level of immunization coverage. Furthermore, the national average figure conceals wide regional disparities. However, as will be seen, spatial patterns in immunization do not follow India's typical features of regional health inequalities.

At the state level, the northeastern states display the lowest prevalence of full immunization, starting with Nagaland (56.6%), followed by Meghalaya (63.2%) and Arunachal Pradesh (63.8%). Children were fully immunized in a proportion above 85% in only four major states: West Bengal, Tamil Nadu, Odisha (topping the list at 90.6%), and Himachal Pradesh, along with smaller regions (Lakshadweep, Ladakh, Jammu and Kashmir, Dadra and Nagar Haveli).

The map of full immunization coverage in the districts of India is shown in Fig. 15.2. Out of 707 districts in India, 14 still record immunization rates below 50%. Most of them are in the Northeast. Intriguingly, the map also shows some isolated districts in Uttar Pradesh, Madhya Pradesh, Gujarat, and Maharashtra, where less than half of the children were fully immunized in 2019–21. Most districts of Uttar Pradesh, Jharkhand, and Bihar record immunization levels below 70%. Numerous parts of India have not benefited from the recent drive towards universal vaccination.

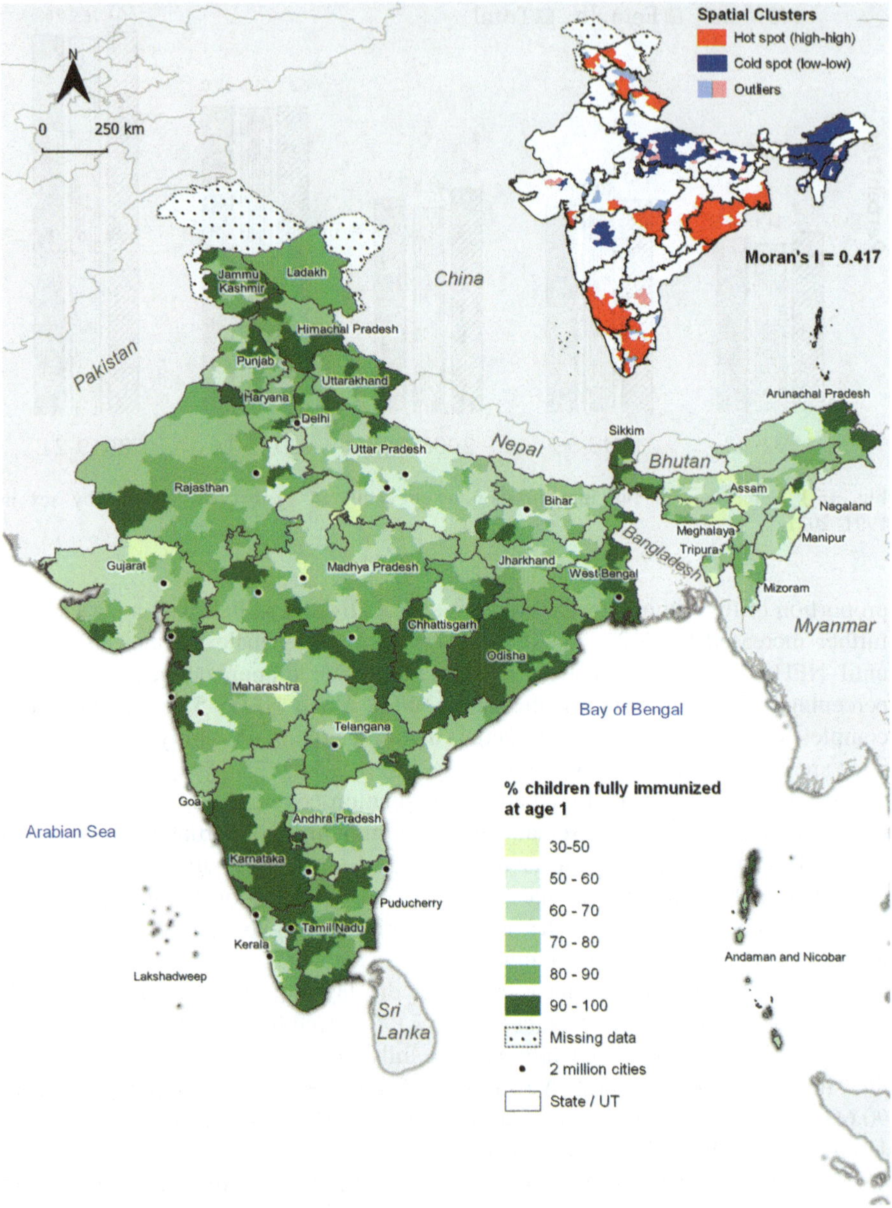

Fig. 15.2 Percentage of children fully immunized at age 1
Source: NFHS-5, 2019–21
The map is for illustrative purposes and may not represent official boundaries

Conversely, immunization rates already exceed 90% coverage in 130 districts. We cannot identify broader regions with high immunization rates clearly. As a result, the geography of full immunization appears somewhat contorted. We observe, for instance, significant disparities in immunization coverage across districts of the same state. For instance, Immunization rates plunge as we move from coastal Maharashtra to inland districts of Marathwada towards the Kongu Nadu region around Coimbatore. Furthermore, the map highlights high levels of regional heterogeneity in other states such as Andhra Pradesh, Odisha, and Gujarat. In addition, substantial variations can sometimes be observed along state borders, such as between Odisha and Andhra Pradesh.

A possible reason for this situation is hesitancy about the immunization drive launched by the government with a new measles-rubella vaccine (Sankaranarayanan et al., 2019). Apart from these, many districts from the empowered action group (EAG) states, such as Uttar Pradesh, Bihar, Assam, Rajasthan, and northeastern states, report a lower level of immunization. Potential explanations for these disappointing figures may be the lower level of education, women's empowerment, accessibility of health centers, and other interrelated factors (Pramanik et al., 2015; Prinjal et al., 2010; Rammahan & Awefeso, 2015). At the same time, it is essential to stress that many districts across Odisha and Chhattisgarh performed exceptionally well regarding vaccination despite their relative geographical isolation and socio-economic backwardness. Programs and policies in these districts appear accordingly to have been especially successful.

We have computed Moran's *I* index for full immunization coverage at the district level in India. Moran's *I* value stands at a low 0.41, one of the lowest levels featured in this atlas, which is not surprising in view of significant variations in immunization levels observed between adjacent districts—the cluster map points to low immunization in most of the northeast but also central Uttar Pradesh. The hotspots of immunization are found in Karnataka and Tamil Nadu, but excluding Kerala, as well as Vidharba, Odisha, and West Bengal. Odisha's unexpectedly advantageous position has already been mentioned. However, Fig. 15.2 also shows that immunization rates are moderate or low in high-performing states like Kerala and point to parts of India's most developed areas, such as Punjab or Kerala. This observation may sound somewhat counterintuitive given these states' otherwise good health performance. These maps may, therefore, indirectly point to measurement issues affecting immunization and be partly interpreted as the product of error due to the small sample size.

As presented in Fig. 15.1, the gap between male and female rates at the national level was not significant, and we found no pattern distinguishing immunization rates by sex across districts of India. The regional distribution of these gender gaps appears to be quite irregular and does not match the maps of son preference examined elsewhere in this Atlas (see, for instance, Chap. 9).

Conclusion

Safe, effective, quality, and affordable essential vaccines are critical targets in achieving health-related sustainable development goals. Childhood vaccination like measles and tetanus is associated with substantially reduced childhood mortality

(McGovern & Canning, 2015). The relationship between vaccination and immunization at the multi-country level reveals that children with an incomplete vaccination schedule have poorer nutritional outcomes (Solis-Soto et al., 2020). In addition, a vaccinated child has improved health, which helps to have improved cognitive skills. Despite such survival and long-term health advantages, more than one-third of the children from India remain unvaccinated or partially vaccinated, contributing to high morbidity and mortality.

Notably, in December 2014, the government of India introduced the mission Indradhanush to vaccinate at least 90% of pregnant women against tetanus and ensure that all children are fully vaccinated. To further intensify the vaccination program, the government also introduced the Intensified Mission Indradhanush (IMI 1.0 and 2.0) to universalize the immunization program. Moreover, the government focuses on improving immunization coverage in rural areas, urban slums, and poor communities. India has made impressive strides in vaccination coverage with the effective implementation of a national immunization program in a short duration. The positive impact of this program is evident in the drop in the number of tuberculosis, diphtheria, and measles cases. A recent study provides insights into approaches for improving vaccination quality through achieving age-appropriate vaccination and considering the socio-demographic variables that adversely impact equity aspects of vaccination (Prinja et al., 2010).

Despite impressive progress in immunization, our study revealed a clear spatial pattern of the immunization coverage gap in the districts of India. The existence of clusters indicates unevenness in immunization coverage. Clusters with a lower level of immunization have been seen in the northeastern states, Uttar Pradesh and Madhya Pradesh, and parts of Gujarat. It is intriguing to notice that immunization coverage is much lower in Kerala than in Tamil Nadu despite its otherwise good healthcare status, which should be investigated further. Andhra Pradesh also has clusters of low vaccination. Vaccination hesitation may play an essential role in these states, as low vaccination coverage is also observed in the COVID-19 vaccination (Srinivas, 2021). At the same time, vaccination coverage in some districts from less advanced states like Odisha or Chhattisgarh is rather heartening and suggests that awareness about vaccination's positive impacts can be raised among privileged and underprivileged groups.

Joint efforts by the government, researchers, and social workers are required to achieve universal immunization coverage. The central and state governments should facilitate the program to reach needy people. The government must ensure the quality of public hospitals with adequate resources, delivering accessible, affordable, and quality healthcare so that more underprivileged sections of society can access immunization at the right time. At the same time, international donor agencies and collaboration can play a crucial role in improving immunization coverage. To conclude, improving the quality of education, health facilities, access to the healthcare system, and increasing investment in the healthcare system can improve India's immunization program.

References

Andre, F. E., Booy, R., Bock, H. L., Clemens, J., Datta, S. K., John, T. J., Lee, B. W., Lolekha, S., Peltola, H., Ruff, T. A., Santosham, M., & Schmitt, H. J. (2008). Vaccination greatly reduces disease, disability, death and inequity worldwide. *Bulletin of the World Health Organization, 86*, 140–146. https://doi.org/10.1590/S0042-96862008000200016

Hinman, A. R., & McKinlay, M. A. (2015). Immunization equity. *Vaccine, 33*, D72–D77. https://doi.org/10.1016/j.vaccine.2015.09.033

IIPS and ICF. (2017). *National Family Health Survey 2015–16 (NFHS-2015-16), India*. International Institute for Population Sciences (IIPS).

IIPS and ICF. (2021). *National Family Health Survey 2019–21 (NFHS-2019-21), India*. International Institute for Population Sciences (IIPS).

Lim, S. S., Stein, D. B., Charrow, A., & Murray, C. J. (2008). Tracking progress towards universal childhood immunisation and the impact of global initiatives: A systematic analysis of three-dose diphtheria, tetanus, and pertussis immunisation coverage. *The Lancet, 372*(9655), 2031–2046. https://doi.org/10.1016/S0140-6736(08)61869-3

McGovern, M. E., & Canning, D. (2015). Vaccination and all-cause child mortality from 1985 to 2011: Global evidence from the demographic and health surveys. *American Journal of Epidemiology, 182*(9), 791–798.

Panda, B. K., Kumar, G., & Mishra, S. (2020). Understanding the full-immunization gap in districts of India: a geospatial approach. *Clinical Epidemiology and Global Health, 8*(2), 536–543. https://doi.org/10.1016/j.cegh.2019.11.010

Pande, R. P. (2003). Selective gender differences in childhood nutrition and immunization in rural India: The role of siblings. *Demography, 40*(3), 395–418. https://doi.org/10.1353/dem.2003.0029

Pramanik, S., Muthusamy, N., Gera, R., & Laxminarayan, R. (2015). Vaccination coverage in India: A small area estimation approach. *Vaccine, 33*(14), 1731–1738. https://doi.org/10.1016/j.vaccine.2015.01.083

Prinja, S., Gupta, M., Singh, A., & Kumar, R. (2010). Effectiveness of planning and management interventions for improving age-appropriate immunization in rural India. *Bulletin of the World Health Organization, 88*(2), 97–103.

Rammahan, A., & Awefeso, N. (2015). District-level variations in childhood immunizations in India: The role of socioeconomic factors and health infrastructure. *Social Science & Medicine, 145*, 163–172.

Sankaranarayanan, S., Jayaraman, A., & Gopichandran, V. (2019). Assessment of vaccine hesitancy among parents of children between 1 and 5 years of age at a tertiary Care Hospital in Chennai. *Indian Journal of Community Medicine, 44*(4), 394–396. https://doi.org/10.4103/ijcm.IJCM_351_18

Solis-Soto, M. T., Paudel, D., & Nicoli, F. (2020). Relationship between vaccination and nutritional status in children. *Demographic Research, 42*, 1–14.

Srinivas, S. (2021). *The curious case of vaccine hesitancy in Tamil Nadu*. Available at https: //www.orfonline.org/expert-speak/the-curious-case-of-vaccine-hesitancy-in-tamil-nadu/

VanderEnde, K., Gacic-Dobo, M., Diallo, M. S., Conklin, L. M., & Wallace, A. S. (2018). Global routine vaccination coverage—2017. *Morbidity and Mortality Weekly Report, 67*(45), 1261.

Wariri, O., Nkereuwem, E., Erondu, N. A., Edem, B., Nkereuwem, O. O., Idoko, O. T., Agogo, E., Enegela, J. E., Sesay, T., Conde, I. S., Kaucley, L., Awuah, A. A.-A., Abdullahi, S., Luce, R. R., Banda, R., Nomhwange, T., & Kampmann, B. (2021). A scorecard of progress towards measles elimination in 15 West African countries, 2001–19: A retrospective, multicountry analysis of national immunisation coverage and surveillance data. *The Lancet Global Health, 9*(3), e280–e290. https://doi.org/10.1016/S2214-109X(20)30481-2

Chapter 16
Hysterectomy in India

Angad Singh and Dipti Govil

Globally, a hysterectomy is the second most frequently performed surgical procedure during the reproductive age after the cesarean section (Anjaneyulu et al., 2016). The operation involves the removal of the uterine corpus with or without the cervix and aims to cure various gynecological complaints, such as uterine cancer and other non-cancerous uterine conditions (fibroids, endometriosis, and prolapse). Many of these health problems are usually benign. For instance, in 2005–06, 81.4% of hysterectomies performed in Germany related to benign diseases of female genital organs (Stang et al., 2011). Hysterectomy artificially ends the reproductive functions and can have multiple adverse effects on women's health—apart from relief from dysfunctional uterine bleeding, pain, discomfort, stress, and improvement in the quality of life. These potential adverse effects include loss of femininity and self-esteem, increased chances of coronary heart disease, obesity, osteoporosis, lack of sexual desire, or depression.

The available research on hysterectomy worldwide stems primarily from clinical settings with a few community-based studies. These studies vary in the sample population and methodologies, making global comparison challenging. The evidence also shows that the prevalence of hysterectomy varies significantly between and within countries. The prevalence is relatively high in high-income countries compared to low- and middle-income countries. Between 20% and 40% of women in high-income countries have had a hysterectomy by age 60 (Rositch et al., 2014).

In contrast, the scenario changes when the uterus is removed for maternity-related causes. A study employing data on women with postpartum hemorrhage from

A. Singh (✉)
Office of Registrar General of India, New Delhi, India

D. Govil
International Institute for Population Sciences, Mumbai, India
e-mail: dgovil@iipsindia.ac.in

C. Z. Guilmoto (ed.), *Atlas of Gender and Health Inequalities in India*, Demographic Transformation and Socio-Economic Development 16,
https://doi.org/10.1007/978-3-031-47847-5_16

193 hospitals in 21 countries in Africa, Asia, Europe, and America found that hysterectomy was more common among mothers in Asia (7%) and Africa (5%) than Europe and America (3%) (Haque et al., 2019). The variation in hysterectomy rates is associated with advanced maternal age, cesarean section, multiple births, insurance status, change in uterine pathology and gender, and healthcare provider training, along with several demographic, social, and economic characteristics (Haque et al., 2019).

The Indian scenario slightly differs from that observed in other countries. A considerable proportion of variation exists in different geographical settings but differs by demographic parameters, economic standing, and social and cultural traits. Community-based studies from India show that the percentage of hysterectomies varies between 1.7 and 9.8 (Desai et al., 2011; Singh & Arora, 2008). Prusty et al. (2018), using data from the District Level Household Survey (2012–13), estimated the prevalence at 1.7 per 100 women, with a range of 0.2–6.3 per 100 women, while more than one-third of these cases had hysterectomy below age 40 years (Prusty et al., 2018). In the low-income settings of Gujarat, the hysterectomy rate was 2.1 per 100 women with a mean age of 36 years (Desai et al., 2017). Another study from Panchkula (Haryana) revealed a higher prevalence among women aged 35 years and above.

These studies have also examined the socioeconomic, demographic, and residence-related correlates of hysterectomies in different settings in India. Education plays a crucial role in deciding about a hysterectomy. In particular, it is observed that less-educated women are more likely to choose a hysterectomy as a solution to their gynecological problems (Lin et al., 2012; Stang et al., 2014). Women from lower-income strata also have a higher chance of having a hysterectomy than their higher-income counterparts (Desai et al., 2017; Lin et al., 2012). Furthermore, health insurance tends to increase the likelihood of a hysterectomy (Prusty et al., 2018), which raises concern about the possibility of misuse of insurance.

The unusual surge in the frequency of hysterectomies in some parts of the country as a routine treatment of gynecological ailments, especially among young women, has brought the issue to public debate. Several researchers and activists questioned the reasons for this increase and have suggested that hysterectomies are, at times, more related to commercial gains than actual medical needs (Acharya, 2017; Chaudhuri, 2013). With this backdrop, we examined how hysterectomy has been expanded across regions and identified some of its determinants.

Materials and Methods

NFHS is the first nationwide survey to provide information on hysterectomy, allowing the estimation of incidence at the national and sub-national levels.[1] Before this, the previous three rounds of NFHSs collected passive information on the

[1] The original NFHS dataset and the spatial analysis methodology are described in detail in Chap. 1.

indicator, where "menopause/had hysterectomy" was one of the answer categories for the questions on menstruation and contraceptive use. Lack of direct information and combined data on menopause/hysterectomy was unsuitable for calculating the estimates; hence, it was not utilized. Another large-scale survey, the District Level Health Survey (DLHS 4) in 2012–13, also collected information on hysterectomies but could not provide nation-level estimates. Several small-scale studies conducted in rural or urban settings by individual researchers across the country offer local-level estimates. Also, in recent years, media reports have highlighted several hysterectomies conducted in various districts, villages, and towns (Ramanan, 2019). These reports and studies, however, do not provide robust national or regional estimates of the prevalence of hysterectomies.

NFHS-5 canvased four questions related to hysterectomy to all women (married and unmarried):

- Some women undergo an operation to remove the uterus. Have you undergone such an operation?
- If yes, how many years ago was this operation (hysterectomy) performed?
- Where was this operation performed?
- Why was this operation performed? Any other reason?

The prevalence of hysterectomy used in our analysis has been derived from the first question by identifying women who had a hysterectomy. Since the incidence rate is relatively low among younger women, the analysis has been restricted to women aged 30 years and above (340,126 women), and the prevalence of hysterectomy is calculated as the number of hysterectomies per 100 women aged 30–49 years.

To assess the determinants of hysterectomy, we selected the following socioeconomic and demographic covariates based on our literature review: five-year age group of the women aged 30–49, place of residence (rural and urban), religion (Hindu, Muslim, and others), caste (scheduled castes, scheduled tribes, other backward classes, and others), and wealth index (poorest, poor, middle, rich and richest), and region (North, North-central, South, East, Central, North-East). Apart from these, parity of women (no children, one, two, and three or more children), the status of female sterilization, and insurance status of the household (not insured, insured).

The analysis has been divided into two sections. In the first section, we examine the district-level situation with the help of mapping and geostatistical analysis. In the second section, we run a logistic regression to identify the determinants of hysterectomy. Appropriate sampling weights were applied to generate representative estimates.

The data on hysterectomy is expected to be of good quality because of strict data quality measures adopted during data collection during the survey. This indicator presents some limitations since it is based on self-assessment/reporting with no verification of medical documents performed during the survey. This situation may lead to underestimating or overestimating the hysterectomy prevalence. Second, the information on hysterectomy is only collected for women in the reproductive ages, excluding women above 49 years of age; therefore, it may again underestimate the prevalence. Finally, we may add that the data on hysterectomies are fragile as there are, on average, only 32 hysterectomies per district.

Results

In India, 3.3% of women aged 15–49 underwent a hysterectomy (3.6% in rural and 2.5% in urban areas); this is within the range of the estimates provided by other Indian studies (Prusty et al., 2018). As expected, the prevalence of hysterectomy increases with age. It ranges from 2.1% for women in their early thirties to 11.6% for those in their late forties. After age 35, a surge in the prevalence of hysterectomy can be observed; it indicates the poor management of pre-menopausal symptoms. We can indirectly compute the age at hysterectomy from the age of surveyed women and the reported operation date. Nearly half of the women underwent a hysterectomy between ages 30 and 40, with a mean age at hysterectomy of 33.8 years in India.

The mapping underlines the considerable variations in the prevalence of hysterectomy among women aged 15–49 across Indian states, union territories, and districts. For example, two South Indian states, Andhra Pradesh (8.7%) and Telangana (8.2%), top the list of higher prevalence of hysterectomy, followed by Bihar (6.0%) and Gujarat (3.9%). Conversely, hysterectomy rates (less than 2%) that are significantly lower than elsewhere are also reported in the Northeast, Lakshadweep, and Delhi.

The district-level map (Fig. 16.1) illustrates the wide disparities in the prevalence of hysterectomy among women aged 15–49, with measured rates varying from 0% to 17%. 21 districts record a moderately higher prevalence of hysterectomies, ranging from 8% to 10%. 18 districts display a high prevalence level, with over 10% of women reporting hysterectomy. Most of the latter districts are spread across Andhra Pradesh, Telangana, and Bihar, as well as in pockets of West India. The sub-regional disparity can also be highlighted with the extreme frequency of hysterectomies reaching 16.7% in Warangal (Telangana), 12.4% in Purba Champaran (Bihar) or 13.1% in Prakasam (Andhra Pradesh).

In contrast, we see large swaths where hysterectomy rates are uniformly below 4%, notably in central India and the Northeast. These areas are predominantly less industrialized, often home to tribal populations, and exposed to natural calamities. Several of the districts in these regions, especially the Northeast, rely on the public health system for healthcare needs, emphasizing the role of the private sector in the rising hysterectomies. Kerala's situation appears to stand out with comparatively fewer hysterectomy cases, whereas the rest of South India tends to record hysterectomy rates higher than the national average.

The spatial analysis underscores the regional homogeneity in the distribution of hysterectomy rates. The LISA map of spatial clusters, presented in Fig. 16.1, points to a rather high value of Moran's I (0.68), suggesting striking distinct spatial patterning. The cluster analysis further emphasizes two primary hotspot regions. The most salient cluster emerges in the Telugu-speaking states of Andhra Pradesh

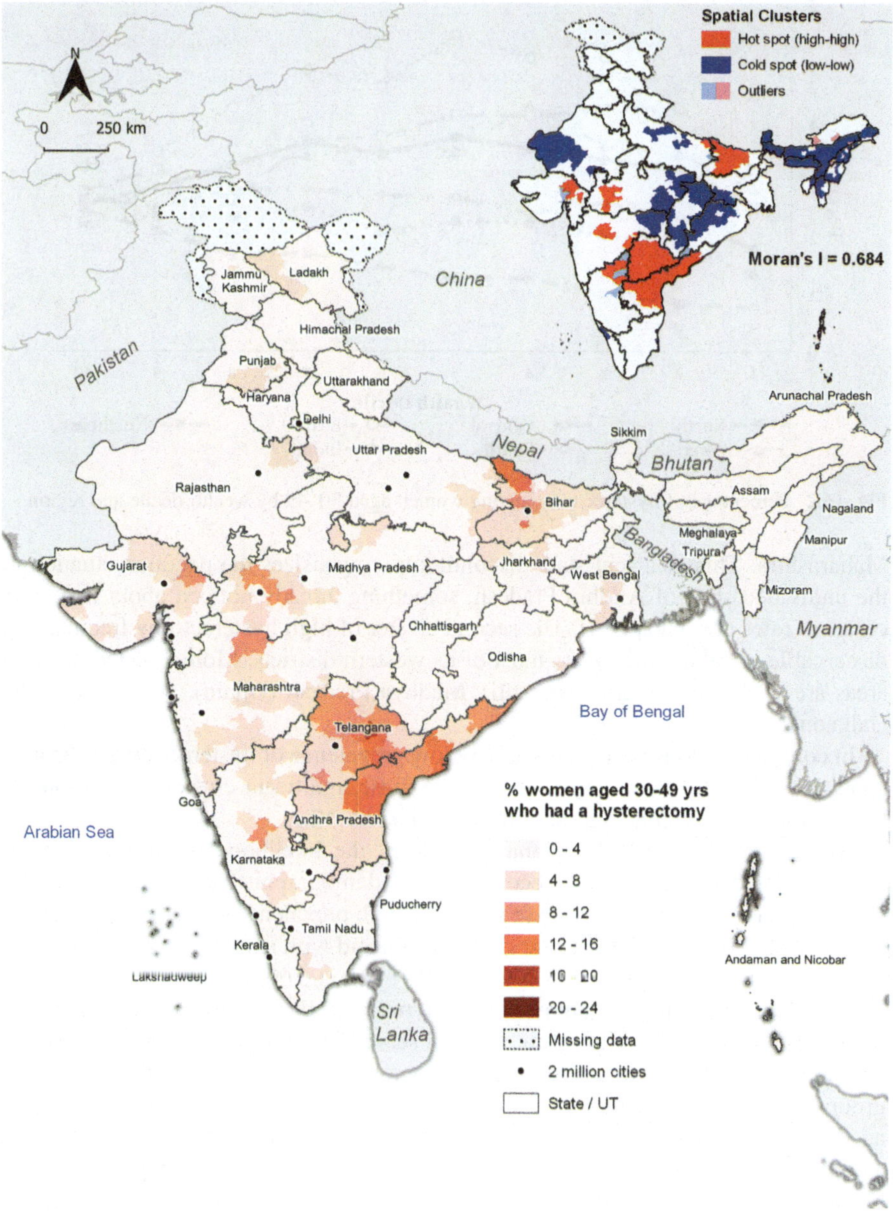

Fig. 16.1 Percentage of women aged 30–49 years who had a hysterectomy
Source: NFHS-5, 2019–21
The map is for illustrative purposes and may not represent official boundaries

and Telangana, extending to nearby Karnataka. This region closely follows administrative boundaries as hysterectomy rates are abruptly divided by a factor of 3 or 4 when we examine rates in the bordering districts of Odisha, Chhattisgarh, or

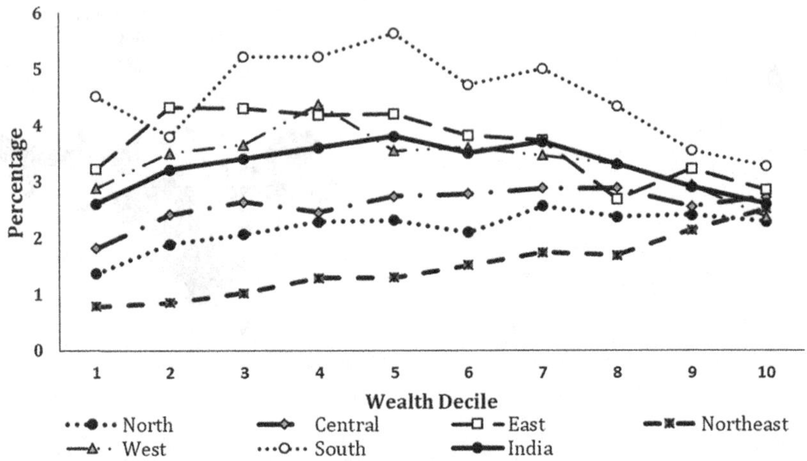

Fig. 16.2 Percentage of hysterectomy among women aged 30–49 by wealth decile and region

Maharashtra. This clear-cut state discontinuity emphasizes the peculiar situation of the undivided state of Andhra Pradesh, something already noticed about its higher cesarean rates (see Chap. 14). The second cluster of high hysterectomy frequency is discernable in Bihar and covers most of its western districts. More isolated hot-spot areas are visible in Gujarat (Aravalli), Madhya Pradesh (Ujjain), and Maharashtra (Jalgaon).

In contrast, regions with an extremely low prevalence of hysterectomies (the cold spots) are more scattered across India. The most significant clusters correspond to the Northeast and Chhattisgarh, with rates close to 0%.

Apart from the marked regional variations, the likelihood of hysterectomy is closely related to various socioeconomic and demographic factors. Other studies document the share of the private sector in the high prevalence of hysterectomy: 62% (Desai et al., 2017), 68% (Shekhar et al., 2019), and with similar patterns across age groups: 65.7% (15–29 years), 71.3% (30–39 years), and 66.6% (40–49 years) (Desai et al., 2019). Interestingly, in most northeastern states, hysterectomies are done in the public sector. Since the highest rates are observed in the three regions (east, south, and west), it was worth presenting the regional variation with other economic groups. Figure 16.2 demonstrates that hysterectomy prevalence among women aged 15–49 increased by wealth decile from 2.6% in the first and poorest decile and plateaued at 3.5–3.8% in the fourth to seventh decile. The percentage of hysterectomy declines in the last three deciles and reaches 2.6% for women in the wealthiest decile. This inverted U-shape is mirrored in several regions where hysterectomy is more common. This feature is especially true for South India, where hysterectomy rates peak at 5.6% among intermediate-income groups. In contrast, regions where hysterectomy is less prevalent, such as the Northeast and North India, display a more linear relationship whereby the frequency of hysterectomy gradually increases by one percentage point or less as we move up the socioeconomic scale.

The logistic regression of the probability of hysterectomy among women aged 30–49 years highlights the most social and economic significant factors behind variations in hysterectomy rates (Fig. 16.3).[2] It corroborates the solid positive link between hysterectomy and age. Likewise, the frequency of hysterectomy rises with parity, with women with two children or more recording the highest odds of hysterectomy. The regional variations examined earlier are confirmed by the multivariate analysis, with the Northeast recording the lowest rates and South and East India the highest.

It also confirms the strong rural gradient of hysterectomy, which appears less frequent in cities and towns despite their better health infrastructures. Intriguingly,

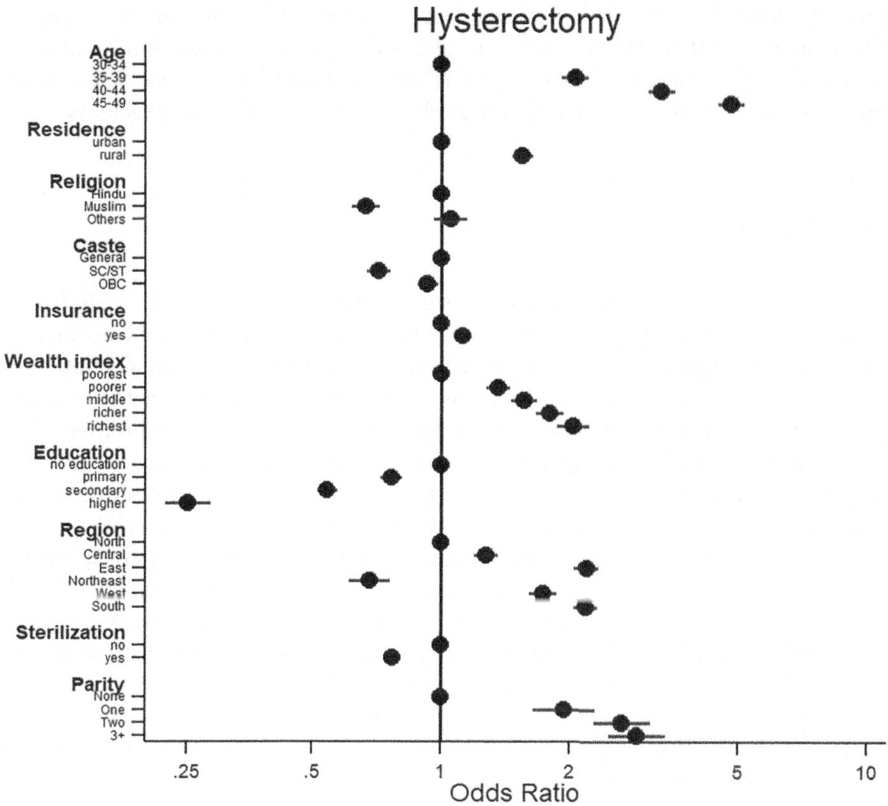

Fig. 16.3 Odds ratios of hysterectomy among women aged 30–49 by selected background characteristics
Source: NFHS 5

[2]Odds ratios measure the strength of the correlation with the outcome variable. Values above (below) one correspond to a positive (negative) association.

the correlations between education and socioeconomic status are inverted. Women from wealthier households experience far more frequent hysterectomies than those from the poorest group. In contrast, education (when socioeconomic status is controlled) reduces the risk of hysterectomy. This result means that affluence *sans* education places women at particular risk of unnecessary hysterectomies. Other interesting social correlates may also be noted. For example, lower-caste and tribal populations record higher hysterectomy prevalence, while rates are the lowest among Muslims.

The analysis confirms that hysterectomy is slightly more common among women from insured households, which suggests an association between unwarranted hysterectomy operations and the profit incentives under the national health insurance scheme and the private health sector. Given this situation, some states restricted publicly funded insurance coverage for hysterectomies in private facilities (Devulanpalli, 2012). Hysterectomy is also linked to or perhaps confused with family planning, especially in rural areas, as evidenced by the fact that women with sterilization have significantly fewer chances to undergo a hysterectomy.[3]

Conclusion

Whether rural or urban, India is witnessing a substantial growth in the number of hysterectomy operations, a trend that may correspond to a growing medicalization of the womb. The map highlights distinct regional inequalities and the concentration of hysterectomy operations in specific areas such as undivided Andhra Pradesh and parts of Bihar and Gujarat. This significant clustering that does not proceed from these regions' specific demographic, social, or economic characteristics requires deeper investigations to understand the root cause of the potential overuse of hysterectomy. Several community-based studies and newspaper articles also report similar rates in these regions. While hysterectomies may often be lifesaving operations, medical professionals agree that some are unwarranted and could be avoided. Hysterectomy is sometimes perceived as a routine operation to remedy common menstrual problems and is considered an easy remedy to prevent menstruation and improve the day-to-day life of working women.[4]

Furthermore, the role of the uterus beyond reproductive functions is often poorly understood by women, and some of them opt for a hysterectomy when they want to stop childbearing, be it for family planning reasons or to get relief from menstruation. Our analysis indicates that women with insurance are more likely to have

[3]For a more detailed analysis based on NFHS-4 figures, see Singh and Govil (2021).

[4]Reportedly, more than half of the women in parts of Beed in Maharashtra did not have wombs, notably because cane-cutting contractors were unwilling to hire menstruating women (Jadhav, 2019). The latest NFHS-5 did not corroborate this high value.

undergone a hysterectomy, but poor education is also a strong correlate of the frequency of hysterectomy.

Though the prevalence of hysterectomy is far less than in many other countries, monitoring the trends in hysterectomy prevalence is of great importance in India. The low mean age at hysterectomy postulates that women may experience menopausal symptoms at a young age, adversely affecting their mental, physical, and sexual health. Educating women on their reproductive rights and providing informed choices and government intervention will help avoid hysterectomies for benign causes. Additionally, in-depth studies on the epidemiology of hysterectomy in India's most affected districts will help to understand the interplay of factors at various levels.

References

Acharya, S. K. (2017). Womb, womanhood and medical ethics: Concern about rising hysterectomy cases in India. *Journal of Family Planning and Reproductive Health Care, 43*(2), 165–166. https://doi.org/10.1136/jfprhc-2016-101649

Anjaneyulu, G., Kumar, M., Deepika, P., Alekhya, R., & Harika, P. (2016). The profile of hysterectomized women from an urban slum of Hyderabad, Telangana state, India. *International Journal of Community Medicine and Public Health, 3*(9), 3633–3636.

Chaudhuri, M. (2013). Women's groups and fertility experts campaign to reduce prevalence of hysterectomy in India. *BMJ, 347*. https://doi.org/10.1136/bmj.f7551

Desai, S., Sinha, T., & Mahal, A. (2011). Prevalence of hysterectomy among rural and urban women with and without health insurance in Gujarat, India. *Reproductive Health Matters, 19*(37), 42–51. https://doi.org/10.1016/S0968-8080(11)37553-2

Desai, S., Campbell, O. M., Sinha, T., Mahal, A., & Cousens, S. (2017). Incidence and determinants of hysterectomy in a low-income setting in Gujarat, India. *Health Policy and Planning, 32*(1), 68–78. https://doi.org/10.1093/heapol/czw099

Desai, S., Shukla, A., Nambiar, D., & Ved, R. (2019). Patterns of hysterectomy in India: A national and state-level analysis of the Fourth National Family Health Survey (2015–2016). *BJOG: An International Journal of Obstetrics and Gynaecology, 126*(S4), 72–80. https://doi.org/10.1111/1471-0528.15858

Devulanpalli, R. (2012, September 28). Secret behind rash of hysterectomies out. *The Times of India*. https://timesofindia.indiatimes.com/city/hyderabad/Secret-behind-rash-of-hysterectomies-out/articleshow/16580758.cms

Haque, I., Das, D., & Patel, P. (2019). Reading the geography of India's district level fertility differentials: A spatial econometric approach. *Journal of Biosocial Science, 51*, 745–774. https://doi.org/10.1017/S0021932019000087

Jadhav, R. (2019, April 8). Why many women in Maharashtra's Beed district have no wombs. *The Hindu*. https://www.thehindubusinessline.com/economy/agri-business/why-half-the-women-in-maharashtras-beed-district-have-no-wombs/article26773974.ece

Lin, L.-P., Hsieh, M., Chen, S.-F., Wu, C.-L., Hsu, S.-W., & Lin, J.-D. (2012). Factors related to hysterectomy in women with physical and mobility disabilities. *Research in Developmental Disabilities, 33*(4), 990–995. https://doi.org/10.1016/j.ridd.2012.01.002

Prusty, R. K., Choithani, C., & Gupta, S. D. (2018). Predictors of hysterectomy among married women 15–49 years in India. *Reproductive Health, 15*(1), 3. https://doi.org/10.1186/s12978-017-0445-8

Ramanan, S. (2019, November 19). Here is why hysterectomy cases in India are rising. *The Hindu*. https://www.thehindubusinessline.com/news/science/here-is-why-hysterectomy-cases-in-india-are-rising/article30017810.ece#: ~: text=A%20new%20study%20has%20indicated,surgical%20procedure%20for%20uterus%20removal
Rositch, A. F., Nowak, R. G., & Gravitt, P. E. (2014). Increased age and race-specific incidence of cervical cancer after correction for hysterectomy prevalence in the United States from 2000 to 2009. *Cancer, 120*(13), 2032–2038. https://doi.org/10.1002/cncr.28548
Shekhar, C., Paswan, B., & Singh, A. (2019). Prevalence, sociodemographic determinants and self-reported reasons for hysterectomy in India. *Reproductive Health, 16*(1), 118.
Singh, A., & Arora, A. K. (2008). Why hysterectomy rates are lower in India. *Indian Journal of Community Medicine, 33*(3), 196–197. https://doi.org/10.4103/0970-0218.42065
Singh, A., & Govil, D. (2021). Hysterectomy in India: Spatial and multilevel analysis. *Women's Health, 17*, 17455065211017068.
Stang, A., Merrill, R. M., & Kuss, O. (2011). Hysterectomy in Germany. *Deutsches Ärzteblatt International, 108*(30), 508–514. https://doi.org/10.3238/arztebl.2011.0508
Stang, A., Kluttig, A., Moebus, S., Völzke, H., Berger, K., Greiser, K. H., & Meisinger, C. (2014). Educational level, prevalence of hysterectomy, and age at amenorrhea: A cross-sectional analysis of 9536 women from six population-based cohort studies in Germany. *BMC Women's Health, 14*(1), 1–9. https://doi.org/10.1186/1472-6874-14-10

Chapter 17
Health Insurance Coverage in India

Bertrand Lefebvre

For the past 20 years, India has led an ambitious policy promoting health insurance. At the national and state levels, programs have multiplied to improve the protection and coverage of the population concerning health expenses. At the turn of the 2000s, the level of out-of-pocket payment was exceptionally high in India, with 74% of the total health expenditures according to WHO (2022) and 32.5 million persons falling below the poverty line in 1999–2000 because of health expenses (Garg & Karan, 2009). The development of health insurance programs targeting the most economically vulnerable groups was seen in India as a priority to meet the Millennium Development Goals (MDGs) and to encourage the development of Universal Health Coverage (UHC). This policy, which materialized in 2008 with the launch of the Rashtriya Swasthya Bima Yojana (RSBY), was not India's first attempt to develop health insurance and social protection. Since the creation of the Employees' State Insurance (ESI) in 1952 and the Central Government Health Scheme (CGHS) in 1954, the central government has aimed to develop social and health protection for its citizens. At the time, these programs were seen as the first steps before an extension to the entire population (Jeffery, 1988). Later, in the 1980s, Community-Based Health Insurance schemes (CBHI) were created to provide better protection for the rural population and the poor (Devadasan et al., 2004).

The 1980s and 1990s were also marked by the insurance sector's liberalization and new private players' arrival (Purohit, 2001). By the mid-2000s, only 5% of households were covered by health insurance (NFHS 3). The low penetration of health insurance at that time could be explained by a lack of financial support from the government, the substantial weight of the informal sector, and the difficulty in developing a regulatory and legislative framework for integrating a fragmented care system (patients, health services). In the 2000s, the development of

B. Lefebvre (✉)
French Institute of Pondicherry, Pondicherry, India
e-mail: bertrand.lefebvre@ifpindia.org

C. Z. Guilmoto (ed.), *Atlas of Gender and Health Inequalities in India*, Demographic Transformation and Socio-Economic Development 16,
https://doi.org/10.1007/978-3-031-47847-5_17

government-sponsored health insurance schemes (GSHIS) was seen as the best way to meet the threefold challenge posed by the Indian health system: improving access to care for the most economically marginalized patients, offering a wide range of accessible care by reaching to the private health sector, and pooling financial resources to ensure the budgetary sustainability of the system (La Forgia & Nagpal, 2012). Today, the NITI Aayog estimates that a health insurance program covers nearly 70% of the population, with 700 million individuals covered by the Ayushman Bharat—Pradhan Mantri Jan Arogya Yojana (AB-PMJAY) and state government extension schemes (Sarwal & Kumar, 2021).

Questions remain about the actual expansion of health insurance coverage in the population, while programs have multiplied at the national level (RSBY, AB-PMJAY) or the state level. Moreover, the growth of government-sponsored programs has not coincided with the same resources or model across India. The NFHS-5 data make it possible to shed some light on the persistent inequalities in the health insurance coverage of the population. They also make it possible to review the sometimes complex trajectories of these national and local programs between complementarity and competition.

Data Source and Methods

The NFHS has been measuring household health insurance coverage since 2005–06.[1] This period was critical as new health insurance programs were being unrolled in India (launch in 2003 of the Yeshavini scheme in Karnataka and of the Universal Health Insurance Scheme) and when governments at the local and national levels initiated plans for ambitious health insurance programs to fight poverty and improve social protection. In addition, Universal Health Coverage was also gaining momentum in global health policies as health insurance programs were being introduced in different regions of the world with promising results (like the 30-Baht scheme in Thailand in 2002).

The information collected in the NFHS questionnaires concerns the presence of a member covered by health insurance and the type of insurance used (NFHS-3 questions 64–65, NFHS-4 questions 54–55, NFHS-5 questions 71–72). The health insurance categories presented in the NFHS cover most national programs (ESIS, CGHS) and increase from 7 to 9 categories, starting with NFHS-4 (2015–16) by incorporating the RSBY and the State Health Insurance Scheme. These different categories highlight the diversity of existing programs and the sector's fragmentation between private health insurance, direct employer reimbursements, subsidized programs, and community-based programs.

There is no data on the actual use of these insurance programs in the NFHS surveys, while questions are asked about the use of and access to health services or

[1] The original NFHS dataset and the spatial analysis methodology are described in detail in Chap. 1.

other public health programs. It should also be noted that it is difficult to compare results from different surveys for each state because of changes in the sampling design in some small states. The recent roll-out of the AB-PMJAY at the time of the NFHS-5 surveys (2019–21) might not have been adequately accounted for in some states. Finally, the health insurance questions are at the household level, not the individual level, preventing a more refined analysis of the coverage inequalities among the population.

Results

At the national level, the latest NFHS-5 results confirm the rise of health insurance in Indian households. From 29% in 2015–16 (NFHS-4), the share of households with at least one member covered by health insurance has now climbed to 41%. Between the NFHS-3 and NFHS-5, the share of households covered by health insurance increased eight-fold nationally. However, there are gaps between rural (42%) and urban (38%) households or between males (30%) and females (33%) aged 15–49 in terms of health insurance coverage. The bottom income quintile remains with the lowest proportion of households covered by health insurance (36.1%), but the increase between NFHS-4 and NFHS-5 was more significant in this quintile than in other income groups (+14.5 pt. vs. 12.3 pt.). A similar catch-up can be observed over this period for the Scheduled Tribes households (+16 pt.), which now have the highest coverage level (46.8%) compared to other groups (SC, OBC, Others).

However, this significant increase over the past 15 years appears to have partly stalled between the NFHS-4 and NFHS-5 rounds. Estimates of health insurance coverage point to diverging regional trajectories, ranging from sustained growth to stagnation or even decline (Fig. 17.1). The impact of NFHS sample size must be

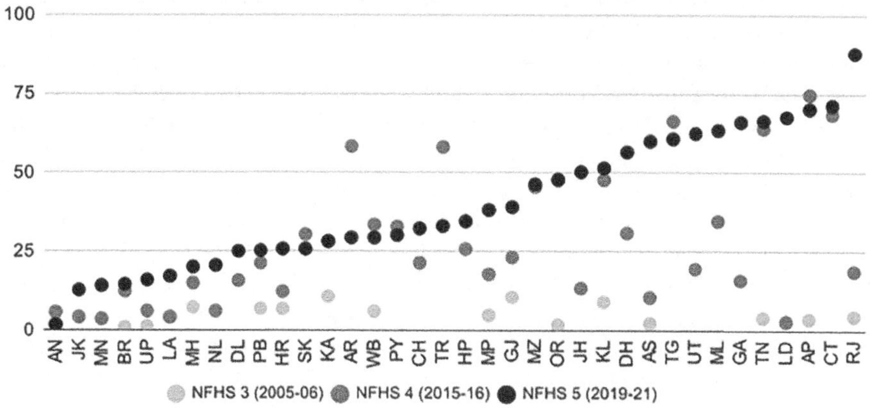

Fig. 17.1 Percentage of households covered by health insurance by state in 2005–21
Source: NFHS 3, NFHS 4, NFHS 5

considered, especially in small states. The sharp decline in household coverage between NFHS-4 and NFHS-5 (−33 pt.) in Tripura state is partly explained by the creation of eight new districts and its effect on district-level sample size in this state (IIPS and IFC, 2021). In Arunachal Pradesh (−29 pt.), the local government-sponsored health insurance scheme (APCMUHIS), launched in 2014, was discontinued at the end of 2016 because of administrative and funding difficulties. It was not until late 2018, a few months before the start of NFHS-5 surveys in Arunachal Pradesh, that a new AB-PMJAY-supported scheme re-emerged for households in the state.

In several Southern states, such as Andhra Pradesh (70.2%), Telangana (60.8%), and Tamil Nadu (66.5%), the already high level of household coverage recorded during the NFHS-4 stagnated or fell back a few points in NFHS-5. Several large states, such as Maharashtra (20%), Karnataka (28.1%), and West Bengal (29.3%), have experienced no significant changes, and their coverage rates remain below the national average. The same observation applies to the heavily populated and poorer states of Bihar (14.5%) and Uttar Pradesh (15.9%), where the proportion of households covered by health insurance remains well below the national average. Other states in the north and south stand out for their robust increase in household coverage between NFHS-4 and NFHS-5. Rajasthan, Goa, Uttarakhand, and Assam present spectacular gains of over 40 points in five years.

Only 318 of 707 districts have values above the mean (42.5%, Median 38.7%). The standard deviation (0.239) and coefficient of variation (0.562) indicate significant differences at the district level. Mapping the share of households with at least one member covered by health insurance by district gives us an even clearer picture of the importance of considering the state level (Fig. 17.2). Along with the analysis of the distribution of values (Fig. 17.3), the district map helps distinguish several broad regional clusters. The high value of Moran's *I* index (0.737) suggests a solid spatial autocorrelation. The distribution of High-High clusters (hot spots) and Low-Low clusters (cold spots) broadly follows state boundaries. Tamil Nadu, Andhra Pradesh, Telangana, and Chhattisgarh districts stand out for having a share of households covered by health insurance ([51–90%]) distinctly above the national mean and median. Local government-sponsored health insurance schemes cover more than 70% of insured households in these states. Launched over 15 years ago, programs such as the Aarogyasri Health Insurance Scheme in Andhra Pradesh or the Chief Minister's Comprehensive Health Insurance Scheme (CMCHIS) in Tamil Nadu have allowed optimal coverage of the population and the territory. The neighboring districts of Kerala, Odisha, and Jharkhand also have household coverage rates higher than the national average but to a lesser degree ([35–70%]). Over 70% of insured households in these states are covered by national health insurance schemes (RSBY or AB-PMJAY). Three other High-High clusters have emerged between the NFHS-4 and the NFHS-5 in Rajasthan, Uttarakhand, and Northeast India (Assam, Meghalaya), again driven by local or national expansion of government health insurance programs that cover more than 70% of insured households. The gap with neighboring states in northern India is particularly notable.

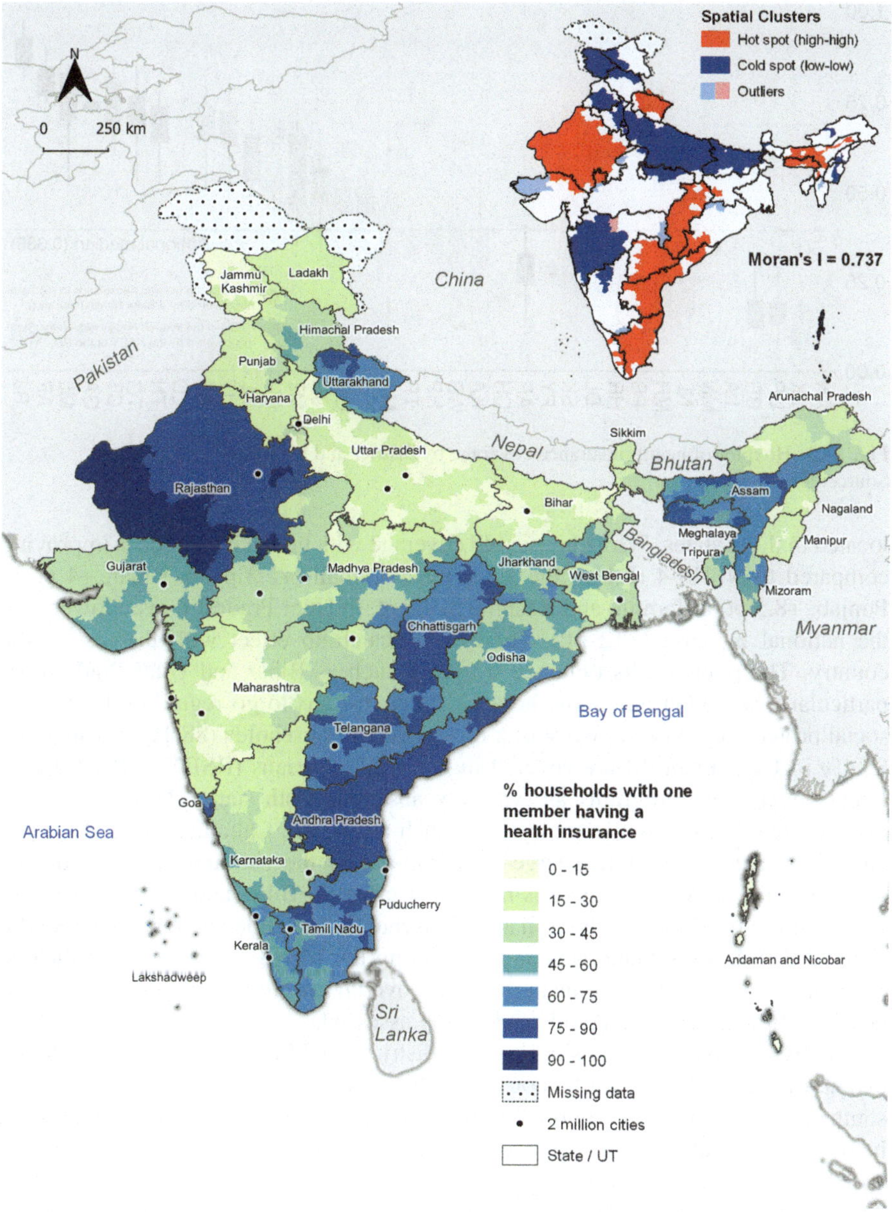

Fig. 17.2 Percentage of households with at least one member enrolled in health insurance
Source: NFHS-5, 2019–21
The map is for illustrative purposes and may not represent official boundaries

A large Low-Low cluster is emerging from Jammu and Kashmir through Punjab, Haryana, Delhi, and Uttar Pradesh to Bihar. No district in this vast cluster reaches the national average ([5–38%]). Thirty-nine of India's 50 worst-performing districts are

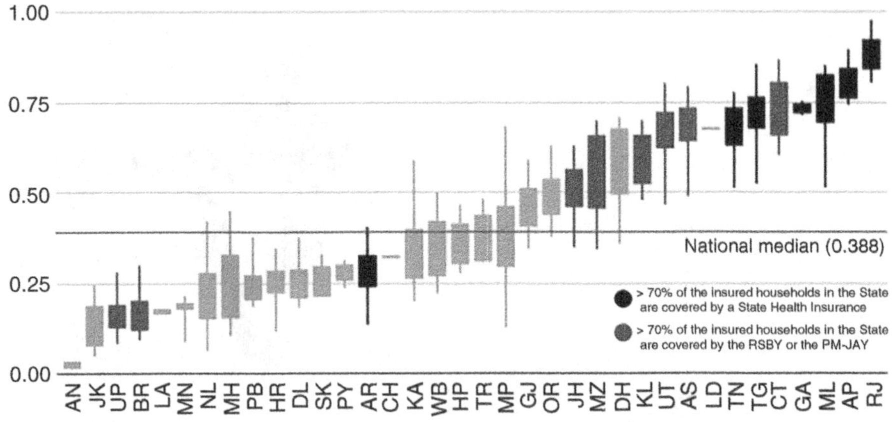

Fig. 17.3 Boxplot of health insurance coverage by district and by state
Source: NFHS 5

located in these states. While household coverage with health insurance is improving compared to NFHS-4 results, the gains remain small (+2.2 pt. in Bihar, +4 pt. in Punjab, +8.5 pt. in Jammu and Kashmir, +9.8 pt. in Uttar Pradesh), even lower than the national increase (+12 pt.). There is no catch-up effect with the rest of the country. The poor results obtained by states such as Bihar and Uttar Pradesh are particularly worrying and show how far India still has to go regarding health and social protection. In these two states, most insured households (88.1% in Bihar and 85.4% in Uttar Pradesh) are covered by national programs (RSBY, AB-PMJAY). Local government programs are virtually absent in both states (less than 2% of insured households). While some states, such as Assam, Chhattisgarh, and Kerala, have been able to support a large-scale roll-out of the national health insurance scheme at the local level, there is no similar effect in Bihar and Uttar Pradesh. In several states like Madhya Pradesh and Himachal Pradesh, the move from the RSBY to the AB-PMJAY scheme was ongoing during the NFHS-5 survey. Nevertheless, the real impact of such a transition on the overall enrollment of households into health insurance schemes could not be fully assessed.

Finally, the particular position of the districts of Maharashtra and, to a lesser extent, of Karnataka should be noted. In contrast to other neighboring states in the south or west of India, the share of households covered by health insurance remains below the national average for most of these districts ([10–59%]). At the time of the NFHS-3 in 2005–06, these states occupied two of the top three spots regarding household health insurance coverage, albeit at low levels (<10% of the households surveyed). In addition, Karnataka supported the development of the Yeshasvini health insurance scheme targeted at informal sector workers. The progress of health coverage in Karnataka and Maharashtra remains below the national trend, while the registration of households living below the poverty line is high in both states.

Discussion and Conclusion

The NFHS-5 data comes at a pivotal time for health insurance coverage in India with the launch of the AB-PMJAY in 2018. It may have come too early to measure the real impact of AB-PMJAY on household health insurance coverage, especially for specific regions in northern India. Based on available results, AB-PMJAY seems to have boosted some small states, especially in northeastern India. As highlighted by some in-depth analysis of the NFHS-4 results (Khan et al., 2021), variations in health insurance coverage can be attributed to specific geographic level effects (State, District, communities) even after adjusting for household demographic and socio-economic differences. The excellent performance of the southern states shows that solid political stewardship coupled with government-led programs can help achieve excellent health insurance coverage results. In states such as Haryana, Maharashtra, and Punjab, where household registration and outreach activities have been left to private insurers and Third Party Administrators (TPAs), health insurance coverage has remained below expectations (Khetrapal & Acharya, 2019; Thakur, 2016; Wagle & Shah, 2017).

The uneven development of the private health insurance sector across India might also explain why the RSBY and other government-sponsored schemes that relied heavily on the involvement of private partners have failed in several parts of northern India. For example, in Kerala, the RSBY has been designed to cover more households beyond BPL ones and to support the redevelopment of public hospitals by bringing more revenues to them and improving the quality of medical care (Palacios et al., 2011). Bridging the gap between national objectives and local health systems realities will be essential for AB-PMJAY's success. Beyond improving household health insurance coverage, monitoring the scheme's usage and impact on OOPs and health outcomes will be essential to assess the AB-PMJAY. Based on the study of state-sponsored health insurance schemes in India, there is a lack of evidence that these schemes make a difference in improving access to health services or offering financial protection (Prinja et al., 2019; Garg et al., 2020).

References

Devadasan, N., Ranson, K., Van Damme, W., & Criel, B. (2004). Community health Insurance in India: An overview. *Economic and Political Weekly, 39*(28), 3179–3183.

Garg, C. C., & Karan, A. K. (2009). Reducing out-of-pocket expenditures to reduce poverty: A disaggregated analysis at rural-urban and state level in India. *Health Policy and Planning, 24*(2), 116–128. https://doi.org/10.1093/heapol/czn046

Garg, S., Bebarta, K. K., & Tripathi, N. (2020). Performance of India's national publicly funded health insurance scheme, Pradhan Mantri Jan Arogaya Yojana (PMJAY), in improving access and financial protection for hospital care: Findings from household surveys in Chhattisgarh state. *BMC Public Health, 20*(1), 949. https://doi.org/10.1186/s12889-020-09107-4

International Institute for Population Sciences (IIPS) and ICF. (2021). *National family health survey (NFHS-5), India, 2019–21: Tripura*. IIPS.

Jeffery, R. (1988). *The politics of health in India*. University of California Press.

Khan, P. K., Perkins, J. M., Kim, R., Mohanty, S. K., & Subramanian, S. V. (2021). Multilevel population and socioeconomic variation in health insurance coverage in India. *Tropical Medicine and International Health, 26*(10), 1285–1295. https://doi.org/10.1111/tmi.13645

Khetrapal, S., & Acharya, A. (2019). Expanding healthcare coverage: An experience from Rashtriya Swasthya Bima Yojna. *The Indian Journal of Medical Research, 149*(3), 369–375. https://doi.org/10.4103/ijmr.IJMR_1419_18

La Forgia, G., & Nagpal, S. (2012). *Government-sponsored health Insurance in India: Are you covered?* The World Bank. https://doi.org/10.1596/978-0-8213-9618-6

Palacios, R., Das, J., & Sun, C. (2011). *Evidence from the early experience of the Rashtriya Swasthya Bima Yojana*. Centre for Policy Research.

Prinja, S., Bahuguna, P., Gupta, I., Chowdhury, S., & Trivedi, M. (2019). Role of insurance in determining utilization of healthcare and financial risk protection in India. *PLoS One, 14*(2), e0211793. https://doi.org/10.1371/journal.pone.0211793

Purohit, B. C. (2001). Private initiatives and policy options: Recent health system experience in India. *Health Policy and Planning, 16*(1), 87–97. https://doi.org/10.1093/heapol/16.1.87

Sarwal, R., & Kumar, A. (2021). *Health Insurance for India's missing middle* [Preprint]. Open Science Framework. https://doi.org/10.31219/osf.io/s2x8r

Thakur, H. (2016). Study of awareness, enrollment, and utilization of Rashtriya Swasthya Bima Yojana (National Health Insurance Scheme) in Maharashtra, India. *Frontiers in Public Health, 3*. https://doi.org/10.3389/fpubh.2015.00282

Wagle, S., & Shah, N. (2017). *Government funded health insurance scheme in Maharashtra: Study of Rajiv Gandhi Jeevandayee Aarogya Yojana*. CEHAT.

World Health Organization. (2022). *Global Health Expenditure database*. Retrieved on January 30, 2022, https://apps.who.int/nha/database

Part IV
Reproduction

Chapter 18
Fertility Differentials in India

Ismail Haque and Md Juel Rana

There have been growing concerns about population, food production, and the environment. Although fertility patterns across the globe have changed markedly over the last few decades and fertility has reached unprecedented low levels, there remain striking differences in level and reproduction patterns across countries and regions. Examining fertility variation between and within countries is crucial to addressing population issues effectively. Most of the countries with higher fertility are coming from the African continent. Asian countries exhibit low to high fertility levels, while South Asian countries have medium to low fertility levels. Among South Asian countries, understanding the fertility pattern of India is crucial due to its vast birth size (about 24 million births every year) and significant variation in fertility indicators by socioeconomic categories and geographical regions.

Since the 1950s, population dynamics in India have witnessed significant changes concerning its socioeconomic development and the early adoption of family planning programs. In the last seven decades, fertility (TFR) has declined from six children per woman in the 1950s to 2.0 in 2020, according to the latest SRS figures. The decadal growth rate has declined from 21.3% during 1991–2001 to 17.7% during 2001–2011. Despite reaching the replacement level of fertility, the population momentum in India will induce a continued increase in population in the next three or four decades. In the past few decades, the fertility transition across the regions of India has been witnessed in various ways. Different states of India have experienced various trajectories of fertility decline that result in diverse geographical variations in the fertility levels in the country. The South Indian states first kicked off the fertility

I. Haque (✉)
Jamia Millia Islamia (A Central University), New Delhi, India
e-mail: ihaque@jmi.ac.in

Md. J. Rana
G.B. Pant Social Science Institute, Prayagraj, India

C. Z. Guilmoto (ed.), *Atlas of Gender and Health Inequalities in India*, Demographic Transformation and Socio-Economic Development 16,
https://doi.org/10.1007/978-3-031-47847-5_18

transition in India, which the North Indian states later followed. Numerous studies have examined factors affecting regional fertility variations (Dyson & Moore, 1983; Murthi et al., 1995). Such sharp regional contrast in fertility indicators still exists across the states (Singh et al., 2017). While some regions like Sikkim, Kolkata, and Kerala experience the lowest-low fertility (Dharmalingam et al., 2014; Ghosh, 2017), several districts from Uttar Pradesh and Bihar are far from replacement level, with a high unmet need for family planning. It is found that the role of socioeconomic development on fertility has reduced over time (Dharmalingam et al., 2014). The regional differentials in fertility remain the central issue in India.

There have been numerous studies addressing trends and socioeconomic determinants of fertility in India, including some that review district-level fertility differentials (Bhat, 1996; Bhattacharya, 2006; Drèze & Murthi, 2001; Guilmoto & Rajan, 2013; Murthi et al., 1995; Chatterjee & Mohanty, 2022). These studies highlight the substantial regional variations in fertility levels across the country. This present study aims to update our knowledge on fertility differential employing more recent disaggregated data derived from the latest NFHS round.

Data and Measurement

Even though India has multiple sources of demographic data, reliable fertility data at the district level is still limited. All the data sources have some strengths and limitations, from coverage of demographic indicators to the feasibility of measurement. After seven decades of India's independence, the coverage and quality of the Civil Registration System (CRS) are not uniform across time and space. Also, irregularities in publishing the CRS data make the researchers rely upon mostly sample surveys, such as the Sample Registration System (SRS). However, the estimates provided by the SRS are available only for a large administrative unit such as the state. While the National Family Health Survey (NFHS-5) and the Census of India give district-level estimates, the latter offers relatively older estimates. The NFHS collects information on children ever born to the mothers from each eligible woman (15–49 years) from the sampled households, which allows us to examine the district-level variation.[1]

The number of children ever born to a woman is the measure of her lifetime fertility until the data are collected. The mean number of children ever born (MCEB) is the indicator of fertility, which comprises the current and completed fertility. Synthetic cohorts are used to compute the Total Fertility Rate (TFR) for a period, typically 3 or 5 years before the survey. In contrast, the completed fertility rate indicates the fertility behaviors of those who have already completed their childbearing. Since the estimates based on women aged 40+ years may fluctuate because of the small sample size and non-representable sample, the MCEB may be a better indicator. The cumulative fertility indicators represented by MCEB offer a more robust estimate to understand the fertility

[1] The original NFHS dataset and the spatial analysis methodology are described in detail in Chap. 1.

status at the survey. Despite a difference in interpretation, the correlation between MCEB and TFR or between the TFR and CBR is high. For example, NFHS-4 data reveal that the estimated MCEB has a high correlation coefficient ($r = 0.90$). The MCEB is a robust indicator of cumulative fertility when computed on smaller, district-level samples. The reason is that the MCEB is computed over a larger number of births. It is based on completed fertility (number of all children ever born) of women aged 15–49 rather than on recent births, as in TFR calculation.

MCEB to women in a specific age group is the average number of children born alive to women in that age group. In estimating the MCEB for all women, age adjustment is required to avoid bias arising from the skewed age distribution by the different age groups in the reproductive period across the districts. For each district of India, the whole reproductive span has been accordingly divided into separate age groups based on the intrinsic age effects on reproductive behaviors and sample size. The women in the reproductive span are divided into seven age groups with an interval of 5 years for age standardization. However, we have divided the women in reproductive span into four age groups, 15–21, 22–29, 30–39, and 40–49 (with an interval of 7, 8, 10, and 10 years, respectively) for two reasons. First, four age groups were prepared, considering the sample size in each age group. Therefore, if we divide the sample into seven quinquennial age groups for each district, the sample may not be available in each age group for all districts. Second, the majority of the births took place in the age groups between 15 and 29 years; this age group is divided into two parts with almost an equal interval (7 and 8 years), while the age group of 30–49 years was classified into two groups with a gap of 10 years. The estimates of each district have been standardized with their standard female population of the same age group for respective states. The standard population has been taken from the Census of India 2011 on the ground that the NFHS-5 has adopted the sample design based on the population enumerated in 2011.

The MCEB also has some limitations as a measure of fertility as it mixes women from different cohorts as well as births from different periods. For the sake of comparison, we standardized the MCEB with the women's age group. The average age-adjusted MCEB covering 707 districts in India is 1.75.

Findings

Out of 15–49 aged women, the mean number of children at the national level is 1.75 children per woman. However, there exist wide variations in the mean number of children across the states: Goa and Sikkim record the lowest mean number of children ever born (1.1), whereas Bihar has the highest mean number of children ever born (2.3), followed by Meghalaya (2.1). District-level estimates are even wider, ranging from 1.0 (Srinagar) to 3.3 (West Khasi Hills in Meghalaya).

Out of 707 districts of India, 607 (86%) record MCEB levels lower than the replacement level (2.1 children per woman). This result indicates that a large majority of districts have reached low fertility, with relatively few districts with above-replacement fertility.

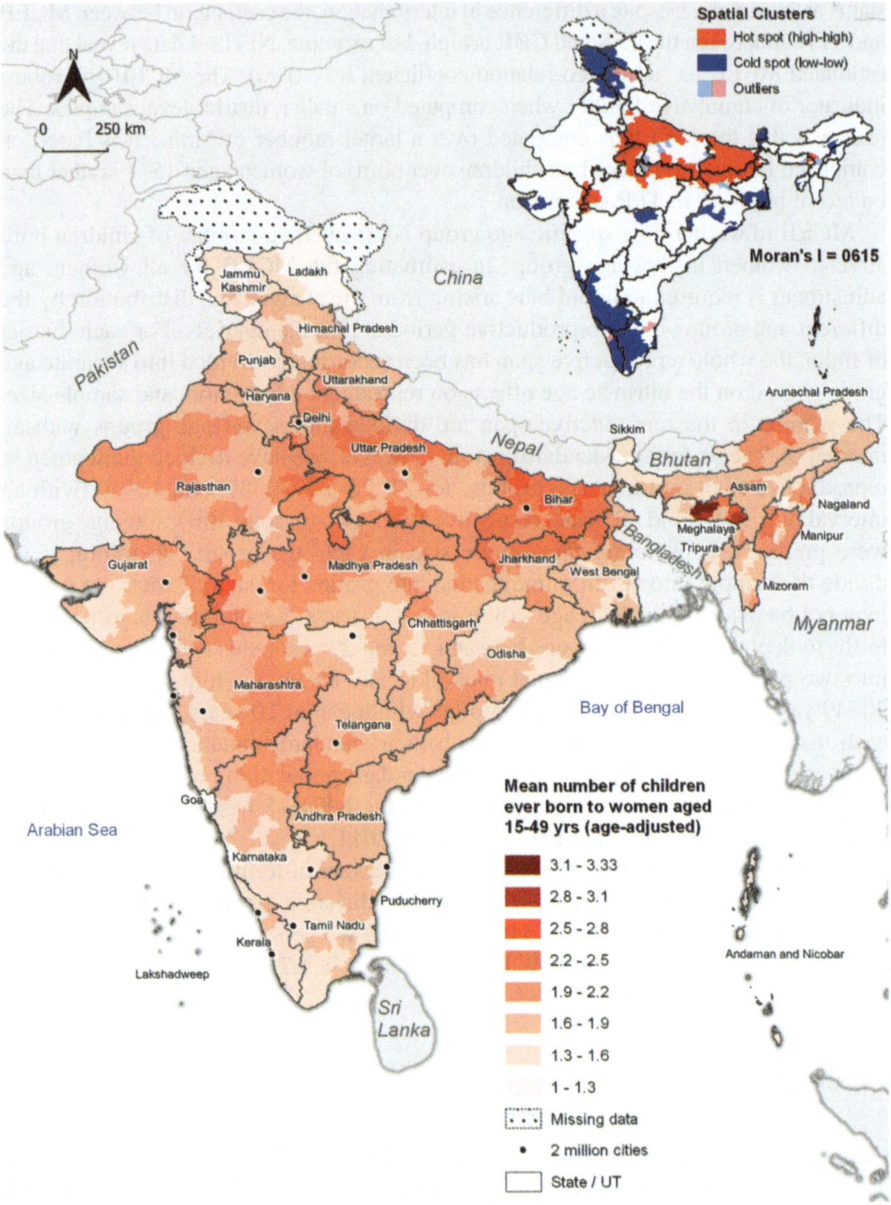

Fig. 18.1 Mean number of ever-born children per woman aged 15–49 years
Source: NFHS-5, 2019–21
The map is for illustrative purposes and may not represent official boundaries

Figure 18.1 displays the spatial variation in age-adjusted MCEB across Indian districts using the NFHS-5. The map shows that high MCEB levels are now mainly restricted to North India. Values above two children per woman are found in Bihar and Jharkhand and parts of Uttar Pradesh, Rajasthan, and Madhya Pradesh.

Relatively high MCEB levels can also be observed in central and east Meghalaya, in stark contrast with other states of the Northeast where fertility is distinctly lower.

As expected, the lowest levels are registered in Kerala, Tamil Nadu, and southwest Karnataka, where the fertility decline started earlier than in the rest of India. However, some of the lowest MCEB levels are also apparent in Punjab, Jammu and Kashmir, and around metropolitan areas such as Delhi, Mumbai, Pune, Kolkata, and Nagpur.

For a more nuanced understanding of the spatial dynamics of fertility patterns, we estimated Moran's I index of spatial autocorrelation. This analysis confirms that the fertility level across Indian districts is characterized by pronounced spatial autocorrelation (Moran's $I = 0.61$). The accompanying cluster map based on the LISA (Local Indicators of Spatial Autocorrelation) helps us better identify the major hotspots and cold spots of fertility in India. The first hotspot of high fertility corresponds to the entire upper and middle Ganga Valley, inhabited by several hundreds of millions of people. This large region starts from east Rajasthan and extends to Jharkhand and Bihar, as well as bordering districts of Madhya Pradesh, Chhattisgarh, Jharkhand, and West Bengal. Interestingly, this region has a central hole and excludes cities of central and eastern Uttar Pradesh (Awadh and Purvanchal) like Kanpur, Lucknow, Prayagraj (Allahabad), and Varanasi districts. This pattern suggests that fertility decline in the Hindi heartland also proceeded from within, puncturing east Uttar Pradesh. We can also identify much smaller hotspots in economically deprived regions along the border of Gujarat and Madhya Pradesh and in eastern Meghalaya.

In South India, we can distinguish the largest cluster (cold spot) of low fertility comprising Kerala, Tamil Nadu, Karnataka, and Goa, excluding north inland Karnataka (Hyderabad Karnataka) as well as northeast Tamil Nadu (Thondai Nadu). Narrower clusters of low fertility are also visible on the map, notably around north Punjab (Doab), Jammu, and Kashmir, as well as adjacent districts of Ladakh and Himachal Pradesh. The southern districts of West Bengal form another distinct cluster that includes Kolkata and its surroundings, the region where fertility is currently at the lowest in India. Even smaller low fertility clusters emerge on the map, notably in Odisha, Sikkim, and around Mumbai or Nagpur. With the ongoing fertility decline, these low fertility clusters will continue to expand towards areas of intermediate fertility.

The distribution of fertility levels across India resembles that of other reproductive health indicators. We may, in particular, juxtapose the map of fertility variations with that of child marriage, low frequency of ANC visits, and poorer menstrual hygiene to stress their shared features (see Chaps. 11, 12, and 13 in this Atlas).

Discussion and Conclusion

The present chapter brings a district-level spatial analysis of fertility indicators, i.e., MCEB. Although India has experienced a rapid decline in fertility, there remain considerable regional variations in reproductive behavior across the country. Also, we observed a strong spatial autocorrelation in the prevalence of MCEB across the districts. In India, the higher fertility areas are often characterized by unwanted fertility due to the unmet need for limiting the number of children and the unmet need for spacing between birth intervals. Higher fertility areas of Uttar Pradesh and Bihar also display a higher prevalence of unwanted childbearing. According to NFHS-5, 9% of currently married women have an unmet need for family planning. The percentage of women with unmet needs for family planning in Bihar and Uttar Pradesh is 13.6 and 12.8, respectively. Previous studies revealed that children of higher birth order are more likely to be unwanted and worse in health and nutritional status. The core concern of the policy should be to minimize unwanted childbearing, which will eventually bring down fertility levels.

Socioeconomic development can be one of the significant causes of fertility decline in India. While high fertility areas are often associated with low socioeconomic status, son preference, and poor healthcare service utilization, low fertility can be explained through the developmental lens. These cold spots are located in particular (1) in southwestern India, covering Kerala, Tamil Nadu, south Andhra Pradesh, southwest Karnataka, Goa, and western Maharashtra; (2) around Punjab, Himachal Pradesh, and parts of Haryana, and (3) in West Bengal and Odisha. However, a recent study examining the spatial correlation of fertility to a range of socioeconomic and demographic factors (Haque et al., 2019) has found that socioeconomic factors are not invariably related to fertility levels across the different regions of India. For instance, many socioeconomic and demographic indicators cannot comprehensively explain the low fertility clustering in the South Indian states of India. Unobserved heterogeneity of the regions and cultural traits may play a significant role in differentiating fertility levels across the districts.

High-fertility clusters have crucial policy implications for the perspective of family planning. In 2016, the government of India launched the "Mission Parivar Vikas" to address the high fertility in districts of India (Government of India, 2016). This program covers 145 high fertility districts (TFR > 3) from seven states of India, such as Uttar Pradesh, Bihar, Rajasthan, Madhya Pradesh, Assam, Chhattisgarh, and Jharkhand. The selected districts have adopted several promotional and provisional family planning schemes. The spatial distribution patterns of MCEB and the identification of hotspots here enable us to revise the ongoing program, Mission Parivar Vikas. More district-specific rather than state-level policy interventions are required to effectively tackle the local need for family planning and other reproductive services. Furthermore, the regional heterogeneity needs to be factored into programming efforts; for instance, a few districts in West Bengal, Gujarat, and Meghalaya display high MCEB, although the overall regional fertility appears low or moderate. Our findings call for the inclusion of these districts with enhancing priority in the ongoing Mission Parivar Vikas. Nevertheless, India may soon also need to confront the issue of ultra-low fertility, already discernable in numerous districts.

References

Bhat, P. N. M. (1996). Contours of fertility decline in India. A district level study based on the 1991 census. In K. Srinivasan (Ed.), *Population policy and reproductive health* (pp. 96–177). Hindustan Publishing Corporation.

Bhattacharya, P. C. (2006). Economic development, gender inequality, and demographic outcomes: Evidence from India. *Population and Development Review, 32*(2), 263–292. https://doi.org/10.1111/j.1728-4457.2006.00118.x

Chatterjee, S., & Mohanty, S. K. (2022). Fertility transition and socioeconomic development in districts of India, 2001–2016. *Journal of Biosocial Science, 54*(1), 135–153.

Dharmalingam, A., Rajan, S., & Morgan, S. P. (2014). The determinants of low fertility in India. *Demography, 51*(4), 1451–1475. https://doi.org/10.1007/s13524-014-0314-9

Drèze, J., & Murthi, M. (2001). Fertility, education, and development: Evidence from India. *Population and Development Review, 27*(1), 33–63.

Dyson, T., & Moore, M. (1983). On kinship structure, female autonomy, and demographic behavior in India. *Population and Development Review, 9*(1), 35–60. https://doi.org/10.2307/1972894

Ghosh, S. (2017). Second demographic transition or aspirations in transition: An exploratory analysis of lowest-low fertility in Kolkata, India. *Asian Population Studies, 13*(1), 25–49.

Government of India. (2016). *Mission Parivar Vikas*. Ministry of Health and Family Welfare. http://www.nhmmp.gov.in/WebContent/FW/Scheme/Scheme2017/Mission_Parivar_Vikas.pdf

Guilmoto, C. Z., & Rajan, S. I. (2013). Fertility at the district level in India: Lessons from the 2011 census. *Economic and Political Weekly, 48*(23), 59–70.

Haque, I., Das, D., & Patel, P. (2019). Reading the geography of India's district level fertility differentials: A spatial econometric approach. *Journal of Biosocial Science, 51*, 745–774. https://doi.org/10.1017/S0021932019000087

Murthi, M., Guio, A.-C., & Drèze, J. (1995). Mortality, fertility, and gender bias in India: A district-level analysis. *Population and Development Review, 21*(4), 745–782. https://doi.org/10.2307/2137773

Singh, A., Kumar, K., Pathak, P. K., Chauhan, R. K., & Banerjee, A. (2017). Spatial patterns and determinants of fertility in India. *Population, 72*(3), 505–526.

Chapter 19
Lowest-Low Fertility in India

Koyel Sarkar

India is entering the last stage of its demographic transition after more than 40 years of fertility decline. A significant contribution to India's final fertility decline is the rising prevalence of childlessness and single-child families. This contemporary development has not received adequate attention so far. The focus of this chapter, therefore, is to examine the lowest-low fertility in India.

Childlessness and lowest-low fertility are features of high-income societies in West and East Asia. Rising economic opportunities, decreasing gender wage gaps, personal aspirations, and individualism among women have led to the breakdown of marriage, a rise in births outside marriages, and small families (Zaidi & Morgan, 2017). While childlessness in low-income countries is also high, albeit at comparatively lower levels, it has received limited research attention, notably regarding its key drivers. A study based on 36 low-income countries argues that childlessness in these countries is primarily driven by two distinct factors: opportunity and poverty (Baudin et al., 2019).

In India, childlessness concerns approximately 7% of all women aged 40 years and above in 2001, and the percentage of childless women marginally increased to 8% in 2011 (Census of India, 2001, 2011). Although India's rate of childlessness is lower than that observed in high-income countries, childlessness in India concerns about 12 million women compared to 1.5 million in the USA. More importantly, India's childlessness rate is way beyond the natural sterility rate, usually uniformly distributed among women aged 25 and above at approximately 1% (Léridon, 2008).

In this chapter, I shed light on the end of the fertility transition illustrated by childlessness and the rising trend of "single childness" (the proportion of women with a single child). The present study offers a comparative overview of

K. Sarkar (✉)
New York University, Abu Dhabi, United Arab Emirates
e-mail: koyel.sarkar@nyu.edu

C. Z. Guilmoto (ed.), *Atlas of Gender and Health Inequalities in India*, Demographic Transformation and Socio-Economic Development 16,
https://doi.org/10.1007/978-3-031-47847-5_19

childlessness in India and single childness across time, geography, and socioeconomic categories. Low fertility and its determinants are of great significance in understanding women's emancipation in a pronatalist and patriarchal society like India (Mitra, 2014).

Definitions and Measures

Some studies in Indian literature have defined childlessness almost synonymously with sterility or infertility (Ganguly & Unisa, 2010), but the phenomenon's reality is probably more diverse. While infertility cases almost invariably lead to childlessness unless medically treated, all childless women are not necessarily infertile. Apart from natural infertility linked to biological reasons, childlessness may also be due to acquired infertility or specific decisions. External, non-biological factors, such as poverty, higher exposure to venereal diseases, and malnutrition, can drive acquired infertility (or involuntary childlessness). It is known in demographic literature as poverty-driven childlessness (Baudin et al., 2019). Childlessness may also result from refusal to bear children or sequential postponement of childbirth because of economic opportunities and other contextual factors—making reproduction unfeasible or undesirable. As a result, it is difficult to determine if this type of childlessness can be termed voluntary or involuntary. For example, if the initial delay in childbearing is a voluntary decision, can the resulting childlessness at a later stage be defined as voluntary or involuntary? The definition of childlessness as voluntary or involuntary is almost impossible in the absence of detailed attitudinal data to reconstruct women's sexual and marital history. A recent study (Baudin & Sarkar, 2021) employing theoretical models on Indian data has shown that childlessness in India is predominantly driven by education and opportunities offered to women and, to a lesser extent, by poverty.

In this chapter, the latest NFHS-5 dataset is used to identify two specific forms of ultra-low fertility: childlessness (percentage of childless women) and single-childness (percentage of women who had only one birth).[1] These indicators are computed on the female population aged 40–49 years, bearing in mind that many younger women have not yet completed their reproductive cycle. The median age at first birth among Indian women is currently 21.1 years, and in the study sample, less than 1% of women had their first births at age 35 or higher. We have accordingly used 40 as the age threshold to analyze low-fertility patterns.

[1] The original NFHS dataset and the spatial analysis methodology are described in detail in Chap. 1.

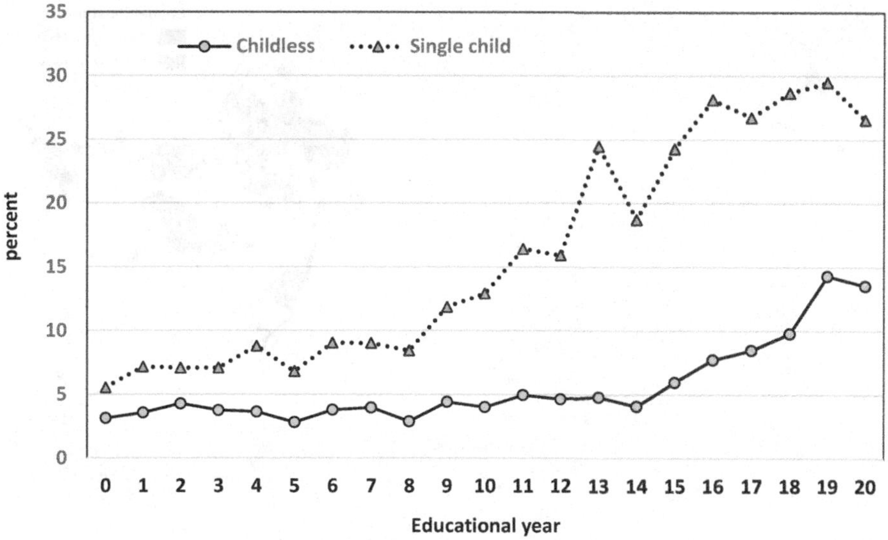

Fig. 19.1 Percentages of childless and single-child women by years of education among women aged 35–49 years

Results

The frequency of childless women shows a regular increase among younger cohorts, nearing 6% among the youngest cohorts born in 1986. This rising childlessness again contradicts the presumed biological factors associated with sterility in India (Ganguly & Unisa, 2010; Unisa, 2010). Today, about 4% of women aged 40–49 are childless, according to NFHS-5 estimates.

The trends for single-childness are similar to those of childlessness and point to an increase among younger cohorts—with 9.7% of women aged 40–49 reporting only one child in 2020–21. Research on single childness in India shows it is usually more common among urban, middle-class, higher-educated, and professionally employed women (Basu & Desai, 2016). Given its growing contribution to below-replacement fertility, the rise in childlessness has not yet received enough attention despite recent sociological research (Bhambhani & Inbanathan, 2018). In the following sections, I present a comparative analysis of childlessness and single-childness among women in India.

Descriptive results from the NFHS-5 data displayed in Fig. 19.1 confirm the J-shape relationship between childlessness and education (Baudin & Sarkar, 2021). Higher education is similarly associated with a rising percentage of single-child women, even if the gap between both series increases with years of education. A similar J-shaped pattern (not shown here) can be found with occupations, with higher status (professional and technical) occupations displaying the highest levels of both childlessness and single-childness. The micro-level analysis below will re-examine the link between low fertility and higher socioeconomic status.

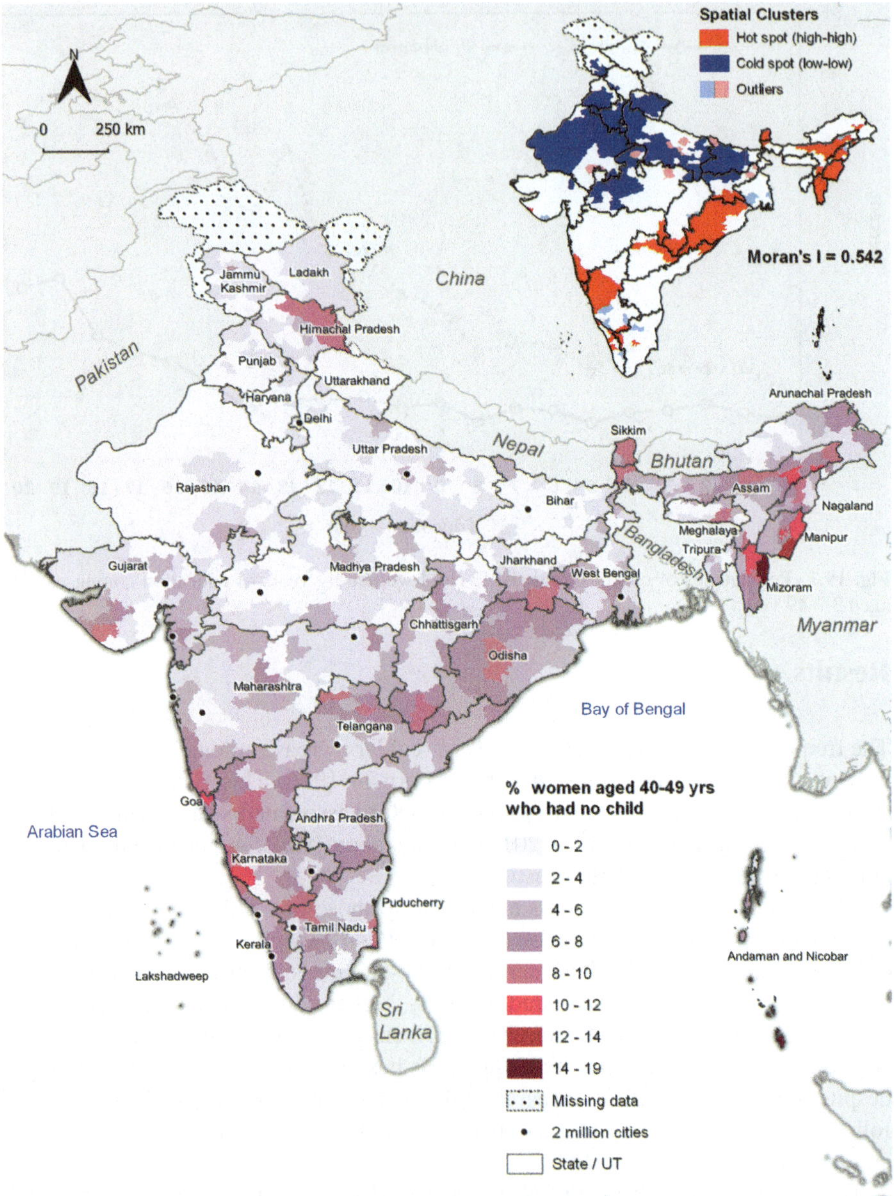

Fig. 19.2 Percentage of women aged 40–49 years who are childless
Source: NFHS-5, 2019–21
The map is for illustrative purposes and may not represent official boundaries

Figures 19.2 and 19.3 provide disaggregated maps at the district level for both childlessness and single-childness. These two maps resemble fertility differentials examined in Chap. 18 of this Atlas. As expected, we recognize the broad North-South opposition typical of India's reproductive system. This correspondence is notably visible

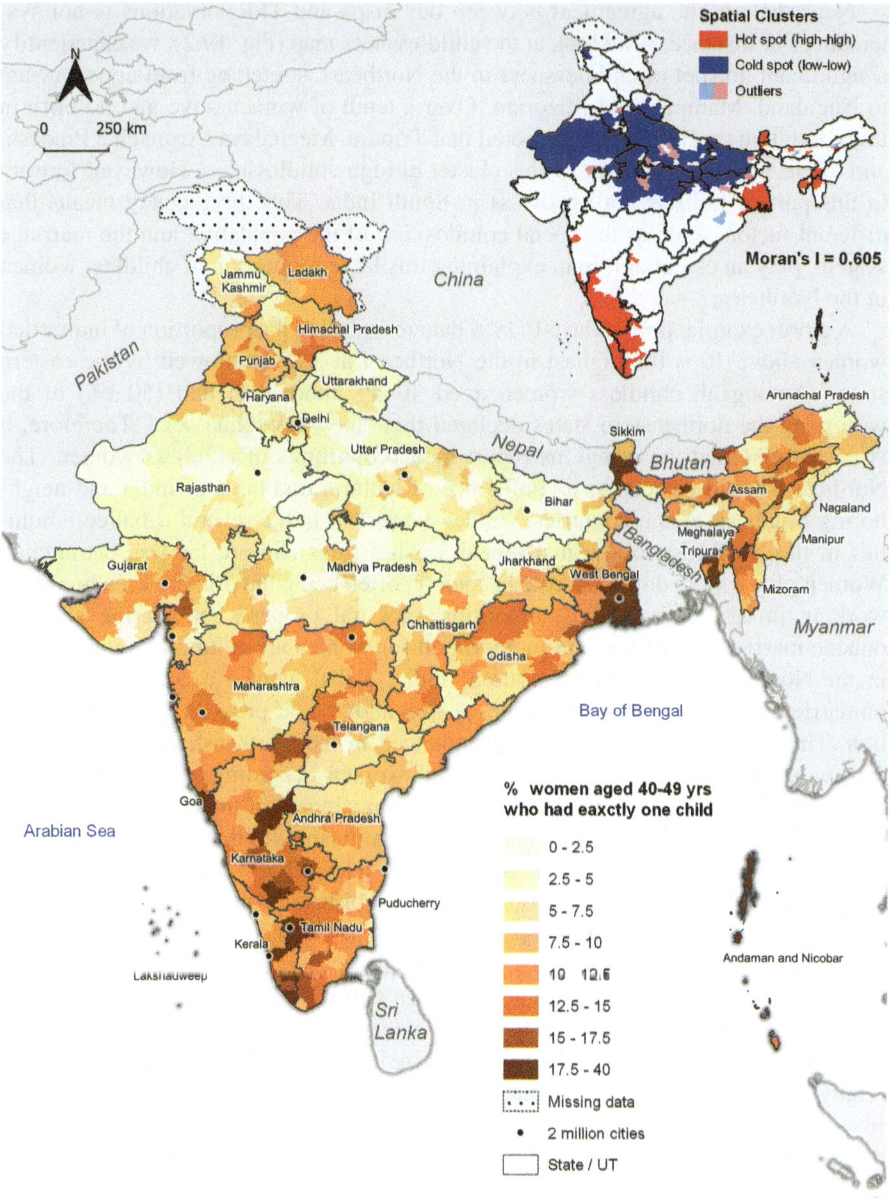

Fig. 19.3 Percentage of women aged 40–49 years who had only one child
Source: NFHS-5, 2019–21
The map is for illustrative purposes and may not represent official boundaries

for the southern states where low fertility is also associated with higher proportions of childlessness and single-childness. Likewise, north-central India (primarily Uttar Pradesh, Bihar, and adjoining districts) concentrates the highest level of fertility and the lowest proportions of childlessness and single-childness.

Nevertheless, the agreement between our maps and TFR variations is not systematic. For instance, if we look at the childlessness map (Fig. 19.2), we can identify a significant hotspot of childlessness in the Northeast, stretching from upper Assam to Nagaland, Manipur, and Mizoram. Over a tenth of women have had no birth in this contiguous region. It may be noted that Tripura, Meghalaya, Arunachal Pradesh, and West Assam are not part of this cluster of high childlessness. However, fertility in this part of India is not as low as in South India. This discrepancy means that different factors, such as the social composition of the population and the marriage system, play an essential role in explaining this large proportion of childless women in the Northeast.

A closer examination of the NFHS-5 data reveals that the proportion of unmarried women above 40 is the highest in the Northeast at 3.2%, followed by the eastern states. Among all childless women aged 40–49, more than half (50.3%) of the women in the northeastern states declared that "they never had sex." Therefore, it is no surprise that these regions report high proportions of childless women. The Northeast should be seen as a confluence of cultural traditions of India and neighboring Southeast Asian countries. Unlike the rest of India, several tribal communities in the Northeast follow matrilineal kinship rules and are far less patriarchal. Women play a more dominant role in society, often being the primary breadwinners, working in agricultural fields, inheriting ancestral property, or bearing children outside marriage. Marriage and motherhood for women are culturally not as crucial in the Northeast as in other regions of India. Tribal women account for 34% of unmarried women in India, a percentage well above their proportion of the population. This imbalance is even more pronounced in the Northeast, where scheduled tribe women account for 62.4% of unmarried women, according to NFHS-5. It is the highest proportion for any social community in any region of India and indicates that singlehood among tribal women contributes significantly to this specific concentration of childlessness in the Northeast. It may be added that women in the Northeast have some of the highest rates of out-of-wedlock births; the proportion of unmarried single child-mothers aged 40–49 years is the highest in this part of India, with rates as high as 3.7% in Mizoram or 2.3 in Nagaland.

Another instance of discrepancies between childlessness and low fertility is the high childlessness observed in Odisha that extends southwards to Telangana. However, this situation can hardly be explained by fertility decline *per se*, which started relatively late in Odisha or Chhattisgarh compared to south or northwest India. Inversely, we may notice that the vast cluster of low childlessness to the west encompasses Punjab, where fertility decline is pronounced and where we would expect a somewhat higher proportion of childless women than elsewhere in India.

We may also observe that hotspots of childlessness in the rest of the country are sparser and cover only fragments of South India. A specific area of higher childlessness is the Konkani region, covering, in particular, Goa and coastal Karnataka; it is another area of late marriage and a higher rate of singlehood. A small cluster of childless women can also be distinguished in northern Himachal Pradesh, which may partly be related to low fertility even if we lack detailed studies on this region. In conclusion, some areas in India exhibit high rates of childlessness despite high fertility, while others exhibit low rates of childlessness and fertility. This result provides suggestive evidence that different mechanisms may affect the prevalence of childlessness, namely poverty and affluence. This may also explain why the overall level of autocorrelation (Moran's *I*) is only 0.54 for childless women, a level lower than for other indicators examined in this Atlas. This lower figure may reflect measurement issues linked to the small number of women aged 40–49 in some districts but also to the combination of the different components of childlessness mentioned earlier in this chapter.

When we examine the distribution of single-child mothers, the correspondence with smaller family sizes is far more robust than with childlessness. The main hotspot is, as expected, South India, covering states such as Kerala or Tamil Nadu, where fertility is far lower than average. This cluster appears almost identical to the low-fertility cluster highlighted in Chap. 18. Interestingly, both Andhra Pradesh and Telangana are not parts of this cluster. Despite its overall low fertility levels, the Telugu-speaking region does not contain any substantial proportion of single-child women; this feature may be related to the frequency of early marriage in this part of South India. This marked heterogeneity within South India was already observed with the map of low fertility presented in Chap. 18 of this Atlas. Similarly, the vast cluster of low values extending from Rajasthan to Bihar closely corresponds to the high fertility region of North India. The measure of spatial autocorrelation (Moran's *I*) is indeed more pronounced at 0.60 for women with one child.

A region of interest for studying single childness corresponds to southern West Bengal, especially in districts around the Kolkata metropolitan area. Urban West Bengal and Kolkata have long been characterized by low fertility. Despite an overall typical age at marriage in West Bengal, Kolkata was among the first areas to report rapid fertility decline since the 1960s (Basu & Amin, 2000), and TFR went down to the lowest level in the country at 1.2 children per woman, according to 2011 census (Guilmoto & Rajan, 2013). The proportion of single-child mothers is the highest in Kolkata, specifically among urban, employed, and educated women (Pradhan & Sekher, 2012). Women's education, economic opportunity, and aspirations contribute to somewhat unique ultra-low fertility levels (Basu & Desai, 2016).

Determinants of Childlessness and Having a Single Child

In the final step of this analysis, I conducted a separate multivariable regression analysis of childlessness and single-childness on all women aged 40–49. Independent variables include education, occupation, religion, caste, and region. Respective odds ratios are displayed in Figs. 19.4 and 19.5.[2]

[2]Odds ratios measure the strength of the correlation with the outcome variable. Values above (below) one correspond to a positive (negative) association.

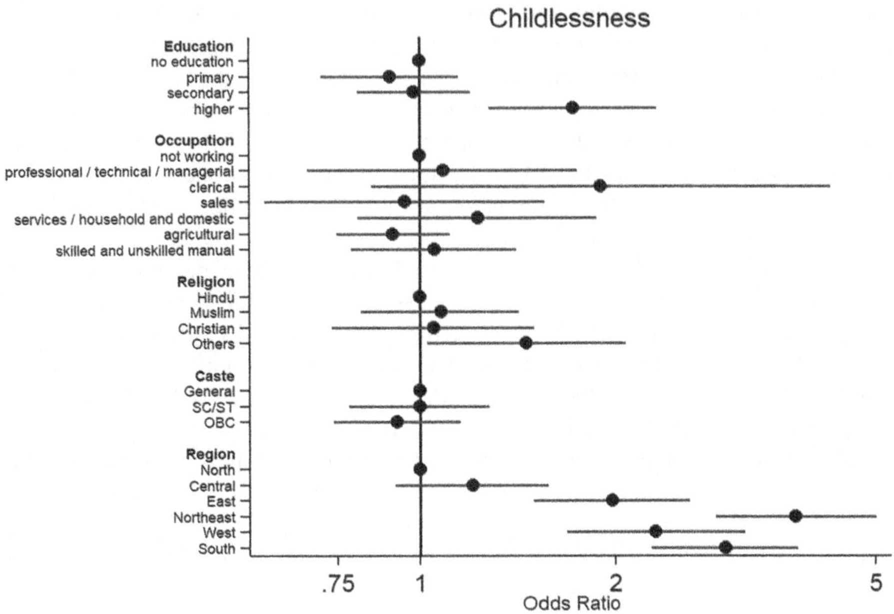

Fig. 19.4 Odds ratios of childlessness among women aged 35–49 years by selected background characteristics

The results are somewhat parallel for both dependent variables. In line with the descriptive results, the dependent variables strongly correlate with education. The most pronounced association relates to the high proportion of women with a single child among those with secondary and higher education. The regional differentials are similar for both variables and reproduce the features detected on the maps of childlessness and single-childness; however, distinct variations in the correlation need to be spelled out.

Childlessness appears more common among working women, especially those in the clerical category, while single-childness is more common among women working in the professional category. Interestingly, we find no association between childlessness and religion or social group; the only correlation is found among Buddhist women, among whom childlessness appears significantly more common. We would need more detail to adequately which type of Buddhist populations are concerned. In contrast, the proportion of women with a single child displays pronounced differentials across socioeconomic and religious groups. For example, the lowest probability of having only one child is associated with women working in agriculture and belonging to Christian, Muslim, and Dalit communities.

When we examine the interaction between regions and socioeconomic factors (detailed results are not shown here), we discover that the effect of education is not identical everywhere in India. We note, for instance, that higher education has the most substantial impact in East India on the risk of having only one child. We also

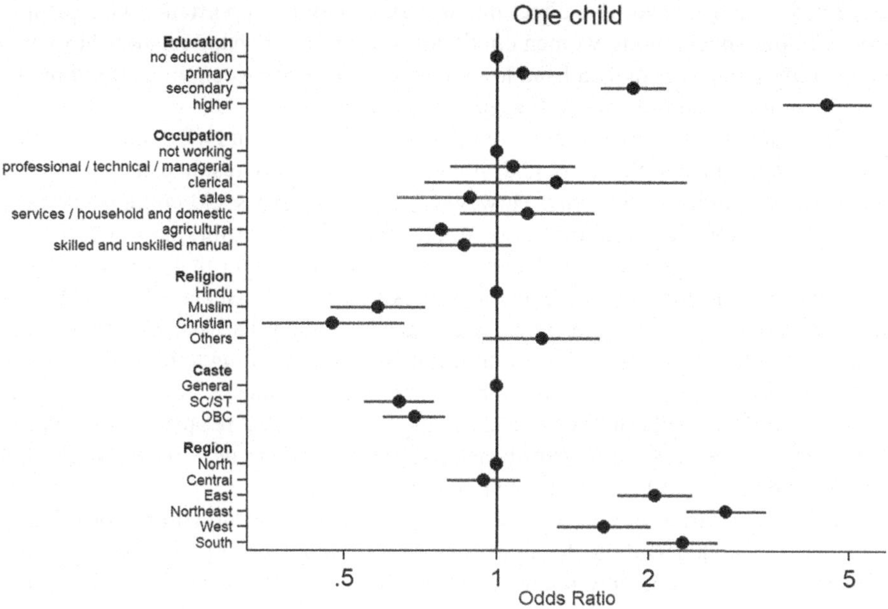

Fig. 19.5 Odds ratios of single-childness among women aged 35–49 years by selected background characteristics

note that even if higher education is connected to childlessness, the link remains the strongest in Northeast India, where better-educated women are the most likely to remain childless. These findings confirm that the overall impact of female education on features of ultra-low fertility (having one child or none) appears significantly marked in east and northeast India compared to the rest of the country.

Conclusion

This study has demonstrated that low fertility among newer generations is on the rise, and having a single child is more common than having no children among women in India. Both childlessness and having a single child are significantly affected by education levels, association with certain socio-cultural groups, and region of residence. Findings show that female educational attainment increases the probability of having no or one child. While the probability of remaining childless follows a J-shape relationship with increasing education, single-childness gets a positive linear relationship. Education attainment is a good proxy for both poverty and opportunity. It can be deduced that having no children or just one child is driven by higher economic opportunities among women. Simultaneously, a small proportion of childlessness is also driven by poverty or no education; this fact is sustained even after adding a direct measure of economic opportunity, i.e., occupation. Childlessness among women continues to impose a J-shape relationship when occupation groups are ranked from low to high. Thus, better economic opportunities among women lead to lower fertility preferences in India.

The analysis has further highlighted that religion, caste, and tribe indicators play different roles in childlessness and single-childness. This result calls for further empirical research on the topic. However, given the high socio-cultural diversity within the regions in India, these two dimensions of low fertility appear to follow region-specific driving factors. I identify two distinct factors that are particularly important behind the varying levels and pockets of childlessness and single-child mothers among women aged 40–49 years across Indian districts. The first major contributing factor is better socioeconomic status corresponding to higher education and economic aspirations among Indian women; it is mostly the case with the southern and in southern West Bengal. The second factor relates to the cultural environment specific to the Northeast, where the importance of marriage and childbearing may not be as prominent as in the rest of India.

The current rise in the proportion of women with one or no child is of primary relevance to understanding the dynamics of declining fertility for the following decades, an issue intimately related to India's demographic growth. Are we going to witness a new reproductive regime dominated by couples opting for one or two children or a further fertility plunge caused by the emergence of singlehood and childlessness among educated women, as observed in East Asia? The response to this question will determine the future course of India's fertility and, ultimately, the number of years until India's population stops growing.

References

Basu, A. M., & Amin, S. (2000). Conditioning factors for fertility decline in Bengal: History, language identity, and openness to innovations. *Population and Development Review, 26*(4), 761–794. https://doi.org/10.1111/j.1728-4457.2000.00761.x

Basu, A. M., & Desai, S. (2016). Hopes, dreams, and anxieties: India's one-child families. *Asian Population Studies, 12*(1), 4–27. https://doi.org/10.1080/17441730.2016.1144354

Baudin, T., & Sarkar, K. (2021). Education and childlessness in India. *Population, 76*(3), 461–486. https://doi.org/10.3917/popu.2103.0491

Baudin, T., de la Croix, D., & Gobbi, P. E. (2019). Childlessness and economic development: A survey. In A. Bucci, K. Prettner, & A. Prskawetz (Eds.), *Human capital and economic growth: The impact of health, education and demographic change* (pp. 55–90). Palgrave Macmillan. https://doi.org/10.1007/978-3-030-21599-6_3

Bhambhani, C., & Inbanathan, A. (2018). Not a mother, yet a woman: Exploring experiences of women opting out of motherhood in India. *Asian Journal of Women's Studies, 24*(2), 159–182. https://doi.org/10.1080/12259276.2018.1462932

Census of India. (2001). *Office of the Registrar General and Census Commissioner, Ministry of Home Affairs, India.* https://www.censusindia.gov.in/2011-common/census_data_2001.html

Census of India. (2011). *Office of the Registrar General and Census Commissioner.* Ministry of Home Affairs.

Ganguly, S., & Unisa, S. (2010). Trends of infertility and childlessness in India: Findings from NFHS data. *Facts, Views and Vision in ObGyn, 2*(2), 131–138.
Guilmoto, C. Z., & Rajan, S. I. (2013). Fertility at the district level in India: Lessons from the 2011 census. *Economic and Political Weekly, 48*(23), 59–70.
Léridon, H. (2008). A new estimate of permanent sterility by age: Sterility is defined as the inability to conceive. *Population Studies, 62*(1), 15–24. https://doi.org/10.1080/00324720701804207
Mitra, A. (2014). Son preference in India: Implications for gender development. *Journal of Economic Issues, 48*(4), 1021–1037. https://doi.org/10.2753/JEI0021-3624480408
Pradhan, I., & Sekher, T. V. (2012). Is urban India moving towards single child families? An analysis of Kolkata City and West Bengal. *Demography India, 41*, 53–69.
Unisa, S. (2010). Infertility and treatment seeking in India: Findings from district level household survey. In *Social Aspects of Accessible Infertility Care in Developing Countries*, Facts, Views & Vision in ObGyn, 59–65.
Zaidi, B., & Morgan, S. P. (2017). The second demographic transition theory: A review and appraisal. *Annual Review of Sociology, 43*(1), 473–492. https://doi.org/10.1146/annurev-soc-060116-053442

Chapter 20
Female Sterilization in India

Raman Mishra

India was the first country to initiate a state-sponsored family planning program in 1952 to lower fertility and population growth rates (ORGI, 2018). The government of India adopted several family planning approaches to curb population growth, starting from the clinic-based approach, extension, cafeteria integrated, target, and target-free systems have been implemented to increase the acceptance of family planning in India (Pradhan & Ram, 2009). Family planning in India and improved socioeconomic status have effectively reduced fertility since independence. There remain sizable disparities across regions and social groups in reducing the unmet need for contraception. Countries with high levels of contraceptive use reflect a mixture of methods. Long-acting or permanent methods (LAPM) play a dominant role and are used by more than one in three married or in-union women worldwide; namely, female and male sterilization, IUDs, and implants accounting for 56% of contraceptive prevalence in 2015 (United Nations, 2015). The reliance on female sterilization in India has its roots in the National Family Planning Programme of the 1970s, which promoted permanent methods of contraception, i.e., sterilization as an effective mechanism for fertility reduction (Säävälä, 1999).

The various rounds of NFHS data show the dominance of permanent methods of contraception in India. Earlier studies show that permanent methods are common in southern India, where states achieved replacement fertility levels much earlier than others (Bose, 1993; Zavier & Padmadas, 2000). The government promoted incentive-based and target approaches to promote sterilization. The coercive nature of the government and the mass sterilization conducted during the Emergency after 1975 did not survive the subsequent fall of the political regime (Basu, 1985).

The government's focus on sterilization is the reason behind the decline in fertility in South India (De Oliveira et al., 2014). In the southern states, especially

R. Mishra (✉)
College of Health Science, Korea University, Seoul, South Korea
e-mail: mishraman@korea.ac.kr

C. Z. Guilmoto (ed.), *Atlas of Gender and Health Inequalities in India*, Demographic Transformation and Socio-Economic Development 16,
https://doi.org/10.1007/978-3-031-47847-5_20

in Andhra Pradesh, the sterilization age is much lower than in the other regions. The long-term consequence of forced sterilization is regret among the mothers if they lose their child later (Singh et al., 2012). Sometimes, women may have to bear medical complications and side effects of sterilization for the rest of their lives. The government has been organizing camps and incentivizing females to opt for sterilization. There have been incidents of female death in one of such camps organized by the government in Chhattisgarh in 2014. It was reported that around 15 females died in that camp (Dahat, 2014). While obtaining consent from the female before sterilization is mandatory, women from underprivileged backgrounds often opt for it because of lucrative incentives and benefits or pressure from health personnel.

Sterilization is also common after women give birth to their last child through cesarean delivery (Bhatia et al., 2020). It is also associated with son preference in India, as sterilization is more frequent after a boy's birth. The decision to opt for sterilization must not be coercive; women must be fully briefed about alternative contraception methods and have the right to choose the best method. The family planning decision should be supported by the male partner as well.

This chapter aims to provide a detailed picture of the distribution of female sterilization across India. Furthermore, we also investigate some of the factors associated with female sterilization at the individual level.

Data Source

Data on sterilization and the associated factors has been collected since the inception of the National Family Health Survey in 1992–93. NFHS collects data from married females aged 15–49 years for sterilization, age at sterilization, side effects of sterilization, compensation received, and knowledge about modern methods.[1]

The current study uses NFHS-5 and rests on a sample size of 521,352 currently married women aged 15–49 years who were interviewed at the time of the survey. Women were asked the following question: "Have you ever used anything or tried in any way to delay or avoid getting pregnant?" and further: "What have you used or done?" (IIPS and IFC, 2017). This chapter's central outcome variable is the self-reported percentage of women using sterilization as a contraception method. Individual-level data were aggregated in percentage for analysis at the district level.

Apart from the spatial analysis, we also conducted a logistic regression to explore factors affecting the probability of female sterilization at the individual level. The predictors used in this multivariate analysis are the age of the women, last birth cesarean, women having health insurance, education, wealth, caste, and religion.

[1] The original NFHS dataset and the spatial analysis methodology are described in detail in Chap. 1.

Results

There is a stark difference in the prevalence of sterilization among females and males. According to NFHS-5, the percentage of sterilized women is 37.9%, while the corresponding figure for men is only 0.3%. The overall contribution to family planning by Indian males is relatively modest. Over time, female sterilization has increased considerably in almost all states of India, from NFHS-1 to NFHS-3, rising from 27% to 38%. However, this percentage dropped to 36% in NFHS-4 and marginally increased to 37.9% in the latest NFHS round. Meanwhile, the percentage of sterilized men has reduced from 3.3% in NFHS 1 to 0.3% in NFHS-5.

Female sterilization emerges as one of the most common methods of contraception in India. During the first round of NFHS-1, southern states like Kerala, Karnataka, Tamil Nadu, and Andhra Pradesh recorded the highest percentages, followed by Maharashtra and Gujarat, as well as Himachal Pradesh and Punjab. A similar regional pattern was found in the second round of NFHS-2, but with the increase in other modern methods of contraception, there was a slight shift away from female sterilization. A different scenario emerged from the third round of NFHS (figures not shown here), with a net decline in Kerala, Maharashtra, and Punjab and a shift towards other modern methods of contraception. However, female sterilization has continued progressing in states like Andhra Pradesh, Madhya Pradesh, Tamil Nadu, and Rajasthan. In the Northeast, female sterilization is far less common than in the rest of India. NFHS-5 shows that female sterilization remains, however, the most popular method of contraception. Sterilization remains extremely common among women who are less educated (48%) or employed (51%).

Among the states, Andhra Pradesh (70.0%) and Telangana (63.8%) have the highest prevalence of sterilization among women. Further, more than half of the women in Puducherry, Karnataka, and Tamil Nadu undergo sterilization during their reproductive age. Interestingly, most northeastern states, such as Manipur, Meghalaya, and Assam, have a sterilization prevalence of 3.7%, 5.6%, and 9.1%, respectively. Sterilization remains relatively uncommon in the other northeastern states as well. In North India, Uttar Pradesh records the lowest rate at 17.0%, but this is also true of Delhi (18.2%) and Chandigarh (19.3%).

Figure 20.1 provides a disaggregated picture of sterilization rates among married women aged 15–49 in the country and reproduces variations observed at the state level to a significant extent. A large proportion of districts (184 out of 707) record rates above 50%, with the highest rates observed notably in Andhra Pradesh and Telangana: over three fourth of women are sterilized in four districts of Andhra Pradesh and Telangana (Nalgonda, West Godavari, Suryapet, and Krishna). This map inevitably resembles that of modern contraception (see Chap. 21 in this Atlas), but it also bears features shared with the map of institutional deliveries (Chap. 14). In contrast, the percentage of sterilized women is much smaller in parts of North India and the Northeast, often reaching values well below 10%. Thus, three districts with less than 1% of women sterilized are East-Kameng (Arunachal Pradesh), Ukhrul (Manipur), and Balrampur (Uttar Pradesh).

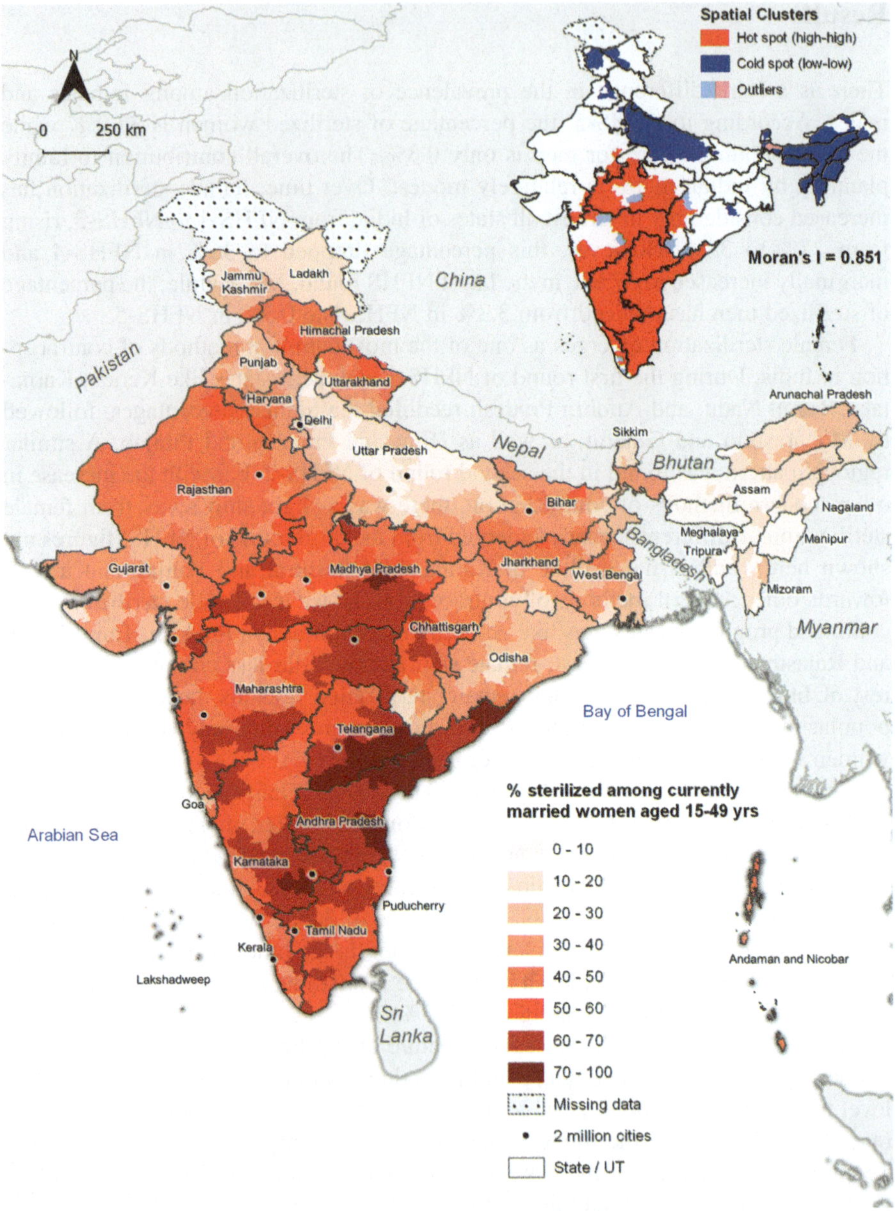

Fig. 20.1 Percentage of married women aged 15–49 years who are sterilized
Source: NFHS-5, 2019–21
The map is for illustrative purposes and may not represent official boundaries

The Moran's *I* statistic computed for female sterilization at the district level is remarkably high at 0.85, one of the highest-measured spatial autocorrelation in this Atlas. This autocorrelation suggests that sterilization as a contraceptive method among women is well-grounded in India and that localities strongly influence each other in their contraceptive preferences. The map of clusters derived from the spatial analysis shown in Fig. 20.1 is, accordingly, straightforward to interpret. It highlights a broad hotspot of female sterilization covering most districts of South India and the Deccan, from Tamil Nadu to Madhya Pradesh. We may, however, notice that many coastal districts in Karnataka, Kerala, and Tamil Nadu are missing from this cluster, even though these areas have some of the lowest fertility levels in India. Women in these districts have probably moved away from sterilization to other modern family planning methods, which probably reflects their high education level and greater awareness of contraceptive options.

Of equal interest for our analysis are the areas with low female sterilization, which comprise two distinct blocks. The first cluster follows the border with Nepal and covers almost entirely Uttar Pradesh. A second distinct cluster emerges in the Northeast, corresponding to almost the entire region. These two clusters correspond to regions where fertility is higher than average and contraception, therefore, is less used, but they may also point to areas with a distinct resistance towards sterilization as a method of family planning.

Apart from the obvious regional patterns, the regression analysis throws more light on some individual determinants of female sterilization. The odds ratios of this regression are plotted in Fig. 20.2.[2] We include the age group as a control variable, with sterilization being more common among older women. We observe that cesarean births are linked positively to sterilization, often performed following the last child. In addition, an equally strong correlation exists between sterilization and health insurance, an association that would require further exploration.

We also examined the association between sterilization and different socioeconomic variables. One of them is the wealth quintile of the woman's household. The regression results show that the odds of being sterilized first increase with socioeconomic status and peaks for the third quintile. Among women from more affluent quintiles, the odds appear to decline and are almost as low for the richer groups as for the poorest ones. So, sterilization appears to be more common among middle-wealth quintile families. Women's education underlines a lesser-known feature, i.e., that secondary and higher education levels tend to strongly reduce the probability of getting sterilized. The lowest odds of sterilization in our regression correspond to women with the highest educational attainment. These two dimensions suggest that the propensity to opt for sterilization follows inverted U (or inverted J) patterns: sterilization rates among the poorest women with no education are low but increase with primary education and better socioeconomic status. Sterilization rates reach a plateau at a certain threshold and revert to lower values below the national average with additional education, notably college-level education. These women typically opt for other contraceptive methods such as condoms, IUDs, or pills.

[2]Odds ratios measure the strength of the correlation with the outcome variable. Values above (below) one correspond to a positive (negative) association.

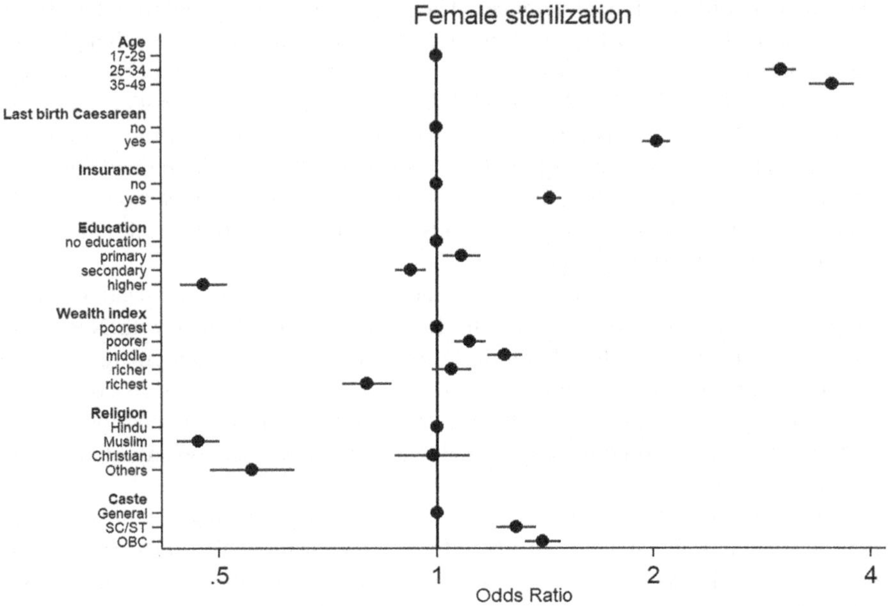

Fig. 20.2 Odds ratios of sterilization among married women aged 15–49 years by selected background characteristics

The regression analysis also suggests that the additional effect of specific social variables, such as the lowest odds of being sterilized, is observed particularly among Muslim women, women of other religions, and other/higher-caste women. In contrast, sterilization appears to be preferred among Hindu women of disadvantaged caste groups such as OBCs, SCs, and STs. It is important to emphasize that these results derived from a multivariate regression are found after controlling the role of all factors.

Conclusion

The analysis presented in this chapter emphasizes the extent of variations in sterilization rates observed across Indian districts. This map does not precisely coincide with the usual map of socioeconomic or educational differentials or fertility differentials in India (see Fig. 18.1 in this Atlas). For instance, low sterilization is a feature of the poorest regions like North-East India, whereas rich states like Punjab do not exhibit higher sterilization rates despite their better socioeconomic standing. However, sterilization is widespread among demographically advanced southern states. This result provides suggestive evidence that the chances of sterilization are influenced by local cultural norms regarding acceptable contraceptive methods. Our analysis also captures India in the middle of a complex contraceptive transition, moving from low contraceptive use among the poorest to high reliance on sterilization among a large majority of the population and finally to a gradual disaffection for sterilization among higher-status groups.

In light of our analysis, we may want to underline the need for the government to promote gender equality in family planning methods to provide high-quality services with follow-up visits. Women should be encouraged to rely on alternative methods of contraception to avoid health complications. It will also reduce the chance of regret linked to sterilization in case of child loss. Relying solely on and promoting female sterilization may not be anymore an ethical practice to facilitate fertility transition. To a large extent, Indian men failed to get involved in contraceptive matters. Only approximately 11% of protected couples rely on male methods such as condoms and male sterilization (IIPS and ICF, 2017). The National Policy for Women of 2016 has already encouraged a shift towards male sterilization. However, the more active promotion of alternative modern methods of contraception should also be considered.

References

Basu, A. M. (1985). Family planning and the emergency: An unanticipated consequence. *Economic and Political Weekly, 20*(10), 422–425.

Bhatia, M., Banerjee, K., Dixit, P., & Dwivedi, L. K. (2020). Assessment of variation in cesarean delivery rates between public and private health facilities in India from 2005 to 2016. *JAMA Network Open, 3*(8), e2015022–e2015022. https://doi.org/10.1001/jamanetworkopen.2020.15022

Bose, A. (1993). *Indian and the Asian population perspective*. B.R. Publishing Corporation; Sales office, D.K. Publishers Distributors.

Dahat, P. (2014). 11 women die after sterilisation surgeries in Chhattisgarh. *The Hindu*. https://www.thehindu.com/news/national/other-states/8-women-dead-in-botched-surgeries-at-chhattisgarh-govt-camp/article6586425.ece

De Oliveira, I. T., Dias, J. G., & Padmadas, S. S. (2014). Dominance of sterilization and alternative choices of contraception in India: An appraisal of the socioeconomic impact. *PLoS One, 9*(1), e86654.

IIPS, and ICF. (2017). *National Family Health Survey (NFHS-4), 2015–16: India*. IIPS.

ORGI. (2018). Special bulletin on maternal mortality in India 2014–16 *SRS bulletin*. Government of India.

Pradhan, M. R., & Ram, U. (2009). Female sterilization and ethical issues: The Indian experience. *Social Change, 39*(3), 365–387. https://doi.org/10.1177/004908570903900303

Säävälä, M. (1999). Understanding the prevalence of female sterilization in rural South India. *Studies in Family Planning, 30*(4), 288–301.

Singh, A., Ogollah, R., Ram, F., & Pallikadavath, S. (2012). Sterilization regret among married women in India: Implications for the Indian National Family Planning Program. *International Perspectives on Sexual and Reproductive Health, 38*(4), 187–195.

United Nations, Department of Economic and Social Affairs, Population Division. (2015). *Trends in contraceptive use worldwide* 2015. ST/ESA/SER. A/349.

Zavier, F., & Padmadas, S. S. (2000). Use of a spacing method before sterilization among couples in Kerala, India. *International Family Planning Perspectives, 26*(1), 29–35. https://doi.org/10.2307/2648287

Chapter 21
Modern and Traditional Contraception Among Indian Women

Aditi Kundu, Bhaswati Das, and Angad Singh

India has had a long history of family planning, starting in the 1950s. The primary focus was to reduce demographic growth by lowering the birth rate. Indian family planning programs were regulated mainly by government policies, and there was little intervention from other bodies, such as Non-Governmental Organizations or private health workers. As a result, the contraceptive prevalence rate (CPR) remained as low as 13% till 1971. Still, the "cafeteria approach" introduced in the late 1960s meant that a wide choice of methods was offered to couples, and the prevalence rate regularly increased since the 1970s to reach 56.3% in 2005–06. According to the NFHS-4 estimates, 53.5% of the currently married women in the reproductive age group (15–49 years) are protected by some traditional or modern method, whether reversible or irreversible. This slight decline observed in NFHS-4 was a source of surprise and stemmed, to some extent, from the decline in the proportion of sterilization. Nevertheless, according to the latest NFHS-5, about 66.7% of the currently married women of childbearing age (15–49 years) use today any contraceptive method (modern or traditional method) to avoid unwanted pregnancy or delay those.

India has implemented several strategies to encourage family planning. A review of the family planning program reveals that India's policy is a target-oriented approach and reward-based. Interestingly, Indian family planning policies have gradually become more female-oriented and poor-targeted. Tubectomies became more popular than vasectomies (Srinivasan, 2017). Oral pills and intrauterine devices started replacing condoms, as males dislike using condoms due to lessening sexual pleasure (Kamal et al., 2013). Still, intrauterine contraceptive devices

A. Kundu (✉) · B. Das
Centre for the Study of Regional Development, Jawaharlal Nehru University, New Delhi, India

A. Singh
Office of Registrar General of India, New Delhi, India

C. Z. Guilmoto (ed.), *Atlas of Gender and Health Inequalities in India*, Demographic Transformation and Socio-Economic Development 16,
https://doi.org/10.1007/978-3-031-47847-5_21

(IUCDs) failed to acquire massive popularity in most Indian states, except states such as Punjab and Haryana. This situation is notably related to the poor health conditions of the women, anemia, and the risk of expulsion of the IUCDs (Ram et al., 2007).

In this chapter, we focus on the variation between modern and traditional methods of contraception. We first examine the spatial patterns of modern contraception and then provide a regression analysis of the main correlates of modern contraception.

Data Source and Methods

The NFHS-5 is by far the largest sample survey, providing detailed insight into the country's contraception data since it covers all types of available contraceptive methods in the most recent time. The survey comprises a detailed section on contraception in the women's questionnaire. Women are asked in particular whether they ever had sexual intercourse and "have ever used anything or tried in any way to delay or avoid getting pregnant." If yes, women are then asked about the methods used. The data is collected on all individual methods: female sterilization, male sterilization, IUD/PPIUD (postpartum intrauterine devices), injectables, pills, condom/nirodh, female condom, emergency contraception, diaphragm, foam/jelly, standard days method, lactational amenorrhea method, rhythm method, withdrawal, other modern methods, and other traditional methods.[1]

It is important to remember that NFHS data are mostly self-reported, with no additional verification. Therefore, communication gaps between the surveyor and the respondent can lead to underestimating contraceptive prevalence. Furthermore, the taboo surrounding discussions about sexual intercourse and contraception can make women shy away from the questions and give shady responses.

Our sample comprises 347,806 married women aged 15–49 who have had sexual intercourse and used any birth control method. This chapter categorizes all contraceptives into a binary category of "traditional" and "modern" contraceptive methods (Festin et al., 2016). A modern contraceptive method can be defined as "a product or medical procedure that interferes with reproduction from acts of sexual intercourse" (Hubacher & Trussell, 2015). This definition lists all fertility awareness-based methods (FABMs) and Lactational Amenorrhea Methods (LAM) as non-modern contraceptives. Modern Contraceptive Methods (MCMs) were "invented so couples could act on natural impulses and desires with diminished risks of pregnancy" (Hubacher & Trussell, 2015). These technological innovations enable couples to have protected sex at any "mutually desired time." MCMs can again be categorized into reversible or temporary, spacing, and irreversible or permanent methods. The spacing methods are hormonal methods (e.g., OCP, injections), diaphragm and barrier methods, male and female condoms, PPIUCD, or foams, creams, and jellies.

[1] The original NFHS dataset and the spatial analysis methodology are described in detail in Chap. 1.

In 2015, the USAID and WHO organized a technical consultation that concluded that a contraceptive method to be labeled as "a modern method" should fulfill a list of characteristics: "a sound basis in reproductive biology," "a precise protocol for correct use," and "existing data showing the method has been tested in an appropriately designed study to assess efficacy under various conditions." LAM is based on the knowledge that prolonged breastfeeding can act as an effective contraceptive method, although it does not involve any medical procedure and has been practiced for ages. We have accordingly classified LAM as a modern method in this study.

Although contraceptives can be categorized differently as "reversible/irreversible," "permanent/temporary," and "long-lasting/short-lasting," most commonly, they are classified as traditional methods and modern methods. This study also follows the same classification even though the present use of these value-loaded words "does not correspond to the temporal or historical context of these words" (Festin et al., 2016). They neither denote less effective nor more effective methods nor can they be perceived as desirable or undesirable.[2]

This chapter lists withdrawal, rhythm, and the standard day method as traditional contraceptive methods. On the opposite, vasectomy (male sterilization), tubectomy (female sterilization), condom/nirodh, female condoms, oral contraceptive pill (OCP), injections, postpartum intrauterine contraceptive device (PPIUCD), diaphragm, foam, and jelly are classified as modern contraceptive methods. Our classification is in line with the National Family Health Survey classification.

For the analysis of the determinants of contraceptive use, we have implemented a logistic regression of modern contraception using the following demographic and socioeconomic covariates: age, place of residence (urban, rural), education levels (no education, primary, secondary, higher), religion (Hindu, Muslim, others), caste/tribe (SC/ST, OBC, others), wealth index (poorest, poorer, middle, richer, richest), parity (no children, one child, two children, three or more children), and India regions as classified in NFHS (North, Central, East, North-East, West, and South).[3]

Results

The rise in contraceptive use and the decline in fertility are not uniform across India. Given the tremendous social and cultural disparity within India, the regional variations observed in the use of contraception are not surprising (see Chaps. 18 and 20 in this Atlas). Similarly, the variations in the type of contraceptive methods (modern vs. traditional contraception) are expected to be affected by both regional and socioeconomic factors.

---

[2] The use of condoms as a barrier method can be dated back to the seventeenth century, and its actual "use effectiveness" is no better than that of a traditional method such as coitus interruptus (withdrawal).

[3] A more detailed statistical analysis of various types of contraception use based on NFHS-4 figures may be found in Singh et al. (2019).

At the national level, 84.6% of married women aged 15–49 used modern contraceptives out of all women who used any birth control method in the same age group. The data point to wide state-level disparities in modern contraceptive use: estimated levels range from a meager 30% in Manipur to extreme values of 99% in Andhra Pradesh, Karnataka, and Mizoram. Overall, southern states record the highest percentage of women using modern contraception.

Figure 21.1 delineates the contours of the modern vs. traditional contraceptive divide in India, resting to a large extent on the north/south differences observed in fertility levels from the 1970s onwards. The value of Moran's Index statistics at 0.74 suggests a strong geographical clustering. The map indicates that modern contraceptive methods dominate almost everywhere in India, with a share of over 95% of women in South India and Deccan states, including south Madhya Pradesh and west Chhattisgarh. This large cluster closely resembles that of sterilization (Fig. 20.1). This cluster notably omits both Kerala and Punjab, where the use of traditional contraception methods is slightly higher and closer to 10–20%. The only other discernable cluster of modern methods is found in Mizoram.

The map also describes what has remained of traditional contraceptive practices. They still account for over 20% in numerous parts of India. The highest reliance on traditional methods is measured in Assam, Manipur, and part of Meghalaya, where most of the 13 districts in which modern methods account for less than half of the contraceptive practice. The cluster analysis reported in Fig. 21.1 highlights several compact areas where the use of modern contraception is consistently below the national average. Traditional methods are notably concentrated in a cluster centered on Assam and extending to Manipur and Tripura, which happened to be Hindu-majority states of the Northeast. We may contrast adjacent Manipur and Mizoram, states with the lowest and highest prevalence of modern contraception, respectively. Apart from the Northeast, the most prominent clusters encompass the tribal and coastal parts of Odisha as well as west Uttar Pradesh, i.e., the wealthiest districts of the latter state. East Uttar Pradesh and Bihar, representing less prosperous and higher-fertility regions, are not part of this cluster and exhibit values closer to the national average.

The multivariate regression analysis confirms this spatial patterning of contraceptive types (see Fig. 21.2). The Northeast stands at the opposite of South India, with the lowest and the highest regional odds ratios for modern contraceptive use, respectively.[4] For instance, reliance on modern contraception regularly increases with age and parity. There are more modest social variations, with Muslims relying less on modern methods. Compared to Hindu women, women of other religions (mostly Sikhs, Christians, and Buddhists) also display lower odds ratios. Finally, socioeconomic status exerts, as expected, a positive impact on modern contraceptive

[4]Odds ratios measure the strength of the correlation with the outcome variable. Values above (below) one correspond to a positive (negative) association.

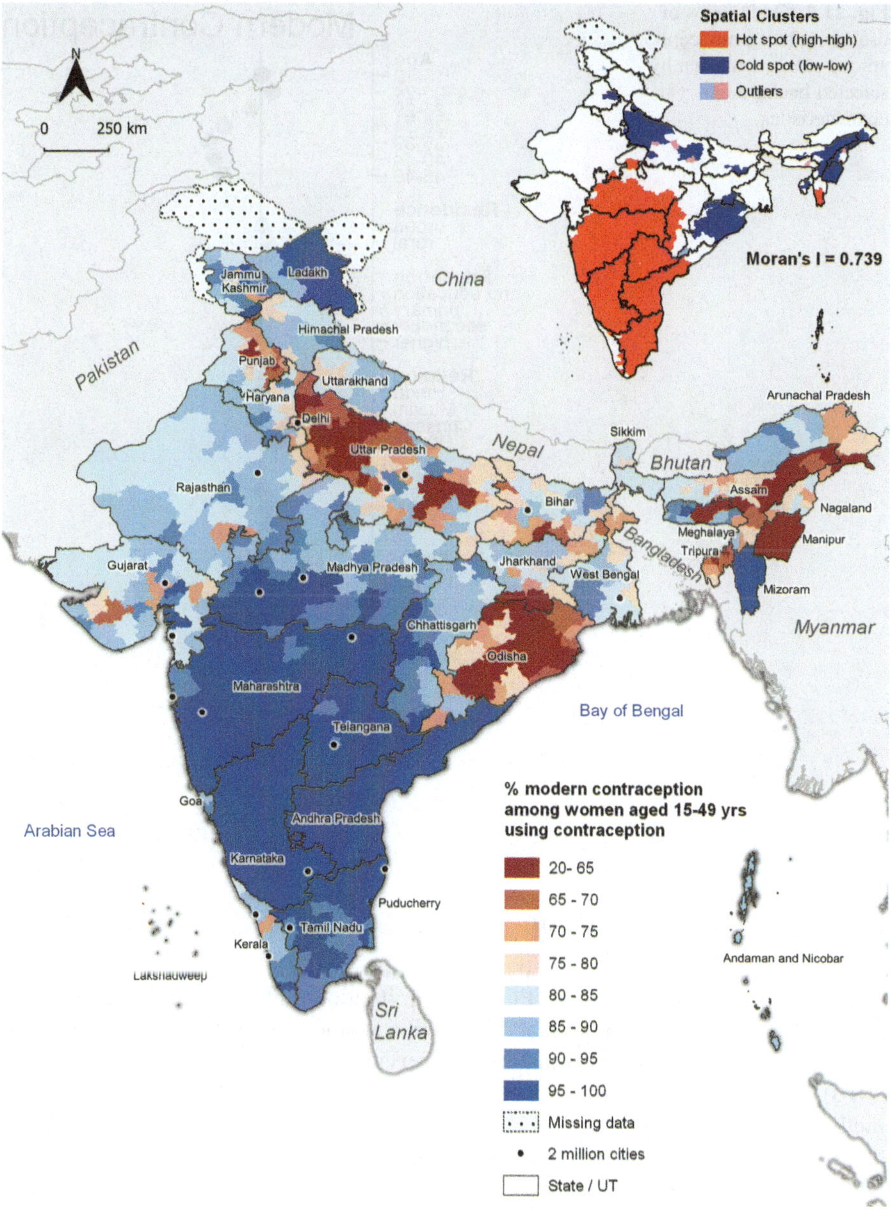

Fig. 21.1 Share of women protected by contraception aged 15–49 years using modern contraception
Source: NFHS-5, 2019–21
The map is for illustrative purposes and may not represent official boundaries

methods. However, this is not the case for education, and the most educated women display, on the contrary, relatively lower use of modern contraception. This result may be partly due to their lower reliance on sterilization (see Chap. 20 in this Atlas).

Fig. 21.2 Odds ratios of use of modern contraception among married women by selected background characteristics

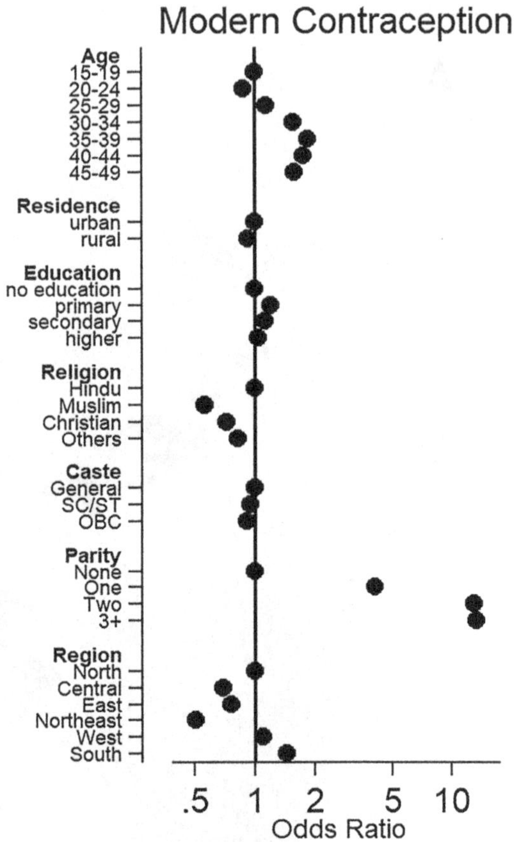

Discussion and Conclusion

The London Summit on Family Planning, in its global meeting held in July 2012, had set the goal that "an additional 120 million women and girls will have access to effective family planning information and services by the year 2020" (Festin et al., 2016). Several authors have argued that dependency on traditional contraceptive methods is like the "last resort for couples" (Ram et al., 2007); that is, it is more of a "lack of choice than a conscious choice." On a different note, many have posited withdrawal and rhythm as a choice of the informed and educated class, the urban elites, and women with some form of authority in the relationship. Indicators of women's empowerment seem to have a significant impact, mainly associated with the level of knowledge, power of making decisions, and attitudes towards domestic violence—and have a positive effect on contraceptive choices.

A previous study shows the two possible situations in which traditional methods are used voluntarily or not. In the first case, a couple consciously chooses to select a traditional method "to avoid pregnancy without compromising on sexual pleasure and health outcomes." In the second case, couples do not have any other option because of the lack of availability of modern methods and are compelled to rely on traditional methods (Ram et al., 2007). These two situations correspond to demand and supply factors, respectively, and correspond in India to quite different population segments.

Contraceptive use increases as the basket of choices expands, both temporally and cross-sectionally. "A wider choice of methods also improves the ability to meet the individual needs of women and couples" (Ross & Stover, 2013). "There is a direct correlation between the number of contraceptive options available and the willingness of people to use them" (Muttreja & Singh, 2018). Although there has been a constant rise in contraceptive use in India, focusing on a single method can push away many willing couples. One method can never serve better in a demographically and socio-economically diverse country like India. The 2017 National Health Policy of India decided to increase the expenditure on family planning to 2.5% of the country's GDP. India's newly launched Parivaar Vikas Programme aims to improve family planning services and access to contraceptives in 145 high-fertility districts of 7 Indian states. These efforts will hopefully also diversify the methods of family planning offered to women.

References

Festin, M. P. R., Kiarie, J., Solo, J., Spieler, J., Malarcher, S., Van Look, P. F. A., & Temmerman, M. (2016). Moving towards the goals of FP2020—Classifying contraceptives. *Contraception, 94*(4), 289–294. https://doi.org/10.1016/j.contraception.2016.05.015

Hubacher, D., & Trussell, J. (2015). A definition of modern contraceptive methods. *Contraception, 92*(5), 420–421. https://doi.org/10.1016/j.contraception.2015.08.008

Kamal, M. M., Islam, M. S., Alam, M. S., & Hasssn, A. E. (2013). Determinants of male involvement in family planning and reproductive health in Bangladesh. *American Journal of Human Ecology, 2*(2), 83–93.

Muttreja, P., & Singh, S. (2018). Family planning in India: The way forward. *The Indian Journal of Medical Research, 148*(Suppl 1), S1–S9. https://doi.org/10.4103/ijmr.IJMR_2067_17

Ram, U., Dwivedi, L., & Goswami, B. (2007). Understanding contraception use among Muslims of India, Pakistan and Bangladesh. *Journal of Population and Social Studies [JPSS], 15*(2), 101–130.

Ross, J., & Stover, J. (2013). Use of modern contraception increases when more methods become available: Analysis of evidence from 1982–2009. *Global Health: Science and Practice, 1*(2), 203–212. https://doi.org/10.9745/GHSP-D-13-00010

Singh, S. K., Sharma, B., Vishwakarma, D., Yadav, G., Srivastava, S., & Maharana, B. (2019). Women's empowerment and use of contraception in India: Macro and micro perspectives emerging from NFHS-4 (2015–16). *Sexual and Reproductive Healthcare, 19*, 15–23.

Srinivasan, K. (2017). *Population concerns in India: Shifting trends, policies, and programs*. Sage Publishing.

Part V
Epilogue

Chapter 22
The Geography of Gender and Health Inequalities in India

Christophe Z. Guilmoto

India has recently recorded significant progress in many economic, demographic, and health indicators. While still lagging compared to some of its neighbors, such as Sri Lanka, Nepal, or Bangladesh, the sustained pace of improvements in the country over the last 20 years suggests that progress will continue in the following decades. For example, as I write, trends measured from the latest National Family Health Survey (NFHS-5) and the few other sources available, such as the report of India's Health and Management Information System (HMIS), confirm non-stop advances in most reproductive health indicators such as antenatal care, institutional deliveries, or child immunization (see Chaps. 13, 14, and 15). In addition, despite the lack of recent census data (the census operations are still adjourned *sine die*), survey-based estimates show that many other social development indicators such as school attendance, fertility, child marriage, nutrition, or health insurance are also improving (see Chaps. 2, 18, 11, and 17).[1]

This optimistic context tends to conceal the extent of gender and health vulnerabilities that represent another fundamental trait of India's contemporary landscape. Such inequalities largely stem from the cumulative impact of distinct factors observed vertically across social groups and horizontally across regions. Income, education, caste, religion, distance to urban areas, and local development levels are the main drivers of these disparities. To take a few examples, we can contrast cesarean rates ranging from 3% in Karauli (Rajasthan) to 77% in Suryapet

[1] See, for instance, the analysis of recent progress based on NFHS rounds published by NITI Aayog (2023). The Multidimensional Poverty Index used in the latter report incorporates several health indicators examined separately in this Atlas: undernutrition, antenatal care, institutional deliveries, and child mortality.

C. Z. Guilmoto (✉)
Centre des Sciences Humaines/IRD (CEPED), New Delhi, India
e-mail: Christophe.Guilmoto@ird.fr

C. Z. Guilmoto (ed.), *Atlas of Gender and Health Inequalities in India*, Demographic Transformation and Socio-Economic Development 16,
https://doi.org/10.1007/978-3-031-47847-5_22

(Telangana); adequate antenatal coverage ranging from 26% among illiterates in Nagaland to 95% among educated classes in Goa; health insurance ranging from 8% among urban women in Bihar to 85% among Andhra Pradesh women without schooling; or proportion of missing girl-only families due to gender bias ranging from 2% in Kaniyakumari (Tamil Nadu) to 87% in Faridabad (Haryana).[2] These extreme values may be typical of Sub-Saharan Africa or staunchly patriarchal countries, on the one hand, and of Southeast Asia and gender-equal countries, on the other. These internal disparities in health, gender, or demographic behavior are unique to India as other large populations like Brazil, China, Indonesia, or the United States are far more homogenous in comparison.[3]

Socioeconomic vs. Regional Inequalities

The range of values reported in India derives from a singular inequality regime that decades of rapid growth may have more exacerbated than reduced. Examples given in the previous paragraph illustrate the extent of social and regional differentials. They also suggest that extreme values are often determined primarily by location rather than social characteristics. For example, under-five mortality estimates range from 3 p. 1000 among Muslims in Kerala to 71 among Dalits in Uttar Pradesh, a value almost 25 times higher. Nonetheless, the discrepancies in mortality rates among children under five are limited in these two states. Mortality differentials by education or socioeconomic status are of the same order. Poor women or children in Kerala thus fare better than elite groups in Uttar Pradesh regarding child survival, and the same observation could be replicated for almost all variables examined in this Atlas.

There is little doubt that social inequalities significantly underpin health inequalities. A disaggregated regional analysis of India's mortality by caste profile confirms this hypothesis (Gupta & Sudharsanan, 2022). More broadly, a recent report lists geography, wealth, caste, and religion as India's primary determinants of inequalities (Oxfam, 2021). A finer sociological granularity would be required to explore and make sense of India's gender and health landscape since discrimination and inequity are implemented locally–within families or communities, in schools, or rural dispensaries. To understand the mechanisms through which gender, income, age, caste, or status determine health outcomes, we need to read the work of ethnographers who better capture the lived experience of sickness, childbirth, or access to medical advice and contraception. I can only encourage readers to delve into in-depth qualitative research focusing, for example, on chronic illness (Kane et al., 2022), healthcare seeking (Pandey et al., 2002), sterilization (Lukšaitė, 2022), health

[2]Figures are from the NFHS-5 state reports or the dataset prepared for the Atlas.

[3]The only nation of comparable heterogeneity must have been the former Soviet Union, where extreme variations were observed, for example, between Central Asian and Baltic republics.

insurance (Ahlin et al., 2016), discrimination in health centers (George, 2019), or childbirth (Pinto, 2022; Jullien & Jeffery, 2021) to quote a few instances of recent - micro-studies. This approach is not what is done in this Atlas based on aggregated data across small regions (districts) from where the grain of gender and health vulnerabilities is missing. The statistical approach allows us to recognize distinct patterns and regularities that local studies cannot restitute. One challenge in comprehending inequality in India is that regional variations outweigh the impact of local status and socioeconomic discrimination mechanisms that operate locally.

While there are vast differences in wealth or caste groups within a region, the bulk of heterogeneity across India relates first to its diverse geography outlined in this Atlas. Each chapter will show the extent of cross-regional variations within the country by plotting district-level estimates of an extensive array of health and gender indicators. Authors frequently highlight social, economic, and demographic differentials in their studies with the help of regression models that incorporate socioeconomic status, education, caste, religion, age, and other standard indicators. These covariates are almost always significantly associated with the primary variable under study. However robust this correlation, social variables never account for the extent of spatial variations depicted on the maps of the Atlas. In other words, the socioeconomic characteristics of women, men, children, or households explain only a limited part of regional differentials observed in India. Instead, these regional variations display unique and lasting spatial features.

Ever since the seminal research by Link and Phelan (1995), we tend to interpret socioeconomic disparities in health through the prism of the theory of fundamental causes. The approach identifies four critical dimensions through which socioeconomic inequalities impact health: the effects of socioeconomic disparities on multiple health risk factors and on multiple morbidity and mortality outcomes, the crucial role played by access to flexible resources (education, financial means, social connections, etc.), and the gradual transition over time of the intervening mechanisms at the root of the socioeconomic inequalities in health.[4] India's health landscape suggests that regional inequalities could be similarly framed. Indicators deployed in the Atlas include an extensive array of both risk factors (from places of delivery to child immunization) and mortality and morbidity outcomes (from child survival to hypertension prevalence), and we may wonder if they move in parallel across the country. In other words, whether the multiplicity of risk factors and health outcomes across social classes highlighted by the theory of fundamental causes applies similarly to regional inequalities. The analysis that follows will attempt to examine this hypothesis.

[4]For a restatement of the theory of the fundamental causes of diseases, see Phelan et al. (2010).

A Synthesis of Health and Gender Spatial Inequalities

Acknowledging the diversity of the configurations depicted by the chapters of this Atlas, I endeavor to provide in this chapter a synthesis of India's health and gender spatial patterns. These two dimensions of health and gender are usually analyzed separately (Balarajan et al., 2011; Dandona et al., 2017; Batra & Reio Jr, 2016) and at the state level or mixed with socioeconomic indicators (NITI Aayog, 2023). Here, I want to build on their numerous commonalities, notably illustrated by reproductive and demographic behavior in which the health and gender dimensions are closely intertwined. Before making claims on India's regional patterning, I want to comprehensively analyze the distribution of the health and gender indicators and then their convergence and divergence. To do this, I will combine the main dimensions drawn from all the analyses prepared by the contributors to this Atlas to delineate the singular patterning of gender and health inequalities in India. This approach borrows from a long tradition of spatial analysis in India inaugurated by Sopher (1972) and recently illustrated (Singh et al., 2021).[5] I also want to examine the hypothesis presented above, whether health risks and outcomes combine regionally in the same way across socioeconomic status according to the theory of fundamental causes of health inequalities.

The analysis rests on indicators computed on the child population and women of childbearing age, as well as more complex indirect estimates relating to the entire household or women's birth history. The confrontation of these indicators brings both expected and unexpected associations: it may sound evident, for instance, that gender bias in fertility behavior correlates with the low frequency of girl-only families; however, a similarly strong linkage between lack of menstrual hygiene and female malnutrition is less obvious. Therefore, rather than relying on a basic visual inspection to compare the maps of various indicators, I submit the dataset prepared for the Atlas to a synthetic statistical analysis of district averages. Interestingly, while this procedure ignores spatial information about these districts, geography will strongly re-emerge from my results.

What follows is primarily an attempt to synthesize all the information derived from the maps included in this volume. The chapters provide a formidable tool to map the diversity in gender and health circumstances across India, but I also need to reorder the diverging geographies that these individual indicators project. However, before doing this, it is essential to consider three caveats of such an analysis.

The first reservation may be that the 28 variables used in this Atlas cannot pretend to cover all dimensions of gender and health in India. The availability of district-level data is limited here to what NFHS-5 can provide. In addition, I have not incorporated district-level figures from sources such as the DHLS or the 2011 census, which are outdated. However, many essential dimensions of gender and health in India are missing from this analysis. For instance, we have no district-level

[5] See also the study by Mohanty et al. (2019) for a comparable exercise conducted around indicators of human development in India.

estimates to capture female autonomy or gender violence and no information on other forms of gender discrimination concerning income, employment, education, political representation, or inheritance. Similarly, we have minimal reliable information on morbidity or access to health facilities.[6] Thanks to new surveys, I hope such information will appear in the coming years at the district level inspired by the most innovative and rich surveys (National Sample Survey, India Human Development Survey, or Longitudinal Ageing Study in India).

The second reservation relates, on the contrary, to the relevance and usability of some indicators derived from the Atlas maps. I did not retain all available variables for the synthetic analysis for two reasons. On the one hand, several variables were characterized by an unknown level of reliability. A preliminary analysis employing geostatistical and statistical tools at the district level highlighted potential irregularities for some variables. These indicators displayed a surprisingly low level of spatial autocorrelation and equally weak or insignificant statistical correlation levels with other standard variables, such as literacy or wealth. These poorly correlated variables were subsequently discarded from the dataset used in the synthetic classification, as it was feared that they would introduce more noise than substance into the analysis. On the other hand, some other variables were strongly correlated. For example, the patrilocal residence index closely followed the proportion of women owning land; similarly, anemia rates measured on women and children are strongly correlated. Including collinear variables in the dataset would bias the analysis toward specific health and gender dimensions. The final dataset used for the analysis in this chapter was trimmed accordingly to avoid redundancies and obvious collinearity.

After assessing the indicators' spatial and statistical reliability and potential redundancy, I decided to restrict the analysis to 24 variables. They represented one (sometimes two) variable(s) from each chapter.[7] I used male mortality to capture the overall mortality level rather than female mortality, as the latter indicator is affected by gender bias. Even if no corresponding chapter was updated with NFHS-5 data, I included a variable on cancer screening. These variables account for the main domains of gender and health covered in this Atlas. Finally, I refrained from incorporating in the analysis any direct or indirect geographical variables (states, geographical coordinates, physical characteristics, etc.) that would have reintroduced spatial patterns through the back door.

A final caveat pertains to the fact that this approach is a pure "ecological analysis" in which districts are the units of the analysis rather than subdistricts, towns, households, families, or women. We are, in particular, trapped by this district-level analysis. Consequently, we cannot capture the grain of spatial differentiation–such as the variations between towns and rural areas or between different terrains (littoral,

[6]The SHRUG Atlas (https://www.devdatalab.org/atlas) prepared by the Development Data Lab offers indicators of health facilities mapped at the village level. Original data come from the Mission Antyodaya, but their coverage appears incomplete.

[7]We use male mortality to capture the overall mortality level rather than female mortality that is affected by gender bias.

hillside, etc.). In addition, the analysis in this chapter should be understood in terms of regional associations but not as proof of correlations at the individual level. For instance, it can be shown that districts with poor levels of menstrual hygiene are also characterized by higher fertility. Still, it does not follow that women using hygienic methods of menstrual protection have fewer children than other women.[8] A more basic cross-tabulation of women's fertility levels by types of menstrual hygiene would be required to confirm this correlation. Some authors in the Atlas have resorted to a formal statistical analysis to sort out the determinants of gender and health indicators and provide more formal proof of the association between the indicators examined in their chapter and the standard socioeconomic characteristics of corresponding women or households. In contrast, the ecological research derived from this Atlas aims at a somewhat different aim: delineating the unique features of regional patterning and interpreting the specific geography of India's health and gender inequalities.

Factor and Classification Analysis

I started with this set of 24 variables from the Atlas and prepared a correlation matrix of district-level averages (results not shown here). Many statistical associations observed between variables at the district level were expected and helped me confirm some of the main dimensions of gender and health in India, such as gender bias (son preference in fertility, deficit of girl-only families, and female land ownership), maternal health services (institutional deliveries, C-section, and antenatal care), and low fertility (ever-born children, early marriage, families with one child or none). Additionally, the correlation matrix pointed to unexpected but significant associations. Several indicators were also found to be poorly correlated or uncorrelated with the rest of the dataset, such as hysterectomy, modern contraception, migrating husband, or neonatal protection against tetanus. Such indicators often appear unconnected to the leading socioeconomic indicators (e.g., social composition, literacy, urbanization) and other health and gender indicators used in the Atlas. While some social and health traits may be perfectly circumscribed to specific regional hotspots,[9] doubts remain on the quality of the measurements of some indicators, notably on self-reported health conditions and morbidity.

Following this preliminary correlation analysis, I launched a factor analysis to see how different indicators were linked (results not shown here). As expected, the first principal component derived from the factor analysis of the dataset was a global dimension of development and relative prosperity, associating, for instance, low

[8]This is a typical example of *ecological fallacy* in which regional associations are incorrectly interpreted as proofs of correlations at the individual level.

[9]The presence of specific outmigration pockets and of isolated matrilineal societies across India is a typical illustration of such phenomena.

fertility, better mother and child health, more frequent use of reproductive healthcare, etc. This coefficient would probably strongly correlate with other unilinear development indicators, such as the recently released Multidimensional Poverty Index that ranks districts from the worst to the best (NITI Aayog, 2023).

Still, the first component derived from the factor analysis accounted for less than a third of the total variance of the district sample. The second significant factor broadly related to gender, while two additional factors were also significant.[10] The intricate combinations of four distinct factors (of various weights) proved challenging to present and interpret coherently. For this reason, and keeping with the geographical approach privileged here, I opted instead for a classification analysis to divide India into smaller subsets of districts. The high spatial autocorrelation indices reported in the chapters of this Atlas suggested that such a classification might lead to the detection of distinct spatial features; this intuition proved correct, as we will see.

Why classify districts? Classification is a standard data mining tool representing a convenient method for reorganizing the large dataset and all the maps assembled for this Atlas. This tool is often employed to shed light on complex spatial configurations, including health outcomes in India (Mutheneni et al., 2018; Anilkumar et al., 2017; Hemalatha et al., 2020). The first purpose of the classification is to offer a robust method to summarize almost 17,000 estimates, i.e., the distribution of 24 variables across 707 districts; this will lead to a concise synthesis of similarities and variations in the dataset. In other words, this dataset exploration aims to extract information, define regions, and provide new instruments to interpret variations and trends in India's current gender and health scenario.

The classification methods begin with analyzing a matrix of inter-district distances with which individual districts will be gradually clubbed into larger groups. I opted for a hierarchical approach comprising a series of nested subdivisions whereby each clustering step depends on the previous one. More specifically, I applied an agglomerative method that starts by clubbing together individual districts one by one. Different ways exist to use distance measurements to perform this clustering, and I apply the most robust here, Ward's method, based on the minimum sum of squares.

One issue never resolved in this classification analysis is identifying the optimal number of clusters. While I did not want a partition into ten or more clusters for pragmatic and heuristic reasons, I still did not know how many clusters to keep. Several methods exist that measure the relative gain in adding a cluster, and I used two of them. The method due to Calinski and Harabasz proved unhelpful; it showed, as expected, a steady decline in the quality of clusters as their number increased, with no noticeable break for the first 15 steps. The alternative rule developed by Duda and Hart was more suggestive (for a description of these methods, see Everitt et al., 2011); their indicator pointed to slightly better clustering for 2, 4, 7, and 9 clusters. I decided to retain seven clusters for the sake of simplicity.

[10] We consider a factor significant when its eigenvalue exceeds 1.5.

Seven Gender and Health Clusters

The advantage of the hierarchical approach employed here is that it is an aggregative process in which the partition can be decomposed step by step. If we start from India as a whole, we can see how it gets gradually subdivided into various clusters. Interestingly, the first partition demarcates a large band of west and north Central India districts from the rest of the country. These 300 districts run from the Pakistani border (from Gujarat to Punjab) to Bihar, Madhya Pradesh to the east, and central Maharashtra and north Karnataka to the south. It makes up a compact set that covers the less developed plains of North India—notably the upper and middle Ganga plains. It excludes hilly states of the northwest (Himachal Pradesh, Jammu and Kashmir, Uttarakhand, and Ladakh). However, it includes a large part of the Deccan plateau, extending to central Maharashtra (Khandesh, Marathwada) and northern districts of Karnataka (North Maidan or Hyderabad Karnatak, recently renamed "Kalyana Karnataka"). As seen further below, this vast region excludes a few districts belonging to eastern Uttar Pradesh (north Purvanchal). In the following disaggregated cluster analysis, this large set of districts has further been bifurcated, resulting in the emergence of three separate clusters, viz. the III.a West India, III.b Rich West India, and IV Ganga clusters. The first partition also led to a vast cluster encompassing East and South India. This second block was also gradually divided as the classification analysis proceeded. It revealed two other large blocks comprising relatively homogenous districts: South India (I.a and I.b clusters) and East and Northeast India (II.a and II.b clusters).

The preliminary distribution of district by state and cluster is given in Table 22.1. The clusters are also displayed on the map of India (Fig. 22.1). To get a sense of the profile of each cluster, their primary health and gender characteristics (average value of the main variables) are provided in Table 22.2. Let us now review each of these seven clusters in detail.

The first two clusters are a familiar feature of India's cultural and social geography, comprising South India's most advanced regions along with the Konkan coast up to Surat and Vidarbha in east Maharashtra. The first distinct cluster, the **South Cluster**, encompasses the southern tip of India (**Cluster I.a**). It includes Kerala, Puducherry, Tamil Nadu, Andhra Pradesh, Telangana, Goa, Lakshadweep, and one coastal district in Karnataka (Udupi). Except for districts along the Konkan littoral, this cluster forms a single block of 96 contiguous districts.

Apart from its distinct geography, this region is the most educated and urbanized of all the clusters and includes many of India's most prosperous districts. However, the Atlas indicators have brought together these districts for different reasons. Regarding child and maternal health, the South Cluster records some of the top results recorded in India. For example, this cluster has the highest share of modern contraception users (and sterilized women), women with a single child or no child, hygienic menstrual protection and antenatal care use, and births delivered in health facilities.

Table 22.1 Distribution of districts by cluster and state

		Clusters							
Cluster		I.a	I.b	II.a	II.b	III.a	III.b	IV	Total
I.a: South	Kerala	14							14
	Tamil Nadu	32							32
	Telangana	31							31
	Andhra Pradesh	13							13
	Goa	2							2
	Lakshadweep	1							1
	Puducherry	2	*2*						4
I.b: Forward	Ladakh		2						2
	Jammu & Kashmir		17		*1*		*2*		20
	Karnataka	*1*	18			*11*			30
II.a: East	Jharkhand			24					24
	Odisha			30					30
	Chhattisgarh			24		*3*			27
	West Bengal			20					20
	Assam			33					33
	Sikkim			4					4
	Mizoram			6	*2*				8
	Tripura			8					8
	Andaman & Nicobar			3					3
	Dadra & Nagar Haveli		*1*	2					3
	Himachal Pradesh		*2*	9			*1*		12
	Uttarakhand			13					13
II.b: Northeast	Arunachal Pradesh				20				20
	Nagaland				11				11
	Manipur				9				9
	Meghalaya				11				11
III.a: West	Rajasthan					33			33
	Madhya Pradesh		*2*	*3*		45		*1*	51
	Maharashtra		*17*			19			36
III.b: Rich West	Haryana						21	*1*	22
	Delhi		*1*				10		11
	Punjab						22		22
	Chandigarh						1		1
	Gujarat		*5*	*1*		*13*	14		33
IV: Ganga	Uttar Pradesh				*12*	*2*	*4*	57	75
	Bihar							38	38
Total		96	67	180	66	126	75	97	707

Note: Numbers in italics refer to the number of districts of each state outside their core cluster. For example, a majority of Karnataka districts belong to Cluster I.b (18 out of 30), but one belongs to Cluster I.a (South) and eleven to Cluster III.a (West)

The highest percentage of households with health insurance (69%) is found in this cluster, which also corresponds to the region where cancer screening is emerging—even if the corresponding rate remains below 6%. Finally, this region is

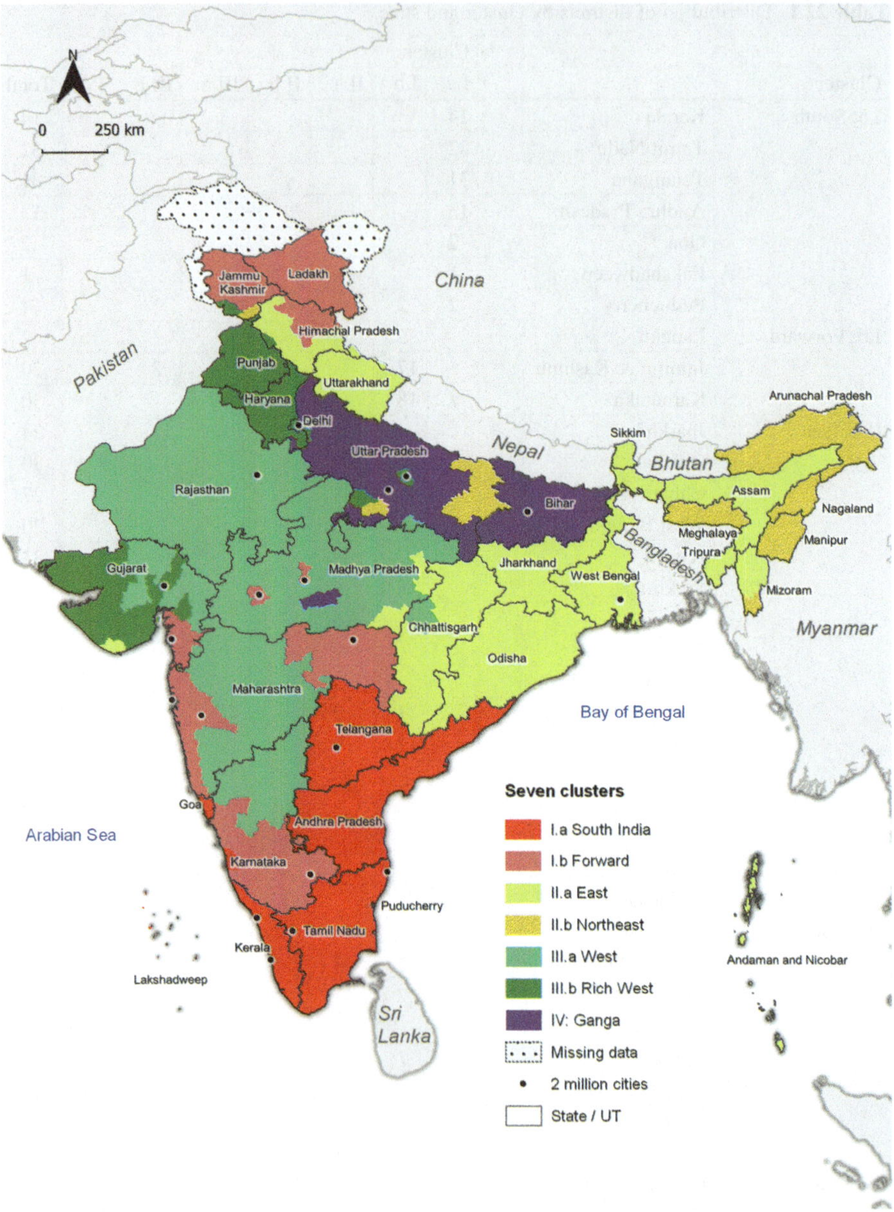

Fig. 22.1 The seven clusters derived from gender and health classification analysis
Source: NFHS-5, 2019–21
The map is for illustrative purposes and may not represent official boundaries

distinguished by the lowest levels of gender bias expressed in fertility preference and behavior (only-girl families). Results are also among the best regarding land ownership by women and non-patrilocal arrangements. It will be apparent in the

Table 22.2 Health and gender profile of the seven clusters

Cluster	I.a South	I.b Forward	II.a East	II.b Northeast	III.a West	III.b Rich West	IV Ganga	India	Chapter
Women underweight	15.2	14.4	19.3	9.8	23.1	14.6	21.9	**17.9**	2
Women overweight*	34.4	26.7	18.7	19.7	16.3	35.8	18.7	**23.1**	2
Vegetarianism among women	2.8	13.7	7.9	3.9	50.3	59.6	31.7	**23.7**	3
Female hyperglycemia	9.4	5.7	7.4	5.3	4.8	6.7	5.4	**6.5**	4
Female hypertension	12.4	11.5	11.4	13.9	9.3	12.7	9.0	**11.2**	4
Anemia among children	59.2	71.7	65.6	51.5	73.2	69.8	69.5	**66.3**	5
Anemia among women*	52.5	58.1	61.4	40.1	56.4	57.8	56.8	**56.0**	5
Male under-five mortality [a]	23.3	18.7	35.7	23.0	41.1	34.3	60.9	**35.5**	6
Female landowners (alone or jointly)	19.6	12.1	9.5	25.5	9.6	9.2	8.7	**12.5**	7
Sons among married children*	89.3	94.4	95.6	80.2	97.6	98.6	96.9	**94.0**	7
Son preference	40.4	45.2	48.9	44.1	64.4	60.9	63.1	**52.9**	8
Avoidance of girl-only families	19.9	37.5	38.6	40.5	64.1	63.0	60.8	**46.3**	9
Migration status of husband	8.3	2.3	7.3	7.1	4.4	3.8	16.9	**7.3**	10
Females married before 18	19.7	12.8	25.2	16.2	27.9	13.0	28.1	**22.0**	11
Menstrual hygiene	93.7	83.9	77.7	80.4	68.9	89.8	65.8	**78.8**	12
At least four antenatal care visits	79.4	79.2	62.5	40.8	60.8	67.6	34.9	**60.8**	13
Neonatal tetanus protection*	91.4	93.6	93.1	82.7	91.9	90.9	91.2	**91.2**	13
Institutional deliveries	98.3	95.8	86.7	71.5	92.1	94.6	80.6	**88.7**	14
Cesarean deliveries (institutional births)	50.5	34.4	21.4	15.9	14.7	29.5	14.5	**24.8**	14
Hysterectomy	5.3	2.4	1.7	1.9	3.2	2.8	3.7	**2.9**	15
Health insurance	68.6	28.1	54.0	31.0	48.3	28.6	16.5	**42.5**	16
Any cancer screening*	5.8	1.2	0.9	1.3	0.9	1.3	1.1	**1.7**	**
Children ever born [b]	1.6	1.5	1.7	1.8	1.9	1.6	2.1	**1.7**	17
Childless women aged 40–49	4.9	4.1	4.9	4.3	2.8	2.4	1.8	**3.7**	18
Women aged 40–49 with exactly one child	10.9	10.1	10.3	7.4	5.7	8.1	3.6	**8.1**	18
Full immunization of children	81.7	85.9	80.1	65.8	77.8	77.2	71.1	**77.6**	19
Female sterilization	58.8	44.5	28.8	14.3	49.3	27.1	22.8	**35.6**	20
Modern contraceptive method	95.4	93.2	78.8	74.1	90.8	79.6	73.2	**83.4**	21

Cluster and national averages are computed over district averages
All variables are in percentages except [a]: per 1000 [b]: children per woman
* Variables not used in the classification analysis; ** No corresponding chapter
See individual chapters for a detailed definition of the variables

following sections that parts of the Northeast (Cluster II.b) perform even better regarding gender indicators.

Are all lights on the green in this South Indian Cluster? Not exactly; the unchecked progress of healthcare, medicalization, and changing lifestyles exert distinct costs. For example, this region records India's highest proportion of women delivering with a cesarean; more than half of the births are surgical deliveries. This figure is significantly above the 15% benchmark recommended by the WHO. It suggests that approximately 40% of non-risk births are delivered by C-sections.[11] We also notice that over a third of women in this region are considered overweight.

Similarly, it records the highest proportion of women (5%) who have undergone a (probably unnecessary) hysterectomy. In contrast to other regions, the South Cluster is marked by the highest rate of diabetes (9%) and a significant proportion of women experiencing anemia. To a large extent, these are typical ailments of affluent India that affect the emerging middle class. The sad news is that the situation in this part of India will probably deteriorate in the coming years without effective policies to curb the rise of overmedicalization and promote healthier diets. It may also be mentioned that the lowest child mortality and the highest immunization rates are not recorded in the South cluster.

The second cluster related to South India is more composite than the first one. I call it the **Forward Cluster** (**Cluster I.b**) to acknowledge its many advanced features regarding gender and health indicators. This cluster is an amalgamation of different sub-regions. Its first and largest component covers the Konkan coast from Bharuch and Surat in the north to Mumbai, Pune, and Dakshina Kannada in the south, stretching to Bengaluru and Kolar along Karnataka's border with Andhra Pradesh and Tamil Nadu. The second component comprises east Maharashtra—Vidarbha districts located around Nagpur—as well as urban districts in nearby Madhya Pradesh (Indore and Bhopal). The third component is in Northwest India and includes most districts of Jammu and Kashmir, Ladakh, and two adjacent districts of Himachal Pradesh.

This dispersed cluster resembles the previous cluster and records some of the best health indicators, as illustrated by satisfactory levels of safe deliveries, antenatal care, child immunization, and contraceptive prevalence. In addition, this region is characterized by India's lowest under-five mortality (19 p. 1000), child marriage rates (13%), and highest rates of protection against tetanus (94%). It corresponds to the most prosperous regions of Karnataka and Maharashtra. A significant difference with the previous South Cluster relates to higher levels of son preference, as notably expressed by gender bias in fertility attitudes and behavior that aligns more with the national average. Anemia is also widespread, in particular among children.

The following two clusters chiefly cover East India. **Cluster II.a** is the largest cluster of the analysis, with 180 districts. I called it the **East Cluster** as it covers a

[11] We assume here that at least 85% of deliveries do not require a cesarean procedure and that all the remaining 15% of births are delivered by C-section.

continuous area starting from Chhattisgarh, Jharkhand, Odisha, and West Bengal and stretching to the east with Sikkim, Assam, Tripura, and Mizoram. In addition, a different regional component of this cluster includes almost 20 adjacent, hilly districts of Himachal Pradesh and Uttarakhand and the Andaman and Nicobar districts.

This cluster represents a less progressive part of India than the previous two clusters examined earlier. Most health and gender indicators in the **East Cluster** lie close to or slightly below the Indian average. Apart from its geography, its main distinctive features relate to its high proportion of underweight women, female anemia, and girls married before 18. This cluster represents a somewhat disparate region and is not characterized by especially low or high indicators. Had I conducted a more detailed cluster analysis, this immense cluster would have been broken up into more homogenous subregions, with the emergence of a distinct cluster restricted to Tribal Central India, viz. Chhattisgarh and Jharkhand. This subregion is particularly fragile because of its land-locked geography. It is notably characterized by the highest level of malaria mortality and the longest distance to cities, two indicators missing from the NFHS dataset.[12]

The **Northeast Cluster** (**Cluster II.b**) was carved out from the previous East Cluster during the classification analysis. It could equally be designated as the mountainous Northeast since it excludes the lowlands of Assam and Tripura and parts of Mizoram. However, it also includes 12 districts of east Uttar Pradesh. Otherwise, this cluster is restricted to Meghalaya, Arunachal Pradesh, Nagaland, and Manipur and contains almost only highland districts with an elevation above 600 m. It should be remembered that local geography and physiography have not been used in the classification analysis. Still, they reappear as we analyze the distinct gender and health features of districts in Northeast India. Cluster II.b is the smallest cluster regarding district number and population size, with only 53 districts in the Northeast (and 13 elsewhere in North India). Because of its geographic segmentation, this cluster is socially heterogeneous and includes many tribal and Christian populations. Other social and economic indicators (wealth index, urbanization) lag India's average levels, except for the higher educational attainment observed in the districts of the Northeast.

We may wonder what makes these few districts so different from the neighboring plains of Assam and Tripura concerning gender or health. The factors behind the divergence from the rest of the Northeast are an unlikely combination of favorable social and gender indicators and alarming health statistics. The gender signature of the Northeast cluster is probably unique in India. First, this region has the highest proportion of women unmarried at age 50 and the highest age at marriage—if we exclude the Uttar Pradesh segment. The difference in this respect with adjacent Assam is pronounced; however, other gender indicators attest to the distinctiveness of this region. The proportion of women reporting land ownership is at its highest

[12]The Malaria Atlas Project has prepared granular maps of malaria prevalence and mortality and travel time to the nearest city. See https://malariaatlas.org

(26%), and the strength of patrilocal residence customs (80%) is the weakest observed in India. As a matter of fact, a few districts in Meghalaya report a remarkably high proportion of uxorilocal arrangements, i.e., families in which the family of a married woman lives with her parents.

The health scenario is mixed in this region. This cluster represents the part of India with the lowest frequency of underweight women (10%), notably compared to the East Cluster, where underweight women are twice as numerous. Simultaneously, the Northeast Cluster does not record a high proportion of overweight or obese women, unlike the rest of India, where prosperity mechanically increases the risk of being overweight. Diabetes and anemia (among children and women) are also distinctly less prevalent. All these traits may be related to local food consumption in a population where vegetarianism (4%) is as low as in the South India Cluster (3%). In addition, under-five mortality is also as low as in South India (23 p. 1000).

This relatively moderate level of child mortality does not square with other health indicators that are less than rosy. This cluster records, in particular, India's lowest rates of protection against tetanus (83%), institutional delivery (71%), and child immunization (66%). Antenatal care, cesarean deliveries, female sterilization, and the prevalence of modern contraceptives are among the country's lowest. These findings point to a significant failure of the health delivery outreach. The lack of urban centers and health facilities, as well as accessibility issues specific to hilly or mountainous peripheral regions, are the primary factors contributing to the challenges in healthcare access in these areas.

The cluster analysis first distinguished a large region to the west, stretching from the Pakistani border to the Deccan plateau. However, further decomposition split this vast region into two components: A wide **West Cluster** (**Cluster III.a**) and a narrower **Rich West Cluster** (**Cluster III.b**).

The **West Cluster** (**Cluster III.a)** is a vast region extending from Rajasthan and adjacent districts in Gujarat to Madhya Pradesh to the east and central Maharashtra (Khandesh and Marathwada) and northeast Karnataka (northern Maidan) to the south. It occupies the largest surface area but is not the most populated cluster, as it covers many low-density districts. This low density stems primarily from the predominance of rain-fed agriculture typical of the Deccan, the absence of major waterways, and low urbanization levels. Except for Jaipur, large urban conurbations, such as Bhopal, Indore, Nagpur, or Pune, belong to different, more advanced clusters. Like the South India Cluster, it is formed of a single block of contiguous districts, but the cluster also cuts across several states like Maharashtra and Karnataka and encroaches upon Gujarat, Uttar Pradesh, and Chhattisgarh.

The West Cluster is a region where demographic, health, and gender indicators are often less favorable than elsewhere in India. For example, we detect India's highest proportion of underweight women and child anemia in the cluster. Early marriage is also widespread, while fertility and child mortality remain high. One distinctive feature of this region relates to gender indicators since son preference appears widespread. Female land ownership is marginal (10%), marriage strictly patrilocal (98%), and son preference intense. The number of observed girl-only families is 64% smaller than expected in this region because of prenatal sex selection and differential stopping (when couples have additional children in the absence of a son).

The **Rich West Cluster (Cluster III.b)** shares numerous features with the previous cluster but corresponds to the more developed and urban parts of Western India. This feature explains why Punjab, Haryana, Delhi, Chandigarh, and the southern districts of Gujarat have detached from a broader West cluster during the classification process. The region's relative prosperity, demonstrated by Punjab's agricultural productivity, Gujarat's industrial development, and Delhi's role as an economic growth driver, enables a comparison with the South and Forward clusters. It shares with them several good health and demographic indicators. In this cluster, we may notice, for example, that child marriage is infrequent (13%), fertility lower than average (1.6 children per woman), modern contraception common (80%), menstrual hygiene widespread (90%), and institutional deliveries almost the rule (95%). In addition, this cluster has not been as affected by overmedicalization (hysterectomy, C-section, female sterilization) as the South Cluster but lags in child immunization (77%) or health insurance (29%).

However, the main difference with the South Cluster emerges from gender indicators. Son preference appears far more prominent in the Rich West Cluster than in the South or the rest of India. For instance, 63% of expected girl-only families are missing, a gap pointing to the strength of prenatal sex selection and gender bias in fertility behavior. This observation probably also explains why the proportion of one-child families and childless women in this cluster is lower than expected, given its low fertility. The birth of a boy is an indispensable component of the couples' reproductive strategies. In addition, patrilocal coresidence (99%) is almost universal. The strong correlation between this gender system and vegetarianism (60%) points to the unique cultural structures characterizing Western India. Therefore, for all its relative prosperity, the Rich West epitomizes the persistence of patriarchy in modern India.

The **Ganga Cluster (Cluster IV)** comprises a pretty compact set of 97 high-density districts in North India. It covers Bihar and Uttar Pradesh entirely, except for districts in northeast Uttar Pradesh and a few more prosperous districts around Noida, Ghaziabad, and Lucknow. It represents the most populated among the seven clusters. Its appellation derives from the fact that it is included in the broader Ganga basin.

Despite its demographic weight and importance in Indian history, this region currently makes up the analysis's poorest and least educated cluster. While densely populated and benefiting from water from the Ganga River and its tributaries, the area has the weakest urban infrastructure in the country. Its heavy reliance on male labor migration is illustrated by the highest proportion observed in this region of married women living without their husbands (17%); rural Bihar and Uttar Pradesh are significant purveyors of migrants in India (see Chap. 10). Besides labor migration, this cluster's regional demographic regime is characterized by its highest fertility (2.1 children per woman), child mortality levels (61 p. 1000), and the lowest female age at marriage–with 28% of women married before age 18. This situation is reinforced by a patriarchal regime illustrated by the strength of patrilocality, staunch son preference, and India's lowest proportion of families with fewer than two children. Despite the absence of deliberate prenatal sex selection, this part of India used to record the top levels of excess female mortality (Guilmoto et al., 2018).

During their reproductive lives, women from this region face several additional health burdens; they notably suffer from the highest reliance on ineffective traditional contraception (27%), the most inadequate antenatal care (35% of births covered), and lack of cancer screening (1%) and health insurance (16%). Other mother and child health indicators, such as safe deliveries, access to C-sections, child immunization, and menstrual hygiene, are all in the red. Other health status indicators also attain below-average values, such as a high proportion of underweight women (22%) and a high prevalence of anemia among children and women.

Spatial Analysis of Clusters

I want to return to the lessons of this classification to understand the spatial patterning of gender and health dimensions in India. It is striking that regional patterns re-emerge from a classification scheme that completely ignores them since the analysis was based on a strictly aspatial dataset. The clusters from the classification analysis consist primarily of compact sets of contiguous districts rather than an assortment of districts dispersed across India. For instance, fewer than ten isolated districts (out of 707) are part of distant clusters. Several (Indore, Bhopal, or Lucknow) are large urban areas, with health and gender indicators markedly more favorable than in their hinterland. As a result, clusters correspond to well-delineated spatial units that can be easily identified and labeled; some also correspond to well-known economic, linguistic, and physiographic regions. Examples of historical regions captured by the cluster analysis include Vidharba, North Maidan, the Brahmaputra Valley, and erstwhile Punjab, but we will see subsequently that they often correspond to current administrative units.

This spatial patterning suggests that India's gender and health geography remains embedded in deep and stable structures. It is probably as much influenced by contemporary socioeconomic dynamics as by inherited geographical constraints, sociohistorical formations, and gender systems. We could assume that India's geography was more segmented a century ago due, for instance, to the lack of unified rule before the colonial period, the relative absence of inter-regional migration, and limited economic exchanges within the country. In theory, rapid social and economic transformations over the last decades should have disrupted this old geography of gender and health inequalities. Likewise, policy interventions and, notably, the large number of all-India schemes that have been introduced should have partly blurred the inherited disparities. The government has indeed launched several programs that directly target many of the health and gender dimensions described in the Atlas.[13] These policy interventions and the gradual economic, social, and political integration should have contributed to a gradual homogenization, the decline of these old regional divisions, and the emergence of a new, more scattered geography articulated around region growth poles. Apart from the cases of some metropolitan areas mentioned earlier, this is not what we observe. The territories of these seven clusters remain spatially highly compact and appear to have resisted homogenization or fragmentation processes.

We do not need spatial autocorrelation tools to demonstrate that clusters are discrete regional formations, the opposite of what a spatially random distribution would resemble. However, one critical spatial feature I want to emphasize relates to the correspondence between clusters and state boundaries. It is striking how individual states fall almost entirely within a given cluster, as for Rajasthan, Punjab, Haryana, Uttarakhand, Bihar, West Bengal, Jharkhand, Assam, Tamil Nadu, Andhra Pradesh, Telangana, or Kerala–to name only the largest units.

I can more formally test the correspondence between clusters and states with a standard Cramér's *V* analysis. This indicator measures the association between two categorical variables in a contingency table and varies between 0 (no association) and 1 (complete association). Suppose we use the distribution of districts by state and cluster (Table 22.1). In that case, Cramér's *V* reaches .86, which indicates that states determine the distribution of individual districts into clusters at a rate of 86%. We may also test the association between states and clusters with multinomial logit regression, in which the 36 states are used to determine the clusters in which India's 707 districts will fall. The pseudo-r^2 of this logit regression is .84, a value almost identical to Cramer's *V*.

While confirming the paramount role of states in determining the cluster in which districts are classified, these results also show that the correspondence is incomplete. A few states are divided into separate segments by cluster analysis, and I will first examine them. Three discrepancies between states and clusters emerge in Karnataka, Maharashtra, and Gujarat. As the map (Fig. 22.1) suggests, the West Cluster penetrates central Maharashtra and north Karnataka from Madhya Pradesh. The resulting division of Maharashtra and Karnataka mirrors internal regional boundaries, with, for instance, Khandesh and Marathwada in the former and North Maidan in the latter being part of the West Cluster. In contrast, coastal and east Maharashtra (Konkan and Vidarbha, respectively) and the rest of Karnataka (South Maidan, Malenadu, and the Konkan littoral) are part of the Forward Cluster. The southward extension of the West Cluster into Maharashtra and Karnataka comprises less developed and more patriarchal areas. It represents a part of the rainfed dryland of the Deccan—areas more prone to drought than the rest of the two states (Rao et al., 2015) that report higher child mortality and female underweight rates. Perhaps more

[13] Chapters in this Atlas notably document various policies rolled out to combat and reduce anemia or hypertension, home deliveries, undernutrition, non-communicable diseases, son preference, unintended births, child marriage, unhealthy menstrual practices, ineffective contraception methods, and the lack of antenatal care, health insurance and child immunization.

importantly, this extension into Maharashtra and Karnataka also diverges from most South India because of its pronounced son preference, larger family size, and more frequent child marriage.[14]

Gujarat's case is another fragmented region, as the state is split into four clusters. The core cluster (Rich West Cluster) covers only the districts of Kutch and Saurashtra and the districts around Ahmedabad, Gandhinagar, and Vadodara; districts to the north are in the same cluster as Rajasthan (West Cluster), while southern districts around Surat belong to a coastal strip that extends to Mumbai and further to Mangalore (Forward Cluster). We may probably interpret this fragmentation as the effect of recent socioeconomic progress in south Gujarat (Rich West Cluster) in line with the parallel development of Punjab and Haryana in North India. Unlike the nearby Forward Cluster, affluent districts in Gujarat have remained patriarchal and represent a typical combination of economic growth accompanied by persisting gender bias.

States at the Core of Inequalities

Returning to the close correspondence between states and clusters, we may focus on the case of cluster boundaries. Let us examine the most remarkable regional correlation of the first South Cluster. This cluster includes all Telangana, Andhra Pradesh, Tamil Nadu, Kerala, and Goa districts. Its boundaries, with three adjacent clusters to the north, strictly follow the borders of these four states—except for the isolated district of Udupi in Karnataka. This cluster reproduces administrative boundaries and merges distinct linguistic areas (viz. Tamil-, Telugu- and Malayalam-speaking districts) into one. Its clear-cut boundaries with the bordering states of Karnataka, Maharashtra, Madhya Pradesh, Chhattisgarh, and Odisha are striking. This grouping does not replicate any previous historical boundaries like those of the Madras Presidency. Instead, it seems to coincide with Dravidian India, plus Goa and minus Karnataka. Today, it also represents a large block of states that have never been ruled by the Bharatiya Janata Party (BJP), the Hindu nationalist party dominating Indian politics for a decade. However, the northern delimitation of the South Cluster seems unaffected by the political geography of Naxalism that affects about 70 districts, notably around Chhattisgarh's Bastar area.[15]

Similarly, the northern segment of the Rich West Cluster overlaps the states of Punjab and Haryana, which were part of the administrative unit (East Punjab) till 1966. The boundaries with Himachal Pradesh, Uttar Pradesh, and Rajasthan are sharply defined. Equally clear-cut borders are visible around the East Cluster, notably with South India, Maharashtra, Uttar Pradesh, Bihar, and several smaller

[14] The share of vegetarian women is also several times as high as in the rest of South India.

[15] More generally, the so-called "red corridor" made of districts affected by left-wing extremism remains invisible on our maps.

northeast states. Instances of overlap between states and clusters, such as along the Chhattisgarh-Madhya Pradesh borders, are few and far between.

States remain the organizing principle behind grouping districts in clusters. Given that the classification analysis excluded any direct or indirect geographical or administrative information and synthesized over 20 variables, these results are somewhat surprising. We might initially fault the survey for this situation by speculating that data collection was biased distinctively at the state level (because of questionnaire translation or separate field agencies), resulting in artificial state-level variations. This hypothesis is contradicted by the merger of several states into the same clusters we have observed (e.g., South Cluster) and the fact that different agencies surveyed large states.

This analysis confirms that these clear-cut divisions across clusters are genuine and correspond to actual variations (or similarities) across state boundaries. The conclusion is, therefore, that belonging to a specific state or a group of adjacent states like Punjab and Haryana is a major determinant of cluster classification and of the overall health and gender profile of Indian districts. As argued earlier, state identity *per se* and the related regional policies may not explain why Uttarakhand and Uttar Pradesh, or Bihar and Jharkhand, belong to different clusters since these two pairs of states were part of the same administrative unit until 2000. Moreover, distinct state trajectories regarding regional socioeconomic change and policy interventions cannot explain why bordering states—such as Andhra Pradesh and Tamil Nadu or Assam and West Bengal—end up in the same cluster. On the contrary, the cluster analysis provides suggestive evidence that states have a strong level of homogeneity regarding gender and health characteristics. Despite several decades of separate political administrations, this homogeneity often extends to contiguous states.

I may offer a few provisional explanations for the robustness of states as a guiding principle of India's health and gender landscape. The first relates to the rapid pace of transformations and potential convergence of neighboring states. However, this regional convergence process whereby, for example, four states in South India would follow the same health and gender path still needs documenting. This observation brings us to a second line of explanations related to stable geographic endowments (rainfall, soil quality, relief, water basins, etc.) at the core of states' singularity. This explanation applies to the Northeast Cluster, a set of hilly districts quite distinct from the adjacent valleys of Assam and Tripura. The West Cluster also encompasses most of India's semi-arid tracts, with a particular agricultural mode of production. An additional set of explanations relates to shared sociohistorical and cultural attributes inherited from the past. For example, regions today most affected by son preference and sex imbalances at birth are typically regions already flagged during the colonial period for the prevalence of sati or female infanticide. Disparities observed today can thus be traced to old gender regimes.

We may further wonder why administrative boundaries, some relatively recent, like the bifurcation of Bihar, appear to correspond to long-term regional demarcation. The only explanation is that contemporary administrative boundaries are *endogenous*. In other words, I take the view that regional political reorganization and the process of redrawing administrative boundaries represent nothing but the recent manifestation of pre-existing socio-historically polities or geographically homogenous regions. The dissolution of the colonial presidencies and Undivided Assam (which comprised the whole Northeast) or the recent bifurcations of Uttar Pradesh, Madhya Pradesh, and Bihar in 2000 illustrate the underlying geographic, social, and economic homogeneity of specific areas were ultimately given political shape through gradual administrative reorganization. It also points to potential administrative changes proposed today (Purvanchal, Maharashtra's division into three states, Saurashtra, or Kalyana Karnataka), which may tally with some intra-variations reflected in the clusters.[16]

Trends and Their Geography

In this chapter, I have tried to explore the extent to which today's gender and health configuration is the product of the dramatic changes observed over the last decades or inherited from the past. We may also wonder whether future transformations will reduce (or exacerbate) the gaps, inequalities, and disparities highlighted in the Atlas. The situation at the beginning of the 2020s profoundly differs from that obtained during the 1990s, as recent decades have brought tremendous transformation to health and demographic behavior in India and have directly or indirectly affected gender contexts. Chapters illustrate these rapid changes, such as the swift progression in the proportion of safe deliveries (jumping from 39 to 89%) or the sustained rise in the proportion of fully immunized children (from 44 to 77%) observed over the 2005–2020 period. The improvements in many health outcomes may be interpreted as direct or indirect benefits of the rapid economic development observed in India till 2015–16. A higher standard of living has notably facilitated greater access to private facilities, even when the costs of health services have kept increasing over the years (see Das & Ladusingh, 2018; Sengupta & Nundy, 2005). These developments have occurred in a post-liberalization era characterized by a steady rise in average income and a sustained reduction in poverty rates. The further penetration of market forces in the lives of Indian citizens has, however, been accompanied by a distinct rise in inequality, as reflected by the increase of the Gini index since the end of the previous century (see also Sarkar & Mehta, 2010).

Direct intervention by the national and regional governments has also been recognized as standing at the core of some of the most striking transitions, e.g., the decline of home deliveries or the emergence of the provision of health insurance. There are also "deeper" trends, such as the reduction of fertility, child marriage, or child mortality, that, once unleashed, carry on somewhat independently of the

[16]The formation of new administrative units may not necessarily correspond to regions of distinct health and gender identity: the new states of Haryana, Telangana, or Ladakh still share most characteristics with their former parent states (viz. Punjab, Andhra Pradesh, and Jammu and Kashmir)

economic context and policy initiatives that triggered them in the first place. However, these health and gender transitions are often incomplete, and my analysis has focused on the vast disparities persisting across districts; this leaves plenty of room for further improvement until poorer states catch up with the rest of India.

There also appear to be many cases of persisting bias or shortcomings in which no significant improvements emerge from the analysis. There is, for instance, little sign of a reduction in gender bias against girls–even if excess female mortality in childhood has significantly reduced over the last 10 years. Similarly, anemia among women remains widespread and has not declined quickly over the last decade. In fact, the apparent stagnation of anemia indicators has recently led the government to drop these questions from the forthcoming NFHS round. While India's anemia levels among women may appear on the high side, child anemia rates are comparable to those estimated in Pakistan.[17] Anemia is otherwise partly linked to iron deficiency among vegetarians, but the link between anemia and diet does not appear very strong in India (Chaps. 3 and 5). Female sterilization also remains the first way for women to avoid unwanted births, while traditional and less efficient family planning methods are still common in North India. Indian women are still a long way from accessing more flexible and less intrusive methods of contraception. These examples suggest that some health and gender indicators have stagnated over decades and seem somewhat impervious to the broader effects of social change and economic development.

More worryingly, the last 20 years have led to examples of deterioration in health practices that may represent an indirect consequence of the epidemiological transition India is going through.[18] The rise of unnecessary cesarean sections and hysterectomies are two blatant cases of "overmedicalization." Overmedicalization corresponds notably to over-diagnosis and over-prescription, the harmful side effects of treatments, and the waste of public or private resources for no valid medical reasons (Kaczmarek, 2019). The overuse of health services is especially disturbing, as it closely follows the diffusion of private healthcare—which was initially supposed to improve the healthcare supply in India. Clinics and practitioners bear a specific responsibility in these developments, even if other factors, such as changing lifestyles, are at play. Another example is the transition from underweight to overweight prevalence (see Chap. 2), a trend associated with the socioeconomic

---

[17] The move to remove anemia from the new NFHS round may be compared to the simultaneous discussion by the government about replacing WHO benchmarks with new "indigenous growth standards" to assess stunting (*Times of India*, 3/08/2023). This is part of a concerted effort to "reverse the gaze" to denounce international standards and to project a more favorable international image of the country (Sanyal et al., 2023).

[18] The epidemiological transition is the structural change in disease patterns characterized by a move from infectious and parasitic diseases (diarrhea, smallpox, malaria, etc.) towards non-communicable and chronic diseases (diabetes, cancer, cardiovascular diseases, etc.). See for an overview of this transition in India (Yadav & Arokiasamy, 2014) and its uneven regional spread (Dandona et al., 2017).

gradient.[19] Another well-known similar story concerns diabetes, the prevalence of which has been increasing rapidly in India ("the diabetes capital of the world") in direct relation to rising incomes, dietary practices, lifestyle changes, and overweight (see Chap. 4 and Ong et al., 2023). Recent data suggest the burden of the disease in India has even been significantly underestimated (Anjana et al., 2023). Such trends lead to the emergence of "double burdens," i.e., situations in which the country may suffer simultaneously from cases of "too few" and "too many." A double burden means that India's public health system has, on one side, to fight the effect of lingering poverty and the lack of access to quality health infrastructures and, on the other side, to come to grips with the overuse and excess associated with the spread of new lifestyles, rising consumption, and overmedicalization.[20] Concurrently, progress toward cancer screening and universal health insurance is comparatively slow. Accordingly, I cannot be utterly optimistic about the future implications of economic and sociopolitical changes on gender relations and health conditions, and monitoring the intensity and geography of new health threats is of primary importance.

By walking readers through various maps, this Atlas has precisely highlighted the unique spatial dimensions that govern regional variations in gender and health across India. Notwithstanding overlaps and inconsistencies across our indicators, a large part of the effort in this chapter was in offering a more synthetic analysis of these ongoing transitions unfolding in twenty-first-century India. A series of neatly defined cluster regions have emerged from the classification analysis, and their spatial patterns are unmistakable. To some extent, these regions echo some familiar maps of gender and development differentials in India. We recognize, for example, the socioeconomic opposition between more prosperous clusters in west and south India and more deprived regions in central India from Rajasthan to Assam, spotlighting the significantly underdeveloped Ganga Valley. Among the more flourishing areas, we also distinguish two distinct pathways: The Rich West Cluster (Punjab, Haryana, Delhi, and parts of Gujarat) and the South India cluster. The latter differs from the former in terms of patriarchal indicators, with the South (and Northeast) clusters standing out as regions where the pressure to marry early and produce sons is much weaker than elsewhere.

A final lesson of this synthesis is that spatial patterns continue to dominate the structure of gender and health outcomes in India, and state divisions (or state clusters) remain the organizing principles of India's gender and health geography. The link between territories and inequalities relates to a broader issue of spatial justice developed by Soja (2013). Such an analysis cannot document the historical

[19] While India's level remains moderate compared to developed countries, it is characterized by one of fastest growth rates in overweight and obesity (World Obesity Federation, 2002).

[20] It should be noted that all these health threats are not purely diseases of affluence. Chapter 16 in this Atlas documents the rise of unnecessary hysterectomies across all sections of the population. Arsenic contamination, linked to increased access to groundwater, is another example of an emerging health challenge that mostly affects rural India, with a strong clustering around Bihar, Uttar Pradesh, and West Bengal (Shaji et al., 2021).

and social dynamics behind the unequal territorial distribution of health and welfare. It should force social sciences to reconsider how space contributes to (re)producing inequalities. The analysis also validates applying the theory of fundamental causes to regional disparities. Health and gender inequalities are indeed reflected in a bundle of risk factors and outcomes that appear to be strongly correlated. These indicators are also linked to socioeconomic status, but as I wrote at the beginning of this chapter, horizontal (regional) variations are more pronounced than vertical variations (across social classes). This finding is probably explained by imbalanced access to flexible resources (money, knowledge, power, etc.), a feature at the core of the theory of fundamental causes (Phelan et al., 2010). The unequal distribution of resources across Indian districts is a well-known phenomenon revealed by marked regional differences in educational attainment, living standards, livelihood practices, or income. In addition, we can also recognize the gradual replacement of mechanisms affecting socioeconomic disparities in the emergence of new health practices (e.g., diabetes or hysterectomy) or the transition from one risk factor to another one (e.g., from underweight to underweight or from home to cesarean deliveries). What probably differs from the theory is that the fundamental causes of health inequalities appear to operate within the clusters identified during the classification analysis rather than uniformly across the country.[21]

This spatial clustering is why we need to place geography at the core of the analysis of the Indian inequality regime and its particular regional configuration. This emphasis is especially relevant given that regional heterogeneity has not diminished despite the rapid pace of demographic and economic change. We are still far from a national convergence and a reduction in regional inequalities. Monitoring future changes in India's gender and health situation is not only about charting the steady progress of health indicators and assessing the impact of new policies and schemes enacted by national and state governments. It is also about mapping the extent of persisting gender and health inequalities and documenting cases of adverse evolution. All these efforts to understand the contours of future changes in the gender and health situation are necessary to make India a healthier, fairer, and more gender-equal place for its citizenry.

References

Ahlin, T., Nichter, M., & Pillai, G. (2016). Health insurance in India: what do we know and why is ethnographic research needed. *Anthropology & Medicine, 23*(1), 102–124. https://doi.org/10.1080/13648470.2015.1135787

Anilkumar, N. A., Gupta, D., Khare, S., Gopalkrishna, D.M., & Jyotishi, A. (2017). Characteristics and causes of malnutrition across Indian states: A cluster analysis based on Indian demographic and health survey data. In *2017 International Conference on Advances in Computing, Communications and Informatics (ICACCI)* (pp. 2115–2123). IEEE.

[21]Besides health outcomes, the inclusion in the analysis of gender as a distinct dimension partly explains the regional clustering of districts.

Anjana, R. M., et al. (2023). Metabolic non-communicable disease health report of India: the ICMR-INDIAB national cross-sectional study (ICMR-INDIAB-17). *The Lancet Diabetes and Endocrinology., 11*(7), 474–489. https://doi.org/10.1016/S2213-8587(23)00119-5

Balarajan, Y., Selvaraj, S., & Subramanian, S. V. (2011). Healthcare and equity in India. *The Lancet, 377*(9764), 505–515.

Batra, R., & Reio, T. G., Jr. (2016). Gender inequality issues in India. *Advances in Developing Human Resources, 18*(1), 88–101.

Dandona, L., et al. (2017). Nations within a nation: variations in epidemiological transition across the states of India, 1990–2016 in the Global Burden of Disease Study. *The Lancet, 390*(10111), 2437–2460.

Das, S. K., & Ladusingh, L. (2018). Why is the inpatient cost of dying increasing in India? *PLoS One, 13*(9), e0203454.

Everitt, B. S., Landau, S., Leese, M., & Stahl, D. (2011). *Cluster analysis* (5th ed.). Wiley.

George, S. (2019). Reconciliations of caste and medical power in rural public health services. *Economic and Political Weekly, 54*(40), 43–50.

Guilmoto, C. Z., Saikia, N., Tamrakar, V., & Bora, J. K. (2018). Excess under-5 female mortality across India: a spatial analysis using 2011 census data. *The Lancet Global Health, 6*(6), e650–e658.

Gupta, A., & Sudharsanan, N. (2022). Large and Persistent Life Expectancy Disparities between India's Social Groups. *Population and Development Review, 48*(3), 863–882.

Hemalatha, R., et al. (2020). Mapping of variations in child stunting, wasting and underweight within the states of India: The Global Burden of Disease Study 2000–2017. *EClinical Medicine, 22*, 100317.

Jullien, C., & Jeffery, R. (Eds.). (2021). *Childbirth in South Asia: Old paradoxes and new challenges*. Oxford University Press.

Kaczmarek, E. (2019). How to distinguish medicalization from over-medicalization? *Medicine, Health Care and Philosophy, 22*, 119–128.

Kane, S., Joshi, M., Desai, S., Mahal, A., & McPake, B. (2022). People's care seeking journey for a chronic illness in rural India: Implications for policy and practice. *Social Science and Medicine, 312*, 115390.

Link, B. G., & Phelan, J. (1995). Social conditions as fundamental causes of disease. *Journal of Health and Social Behavior*, 80–94.

Lukšaitė, E. (2022). "I do not have to hurt my body anymore": reproductive chronicity and sterilization as ambivalent care in rural north India. *Medical Anthropology Quarterly, 36*(3), 312–328.

Mohanty, S. K., Mishra, U. S., & Chauhan, R. K. (Eds.). (2019). *The Demographic and Development Divide in India: A District-Level Analysis*. Springer.

Mutheneni, S. R., Mopuri, R., Naish, S., Gunti, D., & Upadhyayula, S. M. (2018). Spatial distribution and cluster analysis of dengue using self-organizing maps in Andhra Pradesh, India, 2011–2013. *Parasite Epidemiology and Control, 3*(1), 52–61.

NITI Aayog. (2023). *National Multidimensional Poverty Index. A Progress Review 2023*. OPHI, UNDP, NITI Aayog.

Ong, K. L., et al. (2023, June). Global, regional, and national burden of diabetes from 1990 to 2021, with projections of prevalence to 2050: a systematic analysis for the Global Burden of Disease Study 2021. *The Lancet, 402*, 203–234. https://doi.org/10.1016/S0140-6736(23)01301-6

Oxfam. (2021). *Inequality report 2021: India's unequal Healthcare Story*. Oxfam.

Pandey, A., et al. (2002). Gender differences in healthcare-seeking during common illnesses in a rural community of West Bengal, India. *Journal of Health, Population and Nutrition, 20*(4), 306–311.

Phelan, J. C., Link, B. G., & Tehranifar, P. (2010). Social conditions as fundamental causes of health inequalities: theory, evidence, and policy implications. *Journal of Health and Social Behavior, 51*(1_suppl), S28–S40.

Pinto, S. (2022). *Where there is no Midwife: Birth and Loss in Rural India*. Berghahn Books.

Rao, C. S., et al. (2015). Potential and Challenges of Rainfed Farming in India. In D. L. Sparks (Ed.), *Advances in Agronomy* (pp. 113–181). Academic.

Sanyal, S., Arora, A., & Chauhan, S. (2023). *Reversing the Gaze. Re-examining estimates of India's development indicators by international organisation.* Economic Advisory Council to the PM, Working paper series, EAC-PM/WP/14/2023.

Sarkar, S., & Mehta, B. S. (2010). Income inequality in India: pre-and post-reform periods. *Economic and Political Weekly, 45*(37), 45–55.

Sengupta, A., & Nundy, S. (2005). The private health sector in India. *British Medical Journal, 331*(7526), 1157–1158.

Shaji, E., Santosh, M., Sarath, K. V., Prakash, P., Deepchand, V., & Divya, B. V. (2021). Arsenic contamination of groundwater: A global synopsis with focus on the Indian Peninsula. *Geoscience Frontiers, 12*(3), 101079.

Singh, A., Chokhandre, P., Singh, A. K., Barker, K. M., Kumar, K., McDougal, L., & Raj, A. (2021). Development of the India patriarchy index: Validation and testing of temporal and spatial patterning. *Social Indicators Research, 159*, 351–377.

Soja, E. W. (2013). *Seeking spatial justice*. University of Minnesota Press.

Sopher, D. E. (1972). Place and location: notes on the spatial patterning of culture. *Social Science Quarterly*, 321–337.

World Obesity Federation. (2002). *World Obesity Atlas*, www.worldobesity.org

Yadav, S., & Arokiasamy, P. (2014). Understanding epidemiological transition in India. *Global Health Action, 7*(1), 23248.

The manufacturer's authorised representative in the EU is Springer Nature Customer Service Centre GmbH, Europaplatz 3, 69115 Heidelberg, Germany. If you have any concerns regarding our products, please contact ProductSafety@springernature.com

Printed and bound by CPI Group (UK) Ltd, Croydon, CR0 4YY
28/09/2026
02224081-0012